The Tragedy of Childbed Fever

The Tragedy of Childbed Fever

IRVINE LOUDON

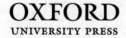
OXFORD
UNIVERSITY PRESS

OXFORD
UNIVERSITY PRESS

Great Clarendon Street, Oxford OX2 6DP

Oxford University Press is a department of the University of Oxford.
It furthers the University's objective of excellence in research, scholarship,
and education by publishing worldwide in

Oxford New York

Athens Auckland Bangkok Bogotá Buenos Aires Calcutta
Cape Town Chennai Dar es Salaam Delhi Florence Hong Kong Istanbul
Karachi Kuala Lumpur Madrid Melbourne Mexico City Mumbai
Nairobi Paris São Paulo Singapore Taipei Tokyo Toronto Warsaw
with associated companies in Berlin Ibadan

Oxford is a registered trade mark of Oxford University Press
in the UK and in certain other countries

Published in the United States
by Oxford University Press Inc., New York

British Library Cataloguing in Publication Data
Data available

Library of Congress Cataloging in Publication Data
Loudon, Irvine,
The tragedy of childbed fever / Irvine Loudon.
Includes bibliographical references and index.
1. Puerperal septicemia—History. I. Title.
RG811.L68 2000 618.7′4′009—dc21 99-33268

ISBN 0-19-820499-X

1 3 5 7 9 10 8 6 4 2

Typeset in Ehrhardt
by Graphicraft Limited, Hong Kong
Printed in Great Britain
on acid-free paper by
Biddles Ltd,
Guildford and King's Lynn

Preface

Although many have written about various aspects of childbed (or puerperal) fever, and especially about Semmelweis, I think I can claim that this is the first comprehensive history of the disease. It covers the two hundred or so years from its first recognition as a separate entity in the eighteenth century, through to the second half of the twentieth, when it rapidly became all but extinct as a life-threatening disorder. In the title of this book I have used the term 'childbed fever' because it is simple, plain, and vivid English, and much easier to pronounce than 'puerperal fever'. Unfortunately, as the reader will discover, the term 'childbed fever' became obsolete quite early in the nineteenth century and 'puerperal fever' became firmly established.

I had never thought of it as a suitable subject for prolonged research until I undertook a study of the history of maternal mortality. Soon, I discovered that my mountain of notes and photocopies on puerperal fever threatened to swamp all other aspects of maternal mortality. It was vast. Indeed, an obstetrician in the 1880s wrote that 'More is said to have been written on this disease than on any other. Dr Fordyce Barker found that within the comparatively short period of twenty years, 1854 to 1874, upwards of 20,000 pages had been published on the subject.'[1] Did the industrious Fordyce Barker really know? Did he really count? There is no way of telling, but I personally doubt if he exaggerated. Furthermore, I would guess that the number of pages had already come close to 10,000 before 1854, and I am certain that far more than 20,000 pages have been published about puerperal fever between 1874 and the present time. So I completed the book on maternal mortality with brief references to puerperal fever,[2] and started on this one.

Such an abundance of sources, much of it repetitive, is not of itself a sufficient reason for a book; but the truth is that the story of this dreadful disease is as gripping and as memorable, if not more so, than the history of any other disease. Moreover, writing this story has provided a unique opportunity for the exploration of changing ideas on the nature of fevers and contagion, the role of hospitals in childbirth, the impact of bacteriology and antisepsis, and the complex pathway that led to immunization and the antibiotics. It has also provided an opportunity to explore some aspects of the history of streptococcal disease as a whole.

[1] C. J. Cullingworth, *Puerperal Fever: A Preventible Disease* (London, 1888), 7.
[2] I. Loudon, *Death in Childbirth: An International Study of Maternal Care and Maternal Mortality 1800–1950* (Oxford, 1992).

In writing this book I have received a great deal of help from many people, and I thank Iain Chalmers, A. Crowther, David Greenwood, Anne Løkke, Jean Loudon, Michael Loudon, Hilary Marland, Joan Mottram, Lisa Öberg, David St George, Gene Stollerman, Anthony Storr, Michael Worboys, and the late A. Barnett Christie. Some have read and provided constructive criticism of various chapters. Others have helped with translation, pointed me towards new sources, most generously given permission to cite their work, or provided much needed assistance in understanding some of the complexities of modern microbiology. I am deeply grateful to Hilary Walford for the skill with which she has copy-edited my typescript. There may still be some errors because there usually are; but they will be mine, not anybody else's.

I. L.

The Mill House
Wantage
Oxfordshire
December 1998

Contents

CONTENTS

List of Figures

List of Tables

Les épidemies puerpérales sont à la femme ce que la guerre est à l'homme. Comme la guerre, elles moissonnent la partie la plus saine, la plus vaillante, la plus utile de la population; comme la guerre, elles frappent les sujets dans la fleur de l'âge . . .

Epidemics of puerperal fever are to women as war is to men. Like war, they cut down the healthiest, bravest, and most essential part of the population; like war, they strike their victims in the prime of their lives . . .

(Jacques-François-Édouard Hervieux, Traité clinique et pratique des maladies puerpérales (Paris, 1880))

1

An Introduction to Puerperal Fever

It was typical of Mary Wollstonecraft (1759–97), the brilliant and radical eighteenth-century author, that she should be robust, independent, and optimistic when she came to the end of her second pregnancy. Her first delivery in France had been easy. The second should be easier still. She 'ridiculed the fashion of ladies who kept to their chambers for one full month after delivery. For herself, she proposed coming down to dinner on the day following . . . [and] she hired no nurse.'[1]

She did, however, hire Mrs Blenkinsop, the matron and midwife to the Westminster Lying-in Hospital, who saw her a few times during pregnancy and came to her house when labour started in the morning of Wednesday, 30 August 1797. Mary Wollstonecraft gave birth to a daughter at 11.20 p.m. By 2 a.m., however, the 'placenta had not yet come away', and the midwife advised William Godwin (Mary Wollstonecraft's husband) to fetch Dr Poignard, physician-accoucheur to the same lying-in hospital. He arrived between three and four hours after the birth and undertook a manual removal of the placenta. Because the placenta was adherent, the operation was unusually difficult, taking several hours, during which Mary Wollstonecraft lost a lot of blood and suffered a series of fainting fits. She was, however, a woman of great strength of character. Considering the ordeal she had been through she was remarkably well by Friday, 1 September.

It was not until the following Sunday that Mary Wollstonecraft had 'a sort of shivering fit'. Her husband was out of the house at the time, but shortly after his return he witnessed the second shivering fit, which was so violent that 'every muscle in her body trembled, the teeth chattered, and the bed shook under her. This continued probably for five minutes . . . She told me after it was over, that it had been a struggle between life and death.'

She continued with a series of shivering fits and a high fever through Monday and Tuesday, and was worse on Wednesday. During this time several friends came and sat with her. She was attended by several medical men, including Dr Poignard, Dr George Fordyce (who was not an accoucheur—that is, an

---

[1] William Godwin, *Memoirs of the Author of 'The Rights of Woman'* (London, 1799). Claire Tomalin, *The Life and Death of Mary Wollstonecraft* (rev. edn., Harmondsworth, 1985).

obstetrician), Dr Clarke of New Burlington Street (who was), and by the surgeon Mr Carlisle, who stayed with her from Wednesday until her death.[2]

Wednesday was a dreadful day, and Godwin, exhausted by worry and watching, lay down on his bed late that night. He was woken early on Thursday morning, 6 September, by Carlisle, who told him his wife was 'surprisingly better'.
By this time the shivering fits had stopped. But on the evening of the same
day Carlisle 'told us to prepare ourselves, for he had reason to expect the fatal
event every moment'. In fact, Mary Wollstonecraft lived through the Friday
and Saturday, although 'her faculties were in too decayed a state, to be able
to follow any train of ideas with force or any accuracy of connection'. She died,
aged 38, at 7.40 on Sunday morning, 10 September 1797.

Her newborn daughter, Mary, survived and, although she was luckier than
many, what happened to her illustrates the tragedy of a death from puerperal
fever. Godwin, who was distraught at the death of his wife and 'bewildered by
the charge of his daughter', found a substitute mother for Mary in his next-
door neighbour, Mrs Clairmont, 'a clever bustling second-rate woman, glib of
tongue and pen, with a temper undisciplined and uncontrolled'. She already
had three children and 'Mary was thrown for sympathy upon the companion-
ship of her father, whose real tenderness was disguised by his frigid manner'.
Small wonder that Mary, whose second name was Wollstonecraft, came to 'idolise
her dead mother, whose memory became a religion to her'. In 1816, at the age
of 19, Mary became the second wife of the poet Percy Bysshe Shelley and in
1818 she published her famous novel, *Frankenstein*. In 1819 she herself suffered
a crushing blow in the death of her son, from which time 'the keynote of her
existence was melancholy'.[3]

Case Histories of Puerperal Fever

This vivid, memorable, and tragic history is known today because of the fame
of Mary Wollstonecraft and her daughter. But it is only one of numerous
eighteenth-century case histories of puerperal fever. A few years earlier there
had been an epidemic of puerperal fever in Aberdeen, which had lasted from
December 1789 to January 1792. It was the subject of a brilliant epidemiological treatise by Alexander Gordon, which is discussed in Chapter 3. The
following case history comes from this treatise.

In the afternoon of 19 August 1790, Gordon was requested by John Low, a
miller, to go immediately to see his wife, who was 'in great danger' following a

---

[2] This was presumably Mr Anthony (later Sir Anthony) Carlisle, surgeon to the Westminster Hospital.
Although it seems that he was a model of kindness and concern in this instance, he later became noted
for his snobbery, conceit, and arrogance and for his implacable opposition to man-midwifery. 'I consider it', he said, 'derogatory to any liberal man to assume the office of a nurse, of an old woman; and
that it is an *imposture* to pretend that a medical man is required at a labour' (I. Loudon, *Death in Childbirth:
An International Study of Maternal Care and Maternal Mortality 1800–1950* (Oxford, 1992), 190.
[3] *Dictionary of National Biography*.

delivery two days earlier. Gordon found Mrs Low in a state of great fever, with a pulse of 140 beats a minute and acute pain in the lower part of her abdomen. She was the fifteenth case out of a total of seventy-seven in the epidemic.

The disorder commenced with a violent rigor at six o'clock in the morning, being about 36 hours after delivery. I had no difficulty in ascertaining the patient's disorder having had previous opportunities of seeing it both in London, and in the course of my practice in Aberdeen . . . And in every respect, the disease answered the description of that known to practitioners by the appellation of the Puerperal Fever, a distemper which so frequently proves fatal to women in childbed, and baffling the skill of the most eminent physicians.[4]

Two days later Mrs Low seemed a little better in so far as her pulse rate had fallen, but she complained of very great swelling and pain of her abdomen. The next day she was in such agony and her abdomen was so tender that she could not bear it to be touched. The 'disease was making rapid progress' and her strength was sinking. The following day, however (the fourth day of her illness), Gordon found:

that the storm had lulled into a calm. The friends received me with transports of joy, vainly thinking that the danger was over. The patient, supposing herself perfectly well, asked my permission to rise; for she seemed to feel no pain, and suffered me to touch and press the abdomen, without showing any signs of uneasiness; a proof that the parts were in a state of gangrene. For this sudden cessation of pain, in the Puerperal Fever is a fatal symptom which announces the approach of death, and denotes that mortification has taken place. The friends, ignorant of this circumstance, were quite overjoyed to see the patient so composed, after such excruciating pain. However, notwithstanding this composure and apparent ease, it was evident from the ghastly appearance of the countenance . . . that death was not far off. Accordingly, in a few hours, the scene was closed.

Although Gordon had given an unfavourable prognosis, 'and desired a consultation', he was blamed for her death—possibly because of the bitter disappointment of death after apparent recovery. In general he found that the epidemic 'exposed me to the unmerited reproaches of the ignorant and illiterate . . . On this as well as on many other occasions, I found that scientific practice and popular opinion very seldom corresponded.'

Some twenty years before the Aberdeen epidemic, there had been an epidemic of puerperal fever at the General Lying-in Hospital in London. The following case histories come from the records of that institution.[5]

[4] Alexander Gordon, *A Treatise on the Epidemic Puerperal Fever of Aberdeen* (London, 1795), 22–7.

[5] Royal College of Obstetricians and Gynaecologists, London, Library. The records of the General Lying-in Hospital in the eighteenth century include three notebooks labelled 'Puerperal Fever', which contain about forty case histories of puerperal fever. It is thought they were written by Dr Christopher Kelly, who was a consultant accoucheur to the hospital and seems to have had a special interest in puerperal fever.

Mrs Drabwell aged 32 to all appearance a strong and healthy woman, was delivered Saturday morning Oct. 21 [1769] between 3 and 4. At 12 that night She had a violent Shivering attended with pain in her Belly, the Nurse gave her a house powder, when she sweated and got easier, and continued to do so Sunday morning but at 1 o'clock noon having a little return of pain a clyster was administered . . . Monday morning. She had a return of pain in her belly but thought fit to conceal it . . . but in the evening the Matron heard her groan, and [I] was informed. She was in great pain in her belly which was very tender. Tuesday 1 o'clock. She has been restless all night, little or no sleep . . . her Belly tender, especially the upper part of it . . . pulse 140 and full. Seven or eight ounces of Blood more were taken which quickened her pulse considerably. Wednesday and Thursday, She grew worse, her Belly became more tense, frequent and involuntary stools, her extremities became cold, and she died on Friday the 6th day from her disease. She was opened that night at 8 o'clock when there was found a great deal of the purulent fluid in the Cavity of the Abdomen, a little pus lying in different parts . . .

Many of the patients in this epidemic died within a week of delivery. For example, 'Rebecca Ingham, 1st child, delivered Sunday Dec 24 1780', became ill on the Tuesday, the third day with 'great tenderness in her Belly, a foul tongue, pulse 120, considerable heat in her skin'. By Friday she was 'Much worse, her belly distended and so exquisitely tender that she can hardly bear the slightest touch', and on Saturday she died, less than a week after delivery.

Puerperal fever could follow an easy straightforward delivery, such as the following case, which was a home delivery by a midwife. Dr Kelly happened to be visiting two doors away when she became ill and he was called in:

Monday March 5 1770 at 5 in the morning, Mrs Babbs of Oxford Road, Aged 26, was delivered of her third child and had an exceeding easy Natural labour . . . The second day at 8 in the morning and when sitting upright in bed, going to Breakfast, she was seized with a Shivering, which was Violent, shook the Bed, and continued half an hour . . . She had at the same time a pain and tenderness in her Belly . . . She died Saturday the 6th day at 8 in the morning.

Amongst the numerous descriptions of this disease, however, few can rival the following vivid account written by Nathaniel Hulme in 1772:

Upon the first, second, or third day after delivery, but most commonly on the second, the patient complains of violent pain and soreness over the whole hypogastric region; that is, from the navel downwards. The tenderness is often so acute that the gentlest touch is almost insufferable. The belly feels commonly soft. Sometimes it will be greatly swelled; but in general, at the beginning of the disease it is not much more tumefied than what may be expected so early after delivery. There is no inflammation or other discoloration to be seen on the abdominal skin.

A general anxiety, or dejection of mind, appears in the countenance, and the eyes participate of the same distress. The face is often flushed, and sometimes there is a deep red, or livid colour, fixed in the cheeks. The skin is generally hot and dry.

The pulse in general is quick and weak, though sometimes it will resist the finger pretty strongly. At the beginning of the disease it seldom beats less than a hundred strokes in the space of a minute; and from this number I have found it run on to one hundred and sixty.

A shortness in breathing, without any wheezing or noise in the breast, generally accompanies the distemper from the beginning . . . I call it a shortness of breathing rather than a difficulty, because a difficulty in breathing may be attended with a full inspiration, and a desire of taking in a large quantity of air; whereas the breathing I here mean to describe is quite the reverse; the inspirations are quick and small, with a fear and dread, as it were, of making a full inspiration, or, in other words, of dilating the thorax. The reason of this, as I apprehend, is not in general owing to any complaint in the lungs or chest (except when the pains extend to the region of the stomach and ribs), but merely to the grand seat of the disorder being within the abdomen, and which, at every inspiration, is squeezed, as it were, between two presses, by the diaphragm from above and the abdominal muscles from below. I almost shudder with horror when I consider the excruciating torments that must rack the distressed patient under these dreadful circumstances.[6]

Most women feared the pain and possible complications of delivery. Once the baby was born, it seemed that all danger had passed. Puerperal fever came totally unexpectedly, and if the mother died the whole family could be destroyed, for her death left a baby and sometimes other children without a mother and a husband without a wife. At best, the husband might remarry and the baby might be cared for by a loving stepmother. At worst, the baby would be sent off to an orphanage, or it might very well die, for it was shown in the 1920s that the risk of a baby dying in the first year of life was four times as high if the mother had died in childbirth than if the mother had survived.[7]

It is these features that single out puerperal fever from other causes of death. The title of this book, *The Tragedy of Childbed Fever*, is no exaggeration. Even medical practitioners in the eighteenth and nineteenth centuries, accustomed to a death rate amongst young people that would horrify their successors today, were openly moved and horrified by this disease. It was, as an American obstetrician remarked about puerperal fever, 'a sort of *desecration* for an accouché to die'.[8]

The Clinical Features of Puerperal Fever

It will be helpful to summarize the main features of puerperal fever as revealed by these case histories.

- Puerperal fever was an exceptionally cruel and dreadful disease that came suddenly and unexpectedly out of the blue and usually when the mother was rejoicing at the successful birth of her baby, and it nearly always began with intense shivering (the rigor) followed by more attacks of shivering, a rapid pulse, and high fever.

[6] Nathaniel Hulme, *A Treatise on the Puerperal Fever* (London, 1772); repr. in Fleetwood Churchill (ed.), *Essays on the Puerperal Fever and Other Diseases Peculiar to Women* (London, 1849), 61–116.
[7] R. M. Woodbury, *Infant Mortality and its Causes* (Baltimore, 1926), 43.
[8] C. D. Meigs, *Females and their Diseases: A Series of Letters to his Class* (Philadelphia, 1848), 576.

- Frequently there was the agonizing abdominal pain of peritonitis, causing so much tenderness that the patient could scarcely bear her abdomen to be touched, or even the weight of the bedclothes.
- Puerperal fever was seen in two forms: epidemics that occurred either in towns or in lying-in hospitals, and sporadic cases. In general, the earlier the onset of the disease after delivery, the worse the prognosis and the shorter the interval between onset and death. Early onset with fatality rates as high as 80 per cent were characteristic of epidemics of puerperal fever. Later onset, a more prolonged illness, and a fatality rate of about 35 per cent were characteristic of sporadic cases.
- The risk of contracting puerperal fever was much greater following surgical intervention, but puerperal fever could follow a perfectly normal delivery. Because surgical intervention occurred in a small minority of total births, however, it is probable that the majority of cases followed a normal rather than an abnormal delivery.
- On some occasions (such as Mrs Low of Aberdeen and probably Mary Wollstonecraft) there was a sudden cessation of pain and fever in the final days of the illness. This was reported so often by different observers that there is no doubt it was a genuine, if occasional, feature of the disease. Indeed, every experienced man-midwife knew that, although the family might rejoice in the belief the patient was getting better, it was a sign not of recovery but of impending death. The pathology of this phenomenon is uncertain, but Gordon's explanation that it was due to intra-abdominal 'mortification' (or gangrene) may contain an element of truth.

How common was puerperal fever? Roughly speaking, there were, in the eighteenth and nineteenth centuries, about 2–3 deaths and 6–9 cases in every 1,000 deliveries. In epidemics, of course, there were far more. But, in general and looked at in the context of total births, puerperal fever was uncommon. But births were very frequent events, and, within childbirth as a whole, puerperal fever was by far the most common cause of maternal mortality, accounting for roughly half of all maternal deaths.[9] Moreover, amongst women of childbearing age, from the time national records began in the mid-nineteenth century up to the late 1930s, maternal mortality was second only to tuberculosis in the leading causes of death. At a rough estimate, there were probably between a quarter of a million and a half a million deaths from puerperal fever in England and Wales during the eighteenth and nineteenth centuries.[10]

[9] Obstetric haemorrhage was usually the second most common cause, and toxaemia/eclampsia the third.

[10] This estimate is based on back projection from the Registrar General's Reports in the second half of the nineteenth century, after making allowance for three factors: (1) the under-reporting of deaths from puerperal fever (see I. Loudon, 'Hidden Maternal Deaths', app. 1 in Loudon, *Death in Childbirth*, 518–24; (2) the evidence that epidemics of puerperal fever were more common in the eighteenth and first half of the nineteenth centuries than the second half of the nineteenth century; (3) changes in the size of the population.

What, then, was the nature or pathology of the disease known as childbed or puerperal fever?

The Pathology of Puerperal Fever

In women of childbearing age, bacterial infection of the genital tract is rare. The acidity of the vaginal secretions, the closed cervix, and the antibacterial properties of the endometrium (the inner lining of the uterus) are effective barriers against infection. During childbirth and the puerperium (the period following delivery) all three barriers are lost, for the vaginal secretions are neutral rather than acid, the cervix is open, and the endometrium is stripped away leaving a raw surface, especially at the site to which the placenta was attached. Under these conditions it is relatively easy for bacteria to gain entrance and become implanted in the uterus. If that occurs, the result is puerperal fever. Puerperal fever is by definition a bacterial infection of the genital tract (usually of the uterus) following childbirth.

The pathological sequence of events following infection was highly variable. At best, the infection was overcome by the body's defence mechanism and all that happened was that the woman developed a slight and transient fever. Alternatively, the infection became localized and formed an abscess that, with or without medical aid, discharged, and recovery usually followed. At worst, the infection spread through the wall of the uterus into the peritoneal cavity, or entered the bloodstream causing septicaemia. If it passed into the peritoneal cavity, the infection could spread downwards and become localized in the pelvis. Usually, however, it spread to infect the whole of the peritoneum causing peritonitis.

Peritonitis was the cruellest feature of the disease. The severity of the pain often increased to such intensity that there are many reports of patients who emitted a continuous cry of agony or alternatively were frozen in speechless terror by the severity of their pain. Charles Meigs of Philadelphia told his students in 1848 that he had seen patients 'who not only suffered intolerable pain, but in whose minds that pain appeared to excite the most unspeakable terror. I think I have seen women who appeared to be awe-struck by the dreadful force of their distress.'[11] It was certainly an extremely common feature in puerperal fever, and possibly more so in the eighteenth and nineteenth centuries than in the twentieth. In 1830 M. Tonnellé of Paris found evidence of peritonitis in 193 out of 222 post-mortem dissections of women who had died from puerperal fever.[12] In a survey of puerperal fever carried out by the North of England Obstetrical and Gynaecological Society in 1925, out of thirty-eight

[11] Meigs, *Females and their Diseases*, 596.
[12] M. Tonnellé, 'Des fièvres puerpérales observées à la Maternité de Paris pendant l'année 1829', originally published as four papers in *Archives Générales de Médecin* (Mar., Apr., May, and June 1830); repr. in 'Critical Analysis', *Edinburgh Medical and Surgical Journal*, 34 (1830), 328–49.

cases that came to post-mortem, twenty-five had evidence of peritonitis.[13] In 1849 Fleetwood Churchill reviewed a large number of reports of cases of puerperal fever. He found that peritonitis was almost invariably present and suggested that a better name for this disease was not 'puerperal fever' but 'puerperal peritonitis'.[14]

Since the 1950s, deaths from puerperal fever are rare in the Western world. Before the introduction of antibiotics, however (and in the case of puerperal fever this means before the mid-1930s, when the sulphonamides were introduced), puerperal fever was an extremely dangerous disease. Death was almost invariably due to peritonitis or septicaemia or a combination of the two. For various reasons the nomenclature of puerperal fever was rather complicated, and it will be helpful to consider this here.

Nomenclature and the Synonyms for Puerperal Fever

The name puerperal (or childbed) fever was used throughout the eighteenth century. It meant the 'fever of the puerperium', the 'puerperium' being the term used to describe the period immediately following childbirth, which was often called the 'lying-in' period in the past, and is called the post-natal period today. In the nineteenth century, although the original name 'puerperal fever' was used most of the time, a large number of synonyms appeared, reflecting the growing importance attached to morbid anatomy.

Broadly speaking, in the eighteenth century diseases were defined in terms of clinical signs and external appearances, in the nineteenth by post-mortem appearances (this is discussed in more detail in Chapter 6). While most diseases were characterized by consistent post-mortem findings, puerperal fever was not. Usually there was obvious pathology in the uterus as well as evidence of inflammation, abscess formation, or thrombosis in the peritoneum, the pelvic cavity, or the pelvic blood vessels or lymphatics. This led to a host of synonyms such as 'metria' and 'metritis' (inflammation of the uterus), 'puerperal peritonitis', 'puerperal pelvic abscess', 'puerperal pelvic cellulitis', 'puerperal pelvic phlebitis' (if the veins were infected), 'puerperal pelvic lymphangitis' (if the lymphatic vessels were involved), and 'puerperal pelvic salpingitis' (if the Fallopian tubes were infected). The terms 'puerperal sapraemia', 'puerperal pyaemia', and 'puerperal septicaemia' were also common in nineteenth-century publications, and, although there were subtle differences in meaning, they meant essentially the same thing: that the infection had entered the bloodstream.

Although this nineteenth-century mania for pathological detail produced some notable advances in the understanding of other diseases, in puerperal fever

---

[13] Royal College of Obstetricians and Gynaecologists, London, Library, Blair Bell papers, catalogue number S.4.

[14] Fleetwood Churchill, 'An Historical Sketch of the Epidemics of Puerperal Fever', in Churchill (ed.), Essays, 3–42, at 31, table.

it tended to cause confusion, with the various synonyms cluttering up the lists of causes of deaths in official and government reports. In practice, however, they soon become familiar, and there is seldom any difficulty in recognizing them for what they were—not different disease entities, but synonyms for puerperal fever.

From the end of the nineteenth century there was a significant change in disease nomenclature. Infective diseases began to be defined (as they are today) by the specific micro-organisms associated with the disease. When it was accepted that puerperal fever was due to bacterial infection of the genital tract, although it was a specific disease in the sense of an infection of the genital tract during the puerperium, it was suspected that puerperal fever could be due to several kinds of bacteria. Was it, therefore, justifiable to call it a fever like measles or typhoid or typhus?

One of the first to deal with this question was a Manchester obstetrician, Arnold Lea, who wrote in 1910: 'The retention of this word [puerperal fever] is undesirable for many reasons . . . it suggests the existence of a specific form of fever in lying-in women comparable to the exanthematous diseases [when] *all cases of fever during the puerperium, unless clearly attributable to some extraneous cause, should be considered as forms of wound infection*' (emphasis in original).[15] He suggested that 'puerperal fever' should be renamed 'puerperal infection', which would have been ideal, but unfortunately his suggestion was not adopted. Instead, the term 'puerperal sepsis' began to replace 'puerperal fever', with two unfortunate consequences.

If 'puerperal sepsis' had been confined to post-partum infection—that is, to puerperal fever in the traditional sense—all would have been well. Unfortunately, because septic abortion was also an infection of the genital tract, and was also due to a variety of bacteria, it was customary in many countries (including England and Wales, but not Scotland) to combine the mortality statistics of these two very different conditions under the single heading of puerperal sepsis. This foolish decision to combine septic abortion and post-partum sepsis in one single category, labelled 'puerperal sepsis', meant it was often impossible to separate the two components. A rise in deaths due to puerperal sepsis might be due to a rise in deaths due to septic abortion, or to post-partum sepsis, or to both, and it is obvious that the social, public-health, and clinical implications of a rise in septic abortion are quite different from those of a rise in post-partum sepsis.

The use of the term 'puerperal sepsis' led to a second source of error. By an act of terminological sloppiness, the habit crept in of using the term 'puerperal septicaemia' as meaning the same thing as 'puerperal sepsis'. 'Puerperal septicaemia' should have been reserved for cases in which septicaemia—infection of the bloodstream—had occurred. That is what it means. Unfortunately, when the Infectious Diseases (Notification) Act of 1899 was introduced, 'puerperal septicaemia' was the name chosen for 'puerperal fever' and listed as

---

[15] A. Lea, *Puerperal Infection* (London, 1910), 9.

such on the forms used for notifying infectious diseases. Many doctors interpreted the term 'puerperal septicaemia' and in the literal sense they were right to do so—as meaning that the only cases of puerperal fever for which notification was compulsory were those in which septicaemia had been proven. Many cases were therefore not notified. As a consequence, deaths from puerperal fever sometimes outnumbered notifications. An obstetrician noted in 1924 that in ninety-three counties and county boroughs in which he had instituted enquiries, there were 310 deaths registered as due to puerperal fever, and only 243 notified cases, giving an impossible case fatality rate of 127 per cent. As he dryly remarked, 'twenty years of compulsion has only secured comic figures'.[16]

Measuring Mortality due to Puerperal Fever

Mortality rates are usually expressed as the annual number of deaths per 100,000 or per million of the *population at risk* of suffering from a particular disease. For a disease such as tuberculosis, the population at risk is usually the whole population, male and female. For certain children's diseases, it is usually the total population under the age of 15. For puerperal fever, it might be thought that the population at risk is women of childbearing age between the ages of 15 and 44. But that fails to take into account falls or rises in the fertility rate.[17] Obviously, the lower the fertility rate, the fewer the pregnancies and the occasions on which women aged 15–44 will be at risk of puerperal infection. The correct method of measurement is the same as the maternal mortality rate, which is the number of maternal deaths per 1,000, 10,000, or 100,000 deliveries.[18] It is most convenient in historical studies to express maternal deaths in terms of 10,000 births; and that is the usage I will follow throughout this book unless stated otherwise.

The Bacteriology of Puerperal Fever

This aspect of puerperal fever is discussed in detail in Chapter 12. Briefly, puerperal fever could be due to a variety of micro-organisms, but a very large

[16] Loudon, *Death in Childbirth*, 51. The idiocy of this situation continued until 1926, when the Ministry of Health changed the definition of puerperal fever from 'puerperal septicaemia' to 'puerperal pyrexia', which was defined as 'Any pyrexia . . . within 21 days of childbirth or abortion . . . of 100.4° F sustained during a period of 24 hours . . . or recurring during this period'. The cause of the fever was deliberately omitted. This resulted in a sudden leap in the number of notified cases. The data on notifications of puerperal fever are about as useless after 1926 as they were between 1899 and 1926.

[17] The birth rate, or crude birth rate, is the ratio of the number of live births to the mid-year total population. The fertility rate is the ratio of live births to women aged 15–44.

[18] Strictly speaking, the maternal mortality rate is not a rate but a ratio, but the use of the term 'maternal mortality rate' persists all the same. Details of the technical problems surrounding the measurement of maternal mortality, which are of little importance to this book, are discussed in Loudon, *Death in Childbirth*, 19–39.

majority of severe cases and deaths were due to one organism, known today as *Streptococcus pyogenes* or as the Group A streptococcus. Puerperal fever was, in effect, a streptococcal disease, and a list of the many other diseases due to the Group A streptococcus can be found in Table 12.3. Mild puerperal fever was often caused by other micro-organisms, but virtually the only one to cause occasional severe or fatal outcomes was *Staphylococcus aureus* (see Table 12.2). As we will see in Chapter 12, the Group A streptococcus occurs in many different serotypes, and there is compelling evidence that the serotypes responsible for puerperal fever were the same as those responsible for erysipelas. This is a theme that will appear so often in the succeeding chapters that it is worth looking at it briefly at this stage.

The Link between Puerperal Fever and Erysipelas

The Group A streptococcus can cause several skin diseases, according to the depth to which it penetrates. Infection of the top layer only (the epidermis) is impetigo. It is not painful nor dangerous, but it is contagious and unsightly. If the infection involves the whole thickness of the skin (the dermis), it produces cellulitis or erysipelas. The distinction between the two is considered definite by some, and blurred by others. Cellulitis is usually the milder form that spreads slowly with a blurred edge between infected and normal skin. Erysipelas spreads more rapidly, is more likely to be accompanied by fever and pain, and has a characteristic raised edge. Cellulitis can appear anywhere on the body. So can erysipelas, but erysipelas has a predilection for appearing on the face. Recently a French dermatologist noted that the term 'cellulitis' was used in English-speaking countries, but was not regarded as a disease entity 'in Latin countries', where the term 'erysipelas' stands alone.[19] Regardless of terminology, however, the important point is that erysipelas can lead to streptococcal septicaemia and for this reason was, and occasionally still is, potentially very dangerous. In the second half of the nineteenth century there were, on average, about as many deaths a year from erysipelas as there were from puerperal fever.

If skin infection by the Group A streptococcus penetrates below the level of the skin, involving subcutaneous tissues such as ligaments, fat, muscle, and even bone, it becomes that very dangerous and frightening disease known as necrotizing fasciitis. This is always an uncommon disease, but there is evidence of an increase in incidence in developed countries since 1980. Necrotizing fasciitis is a modern name. The disease was previously known as 'phagadena' ('phage' meaning to eat because the infection 'eats away' infected tissues), or as gangrenous erysipelas. The most common cause of necrotizing fasciitis is the Group A streptococcus, but other organisms may be involved. In Chapter 4 we

---

[19] E. M. Grosshans, 'The Red Face Erysipelas', *Clinics in Dermatology*, 11 (1993), 307–14, at 311.

will be recounting an extraordinary epidemic of necrotizing fasciitis, ordinary erysipelas, and puerperal fever that occurred in the USA in the mid-nineteenth century.

Evidence of the close link between erysipelas and puerperal fever comes from several directions, but especially from case histories, such as the following account by Sir James Young Simpson. The story began with a carpenter who snagged the edge of his hand while placing a corpse in a coffin:

A severe attack of erysipelas followed. Subsequently his wife had a similar attack of erysipelas. Their daughter, living with them and in the seventh month of her pregnancy, was then taken with an attack of fever. In a day or two she gave birth to a dead child, whose body had all the appearance of being affected with erysipelas. The mother herself died within twenty-four hours with the symptoms of malignant puerperal fever . . .

The family doctor, Dr Hill, who attended this family, was 'on his road home from visiting the patient [when he] was called to a case of labour, and this other was also attacked with puerperal fever'.[20]

Mothers who were exposed before or after delivery to a case of erysipelas in their own home were at grave risk of dying of puerperal fever. Infants born to mothers who developed puerperal fever often died of erysipelas. Doctors who attended cases of erysipelas before attending a confinement often transferred the infection to their maternity patient, who then developed puerperal fever. Midwives and doctors who attended cases of puerperal fever were sometimes infected and developed erysipelas on their arms, and doctors who carried out post-mortem examinations on cases of puerperal fever were at risk of dying of erysipelas and septicaemia. Likewise, in hospitals with maternity departments, an outbreak of erysipelas on a surgical ward was apt to be followed by an outbreak of puerperal fever on the maternity ward. Town epidemics of puerperal fever were sometimes accompanied by an outbreak of erysipelas in the local hospital. It is probable that both the surgical and maternity cases were manifestations of a high carrier rate of virulent streptococci in the local population. The significance of the link between these two diseases will be discussed in Chapter 12.

Overview

This story of puerperal fever is arranged in roughly chronological order so that ideas can be traced as they emerged, were accepted or rejected, replaced, and sometimes rediscovered. The chapter that follows this introduction, Chapter 2, deals with the earliest ideas about puerperal fever, when it was first recognized as a distinct entity in the eighteenth century. Chapter 3 is about Alexander

[20] J. Y. Simpson, *Selected Obstetrical and Gynaecological Works of Sir James Y. Simpson Bart.*, ed. J. Watt Black (Edinburgh, 1871), 506.

Gordon of Aberdeen, who, at the end of the eighteenth century, wrote a brilliant treatise, which provided the first clear and irrefutable evidence that puerperal fever was a contagious disease, closely linked with erysipelas and transmitted from one woman to another by midwives and doctors.

Chapter 4 is an account of the least-known aspect of puerperal fever—the epidemics in towns that were a striking feature of the first half of the nineteenth century. The much better-known epidemics of puerperal fever occurred in lying-in (maternity) hospitals, and these are the subject of Chapter 5. Throughout, the history of puerperal fever is set in the context of the history of changing ideas on the nature, cause, prevention, and treatment of infectious diseases in general, and of the often vigorous and sometimes furious debates that surrounded a subject greatly favoured by medical historians: the problem of contagion, which is discussed in Chapter 6.

Chapter 7 deals with the most famous name in the history of puerperal fever, and indeed one of the famous names in the history of medicine: Ignaz Semmelweis, who worked at the Vienna maternity hospital in the mid-nineteenth century. Throughout the twentieth century he has been idolized by most historians, but I believe his importance has been exaggerated. It is the fascinating story of a man who made some highly original observations, but whose character was deeply flawed. Semmelweis died under mysterious circumstances in a common lunatic asylum. He was then almost totally forgotten until some twenty years after his death, when, quite suddenly, he was posthumously elevated to the status of an unjustly forgotten genius and a martyr, for reasons discussed at the end of Chapter 9.

Chapter 8 deals with the impact of the discovery of bacteria on ideas about puerperal fever, with special reference to Pasteur, and Chapter 9 describes the impact of the antiseptic method of Lord Lister on mortality due to puerperal fever. In Chapter 10 we come into the twentieth century and see that the period up to the mid-1930s was one of relative stagnation as far as puerperal fever was concerned, apart from some important research on the biology of the streptococcus. Chapter 11 is devoted to the story of the first effective treatment of puerperal fever: the introduction of the sulphonamides in the mid-1930s (penicillin came later). Within a period of twenty years puerperal fever had almost ceased to be a disease of any consequence.

Chapter 12 is an overview of the whole story of puerperal fever in which I attempt to fuse historical data with modern knowledge derived from microbiological research on the Group A streptococcus, and in particular with research since the 1980s, which has enabled us to understand much more than we did about the history of puerperal fever. This final chapter is more statistical and 'technical' than any of the previous chapters, but I have tried to write for readers with no special knowledge of medical and bacteriological matters.

2

Puerperal Fever in the Eighteenth Century

In the late eighteenth century, the naval physician Thomas Trotter (1760–1832) observed: 'The name and definition of a disease are perhaps of more importance than is generally thought. They are like a central point to which all converging rays tend: they direct future inquirers how to compare facts, and become, as it were, the base on which accumulating knowledge is to be heaped.'[1] This is certainly true of puerperal fever, which is probably as old as childbirth itself, for it was not until somewhere between the late seventeenth and the mid-eighteenth centuries that it came into existence in the sense of being named and recognized. It is true that from antiquity one can find passing references to disorders of lying-in women, some of which may well have been descriptions of puerperal fever, but scarcely anything of note was published on puerperal fever before the eighteenth century.[2] What references there are before 1700 are of little more than antiquarian interest and we know nothing of its prevalence or mortality in earlier times.

The First Appearance of the Term 'Puerperal Fever'

François Mauriceau (1637–1709), the greatest authority on childbirth in the seventeenth century, is believed to have been the first to describe epidemic puerperal fever, but he mentions the disease only briefly in his *Traité des maladies des femmes grosses* and dismisses it in a few uninformative sentences.[3] Thomas Willis (1621–75) was the first to use the term 'febris puerperarum' in

---

[1] T. Trotter, *Medicine Nautica* (3 vols.; London, 1797–1803), iii. 467. Trotter was actually talking about what seemed to him to be a new disease, which he called the 'Malignant Ulcer', which was probably the disease known today as necrotizing fasciitis.

[2] Lists of such references were compiled by a number of nineteenth- and twentieth-century authors, such as, for instance, Hervieux (1879) and Burtenshaw (1904), both of whom started with descriptions by Hippocrates and Galen. See J.-F.-E. Hervieux, 'Revue historique et critique des principales doctrines qui ont régné sur ce qu'on a appellé la fièvre puerpérale', *L'Union médicale*, 2nd ser., 30 (1886), 66–71, 84–7, 97–106; J. H. Burtenshaw, 'The Fever of the Puerperium (Puerperal Infection)', *New York Journal and Philadelphia Medical Journal*, 79 (1904), 1073–9, 1134–8, 1189–94, and 1234–8; 80 (1904), 20–5.

[3] F. H. Garrison, *An Introduction to the History of Medicine* (4th edn., Philadelphia, 1929), 277. F. Mauriceau, *Traité des maladies des femmes grosses* (Paris, 1668).

1676,[4] but the Anglicized version, 'puerperal fever', did not appear until 1716, in an essay on fevers by the physician Edward Strother. This is a curious work, for it opens with a long section on the importance of mathematics before it comes to the fevers, which are defined as a group of disorders in which there is 'An unusual or Preternatural Heat along with a Frequency and Quickness of the Pulse'.[5]

Strother divided fevers into groups such as the 'Ardent' and the 'Slow and Hectic', and described them in considerable detail. At the end of the book, he compiled an appendix consisting of a list of fevers with brief definitions of each. In the middle of this list, two fevers come side by side:

The LACTEAL FEVER, a fever coming on the Third Day after Labour from the Milk in the Blood . . . The PUERPERAL FEVER . . . [which] have pains in the Abdomen Hypogastrica and Loins. I suspect it to be Inflammatory mostly. 'Tis from the Lochia suppressed.[6]

This is the sole reference to puerperal fever. There is no indication that he regarded it as an important, still less a specific disorder. It was an inflammatory fever that sometimes followed childbirth. That was all.

It was not until the mid-eighteenth century that puerperal fever first began to be recognized as a common and dreadful disease, as fatal if not more so as any other kind of fever, and quite distinct from other fevers. Although there was much dissent over the nature and the 'seat' of the disease, a small minority was of the opinion that it was an ordinary common fever, sometimes found in lying-in women because childbirth had increased their susceptibility to fevers. By the late eighteenth century, puerperal fever for the majority of physicians was a specific disease, an entity confined to lying-in women. As Hulme said in 1772: 'it is a disease *sui generis*, of a nature peculiar to itself, and as simple and regular in its appearance, for the most part, as any distemper incident to the human body . . .'.[7] It was also the most serious, deadly, and terrifying of all the complications of childbirth and the most common cause of maternal deaths.[8]

---

[4] Burtenshaw, 'The Fever of the Puerperium', 1076, and Garrison, *History of Medicine*, 263. But according to F. Winckel (*The Pathology and Treatment of Childbed* (London, 1876)), the term was first used by Morton and only afterwards by Willis.

[5] Edward Strother, *Criticon Februm, or a Critical Essay on Fevers* (London, 1716), 74. It is interesting in passing to note an early reference to thermometry. Strother suggested that a thermometer might be a means by which the heat of a fever could be distinguished from 'The Natural Warmth' of the body, thus allowing 'Perfect Judgement' in fevers. It can be found on p. 82, where the author states that the 'Natural Heat can not otherwise be demonstrably determined, than by the Person's having often before such a seizure try'd with a Thermometer the Standard of their Natural Warmth; but this not being as yet practised (which I look upon as being a fault) . . .'. [6] Ibid. 207–8.

[7] Nathaniel Hulme, *A Treatise on the Puerperal Fever* (London, 1772), repr. in Fleetwood Churchill (ed.), *Essays on the Puerperal Fever and Other Diseases Peculiar to Women* (London, 1849), 61–116, at 69.

[8] In passing it should be noted that the word 'puerperium' denotes the 'lying-in period'—that is, 'the period of confinement, after labour'; hence of course, puerperal fever. But 'puerperal' was often used loosely as an alternative to 'maternal', as, for instance, when authors used 'puerperal mortality' not in the strict sense of maternal deaths occurring after labour, but as a synonym for 'maternal mortality' including maternal deaths that occurred during pregnancy or labour.

The Recognition of Puerperal Fever as a Separate Disease

Why did puerperal fever receive so little recognition until the eighteenth century? Was such late recognition due to the growth of medical knowledge and nosology leading to a more sophisticated description and classification of fevers? These factors may have played a part, but the main reason is quite simple.

Until the 1740s in Britain (and about fifty years earlier in some parts of France) the management of normal as well as abnormal childbirth was not an accepted part of medical practice. In so far as medical practitioners were involved in childbirth, it was, with very few exceptions, only when they were called by a midwife to attend complicated deliveries that lay beyond her powers. Normal childbirth belonged to women: to the parturient mother, the midwife, and the group of friends or 'gossips' who were chosen by the mother to keep her company in her labour. Medical practitioners were not involved. It was not their province, and most midwives, or so it was said, seldom recognized puerperal fever for what it was. One London accoucheur complained in 1772 that 'Nurses and women in general seem, in a great measure, ignorant of such a disease as this being incident to lying-in persons. I dare venture to say that the very name of it is as much a stranger to most of them as if no such malady existed; and yet there never was a time when this disease did not exist.'[9] Another explained in 1793 why puerperal fever had been neglected: 'The reason for this apparent negligence is that in most countries the practice of midwifery, and the subsequent treatment of lying-in women, has been committed to women, the nature of whose education did not lead them to make, or record, observations.'[10] In the UK the regular involvement of medical men in normal as well as abnormal childbirth dates from the mid-eighteenth century. By the end of the century, midwifery had become an integral part of the practice of almost all the numerous surgeon–apothecaries, the predecessors of the general practitioners and the same in all but title.[11]

But the major reason for the sudden recognition of puerperal fever was the appearance of the lying-in hospitals, which were plagued by puerperal fever from the time they were first established until the very end of the nineteenth century. The physicians appointed to lying-in hospitals, who were also the authors

---

[9] Hulme, *A Treatise on the Puerperal Fever*, in Churchill (ed.), *Essays*, 76. The diary of a midwife in Maine, USA, during the late eighteenth and early nineteenth centuries shows that she had several cases that can be identified almost certainly as puerperal fever. But it seems she did not recognize puerperal fever as a specific disorder of the lying-period. Neither the name 'childbed fever' nor 'puerperal fever' appears in her records. See L. T. Ulrich, *A Midwife's Tale: The Life of Martha Ballard, Based on her Diary, 1785–1812* (New York, 1990).

[10] John Clarke, *Practical Essays on the Arrangement of Pregnancy and Labour and on the Inflammatory and Febrile Diseases of Lying-in Women* (London, 1793; 2nd edn., 1806), 47.

[11] See I. Loudon, 'The Nature of Provincial Medical Practice in Eighteenth-Century England', *Medical History*, 29 (1985), 1–41; 'The Concept of the Family Doctor', *Bulletin of the History of Medicine*, 58 (1984), 347–62; 'Obstetrics and the General Practitioner', *British Medical Journal*, 301 (1990), 703–7.

of most of the treatises on puerperal fever, saw far more cases in a year, if not in a few months, than a physician whose practice was confined to home visits would see in a lifetime. Indeed, puerperal fever threatened to undermine the whole charitable purpose of hospitals that had been erected to help, not to kill, poor childbearing women. Hirsch, the nineteenth-century author of the magnificent *Handbook of Geographical and Historical Pathology*, pointed out in 1881,

The important place which puerperal fever now takes in the statistics of sickness and mortality of civilised countries dates no farther back than the end of the seventeenth or beginning of the eighteenth century, or from the period when the first maternity hospitals or other institutions for the reception of the lying-in were established.[12]

There are only rare instances of occasions when puerperal fever is mentioned by name by English practitioners before the establishment of lying-in hospitals. William Brownrigg MD FRS (1712–1800) is one. Brownrigg, a physician in Whitehaven, Cumberland, whose casebook has survived and who was highly educated and widely read, described and named six cases of puerperal fever in 1737–8, of whom five died.[13] It is unlikely, however, that the general run of provincial medical practitioners had heard of puerperal fever as early as the 1730s. Indeed, as we will see in the next chapter, it seems that the disease was unknown in Aberdeen as late as the 1780s.[14]

Broadly speaking, then, the recognition of puerperal fever in Britain was at first largely confined to London accoucheurs who held appointments at lying-in hospitals. Faced with recurrent epidemics of the disease, they had, as it were, to start from scratch, relying on clinical observation and personal experience, for there was no canon of accepted work on 'the fever of childbed' and virtually no guidance from ancient authority. Not that they saw this as a disadvantage. On the contrary. In a passage that characterizes late-eighteenth-century medicine, John Leake, physician–accoucheur to the Westminster Lying-in Hospital, wrote in 1772 that:

Nothing has been so great an obstacle to the improvement of science as the partiality and obsequious regard which men have been apt to pay to great authorities . . . Of late, indeed, medical writers have happily withdrawn themselves from the fairy-land of hypothesis and conjecture, and instead of deviating from the solid path of nature,

---

[12] A. Hirsch, *Handbook of Geographical and Historical Pathology* (2nd edn., 1881), trans. C. Creighton, (3 vols.; London, 1883), ii. 419. In choosing the late seventeenth and early eighteenth centuries, Hirsch had continental lying-in hospitals in mind. They preceded English ones by some fifty years.

[13] J. E. Ward and J. Yell (eds.), 'The Medical Casebook of William Brownrigg MD FRS (1712–1800) of the Town of Whitehaven in Cumberland', *Medical History*, suppl. no. 13 (London, 1993). The one woman who survived, Mrs Drewitt, is a doubtful case of puerperal fever, because the symptoms do not suggest puerperal fever and the illness did not commence until three weeks after the birth of the baby.

[14] My own research into casebooks and other manuscript sources of the mid-eighteenth century, which included cases of midwifery, did not reveal a single instance of the term 'puerperal fever' (I. Loudon, *Medical Care and the General Practitioner, 1750–1850* (Oxford, 1986)).

as many of them had formerly done, are now principally guided by observation and experience.[15]

The same sentiments were expressed even more forcibly in 1795 by Alexander Gordon, whose work is the subject of the next chapter: 'I combat opinions on the certain ground of practice, and not on the uncertain ground of theory; for which reason, the highest authority upon earth could not persuade me to admit a doctrine which disagrees with my own experience.'[16] In this frame of mind, they observed cases, 'opened bodies', and kept careful notes. While there was general agreement on puerperal fever as a separate entity, on the details there was a great deal of dissension. No sooner had one author published a work in which he presented his views on the causes, pathology, and the correct form of treatment than another published opposite views of equal cogency. It was a feature that drove John Leake to exclaim, 'Which way are we to turn, where rocks lie on one side and quicksands on the other?'[17] What, then, were the views of the authors of these eighteenth-century treatises that laid the groundwork for future investigations and theories?

Early Views on the Nature and Causes of Puerperal Fever

Continental authorities in the early eighteenth century[18] believed puerperal fever was due to the suppression or retention of the lochia—the lochia being the uterine discharge following childbirth.[19] This idea, however, was gradually replaced by the theory of 'milk metastasis', or 'the translation of the milk',[20] a theory that was apparently confirmed in the winter of 1746 when there was an outbreak of puerperal fever in the lying-in wards of the Hôtel Dieu in Paris in which almost every woman who contracted the disease died of it. On opening the bodies, it was seen that the intestines and omentum were covered with a substance that appeared to be putrified milk, which, it was assumed, had been carried in the bloodstream from the breasts to the peritoneal cavity.[21]

---

[15] John Leake, *Practical Observations on the Child-Bed fever* (London, 1772), repr. in Fleetwood Churchill (ed.), *Essays*, 117–204, at 121.

[16] Alexander Gordon, *A Treatise on the Epidemic Puerperal Fever of Aberdeen* (London, 1795), 59.

[17] Leake, *Practical Observations*.

[18] In this and subsequent sections of this chapter I have used both original publications wherever possible. I have also used Fleetwood Churchill's convenient collection of eighteenth-century treatises on puerperal fever published as *Essays on the Puerperal Fever and Other Diseases Peculiar to Women* (London, 1849) for the treatises of Joseph Clarke, Denham, Hulme and Leake, and the modern edition of Charles White, *A Treatise on the Management of Pregnant and Lying-in Women* (London, 1773), which was republished in 1987, with an introduction by Lawrence D. Longo, by Science History Publications, Canton, Mass.).   [19] Hervieux, 'Revue historique et critique', 66–71 n. 2.

[20] It is interesting that Brownrigg of Whitehaven appears to have subscribed to supression of the lochia as the primary cause of puerperal fever, although he also believed 'the fever is partly caused by her milk' (Ward and Yell (eds.), 'Medical Casebook', the case of Mrs Hudlestone, pp. 100–2).

[21] Metastasis refers to the transfer of disease from one organ or part of the body to another not directly connected with it. The transfer is usually through the bloodstream. It has now become synonymous with the spread of cancer, but it is still perfectly correct to use it to describe the transfer of infected or other material involved in disease processes.

It was an attractive idea, for it linked together the two fevers, 'milk fever' or 'lacteal fever' (in modern terminology acute mastitis) and puerperal fever. What the French doctors were seeing at post-mortem was, of course, not milk but streptococcal pus; but they clung firmly to the putrid-milk theory until it was shown to be false by Bichat in 1801.[22]

In Britain, few accepted the milk-metastasis theory. Thomas Denman, one of the most famous accoucheurs of his day, referred to it in his essay on puerperal fever published in 1773 and said he belived it was groundless. Instead he pointed out that many opinions existed: some accoucheurs thought puerperal fever was a miliary fever (miliary fever was a form of typhus), others that it was an inflammation of the uterus, and some believed it was confined to the bowels.[23]

Nathaniel Hulme (1772) believed the immediate cause of puerperal fever 'is an inflammation of the intestines' and the chief proximate cause 'the pressure of the gravid uterus against the intestines and omentum—the faeces being long pent up by the pressure of the gravid uterus, become putrid . . .'. In short, the diseases stemmed from the putridity of the bowels.[24] Thomas Kirkland (1774) was exceptional in not believing that puerperal fever was a single specific disease, but a number of different fevers for which there were many causes, an idea that was revived briefly in the mid-nineteenth century.[25]

John Leake, a London physician–accoucheur with a hospital appointment, was uncertain about puerperal fever. On the whole, he was inclined to think it was an inflammation of the omentum. He described how the opening of the bodies of women who had died of puerperal fever led 'to a putrid flatus, intolerable to the smell, [that] issued forth with a hissing noise, and the prominence of the belly immediately subsided'. This flatus came not from the bowel but from the peritoneal cavity and the putrid omentum.[26] Joseph Clarke concluded in 1793 that puerperal fever 'consists in an inflammation of the peritoneum; and hence, the nosological name of peritonitis has been given to it by Dr Forster'.[27]

As many observed at the time, anyone seeking guidance from these treatises would have found a great deal of confusion. Almost no one in Britain supported the theory of 'milk metastasis', but some still favoured the suppression of the lochia or the menses. A few thought puerperal fever was a form of typhus or erysipelas that became transformed into puerperal fever when it affected lying-in women. From the anatomical point of view, some thought the seat of the

[22] Hervieux, 'Revue historique et critique', 70.
[23] Thomas Denman, *Essay on the Puerperal Fever* (London, 1768; 2nd edn., 1773); repr. in Churchill (ed.), *Essays*, 43–60.
[24] Hulme, *A Treatise on the Puerperal Fever*, in Churchill (ed.), *Essays*, 103.
[25] Thomas Kirkland, *A Treatise on Childbed Fevers, and the Methods of Preventing Them* (London, 1774).
[26] Leake, *Practical Observations*. Leake, incidentally, began his treatise by accusing Hulme of plagiarism. Hulme had attended Leake's lectures, and Leake maintained he had copied down the lectures and published them as his own ideas.
[27] Joseph Clarke, 'Observations on the Puerperal Fever etc.', *Edinburgh Medical Commentaries*, 15 (1790), 299 ff.; repr. in Churchill (ed.), *Essays*, 351–62, at 356.

disease was the uterus, others the omentum, and most the peritoneum. The notion that puerperal fever was a form of peritonitis gradually gained ground, until, in the 1830s, Gooch went so far as suggesting it should be renamed 'puerperal peritonitis'.[28]

Almost everyone agreed puerperal fever was 'epidemical', for it was known to be a seasonal disease with a winter peak, usually in February.[29] This appeared to support the theory of the 'epidemic constitution' of the atmosphere, in the sense that Sydenham used the term as the crucial factor in determining what kind of fever prevailed at certain seasons. This notion was held by most London accoucheurs, such as Nathaniel Hulme and John Leake.[30] There were several difficulties, however, in accepting epidemic constitution as a major factor. Epidemics in hospitals and towns should have occurred at the same time. Often, however, they were independent of each other. Further, hospital epidemics were only slightly seasonal in onset.

There were other ideas. Some held that pregnancy and childbirth induced a state of 'irritability' or susceptibility to fevers—an idea that came to the fore in the mid-nineteenth century. Others believed that the birth of a baby led to a flood of blood into the emptied abdominal cavity, with gross disturbance of the circulation. Others dwelt on the proximity of the bowel to the uterus and the way they were pressed tightly against each other during pregnancy. Tight stays were also blamed in this, as in other diseases. In short, there was a multiplicity of theories on the 'seat' or nature of puerperal fever and on the underlying causes of the disease.

Charles White and the Prevention of Puerperal Fever

When he surveyed these muddled and contradictory treatises of the 1760s and 1770s, the surgeon Charles White of Manchester saw the need for a work based on clear and definite opinions. A practical man, interested in therapy rather than theory, he decided to write a treatise on the correct management of the lying-in period. Significantly, he did not call his work a treatise on puerperal fever, but *A Treatise on the Management of Pregnant and Lying-in Women*, and it was published in 1773.[31]

It is a work that has received much more attention from historians than its predecessors, partly, perhaps, because of its air of authority. White held strong

---

[28] R. Gooch, *An Account of Some of the Most Important Diseases Peculiar to Women* (London, 1831; 2nd edn., 1838), 2.

[29] This was indeed correct. In temperate zones streptococcal infections are still strongly seasonal, reaching a peak in late winter with the lowest level in August. See B. B. Breese and C. Breese Hall, *Beta Hemolytic Streptococcal Diseases* (Boston, 1978), 40, graph.

[30] Hulme, *A Treatise on the Puerperal Fever*; Leake, *Practical Observations*.

[31] Charles White, *A Treatise on the Management of Pregnant and Lying-in Women*, and *An Appendix to the Second Edition of Mr C. White's Treatise on the Management of Pregnant and Lying-in Women* (London, 1777).

views and expressed them firmly. He was sure that puerperal fever was caused by the spread of putrid matter from the bowel to the womb, by the suppression of the lochia, and most of all by the putridity of the atmosphere in the lying-in room where the air was 'vitiated air' because of closed windows, a large fire to prevent the patient 'catching cold', soiled bedclothes, the unemptied close-stool, and a crowd of women in attendance.

In the opening pages White provides a memorable account of the way that 'nurses' (the term was used by everyone to include midwives) managed their patients during their lying-in. Even if labour was quick and normal, nurses insisted that the patient was kept lying perfectly flat in bed for several days:

She is covered up close in bed with additional cloaths, the curtains are drawn round the bed, and pinned together, every crevice in the windows and door is stopped close, not excepting even the key hole, the windows are guarded not only with shutters and curtains, but even with blankets, the more effectually to exclude the fresh air, and the good woman is not suffered to put her arm or even her nose, out of bed, for fear of catching cold. She is constantly supplied out of the spout of a teapot with large quantities of warm liqours . . .[32]

If the woman had a shivering fit—the first ominous sign of puerperal fever—the nurses thought that for all their efforts she had caught cold, and they piled on more blankets, stoked up the fire, and plied her more and more with hot spiritous liquors.

All this was anathema to Charles White, who waged war against such traditions with a vigour that must have shocked and astonished the nurses, and may well have lost him some patients. He threw open the windows of the lying-in room, put out the fires, kept his patients cool, and banished everyone from the lying-in room except those who were essential for the care of the patient. He instructed his patients to sit up high in bed to encourage drainage of the lochia, and he insisted on the absolute cleanliness of the bedlinen and the banishment of all smells and vapours that created the putrid miasmas, the prime causes of puerperal fever.

Charles White's treatise was revolutionary in its attack on long-standing tradition, its clarity, and its dogmatism. For the practitioner seeking guidance, it must have seemed at the time the best of all the treatises published in the 1770s. Some modern writers have exaggerated the importance of White by portraying him as an early advocate of antisepsis and asepsis.[33] That is nonsense. It never occurred to White that the disease entered the uterus through the birth canal, or that scrupulous cleanliness of the hands or obstetric instruments of

[32] White, *Treatise* (1773), 3.

[33] In 1922 J. George Adami, Vice-Chancellor of the University of Liverpool, made extravagant claims for Charles White, whom he saw as one of the founding fathers of the Manchester medical school, claiming that White practised antisepsis and was far ahead of his time. It was perhaps a case of strong north-west England local loyalties getting in the way (J. George Adami, *Charles White of Manchester (1728–1813), and the Arrest of Puerperal Fever* (Liverpool, 1922)).

the birth attendant was a factor of any importance. White's insistence on fresh air and cleanliness was based solely on his certainty that it was the only way to prevent putrid miasmas.

The Treatment of Puerperal Fever

Broadly speaking, the treatment of puerperal fever in the eighteenth century consisted of either medicines or venesection or both. It would be possible but historically unprofitable to list all the suggested forms of medical treatment and their respective supporters. The number was legion, and extravagant claims were made. For instance, in the 1770s the maternity wards of the Hôtel Dieu in Paris suffered epidemics of puerperal fever in which nearly every patient died. Dr Doulcet tried the effects of doses of ipecachuana, and claimed this was so successful that he saved the lives of 200 women with this form of treatment.[34] The French government ordered the Royal Medical Society of Paris to invest-igate these claims and a translation of the resultant report made ipecachuana briefly fashionable in England.[35]

Unfortunately, as so often happens with spectacular claims, the treatment mysteriously failed to work in other people's hands, and it soon died out. Similar claims were made for a wide variety of medicines. William Butter of Derbyshire published a short series of cases of puerperal fever cured by such simple medicines as 'rhubarb and cordial confection'. They never failed, he said, and he rejected the use of the lancet as unnecessary and sometimes dangerous. Many of his contemporaries, however, believed that what Butter had described was not puerperal fever at all, but a simple mild intermittent fever. That was why his patients recovered. Almost certainly they were correct.[36]

As far as treatment was concerned, the main issue was whether or not to bleed in puerperal fever. Charles White was in favour of bleeding on some occasions but not on others.[37] Leake was in favour of early and copious bleeding in all cases.[38] Joseph Clarke of Dublin, on the other hand, had never seen any bene-fits from bleeding and thought it harmful.[39] Denman, with uncharacteristic indecision, was against bleeding in the first edition of his *Essay on the Puerperal Fever* in 1768, unless there was clear evidence of an inflammatory process. In the second edition of 1773, however, and in the chapters on puerperal fever

---

[34] Clarke, 'Observations on the Puerperal Fever etc.', in Churchill (ed.), *Essays*, 353.

[35] John Whitehead, *A Report made by Order of Government, of a Memoir, Containing a New, Easy, and Successful Method of Treating the Child-Bed or Puerperal Fever, Made Use of by the late M. Doulcet* (London, 1783).

[36] William Butter, *An Account of the Puerperal Fevers as they Appear in Derbyshire and Some of the Counties Adjacent* (London, 1775). It is possible that the cases seen by Butter were due to very mild strains of the streptococcus, but it is more likely that they were due to some other organism or some other disease, and not puerperal fever.   [37] White, *Treatise* (1773), 11.

[38] Leake, *Practical Observations*, repr. in Churchill (ed.), *Essays*, 118.

[39] Joseph Clarke, 'Observations on the Puerperal Fever', repr. in Churchill (ed.), *Essays*, 361.

in later editions of his textbook of midwifery, he had changed his mind and recommended early and copious bleeding as a general rule.

Once again, these citations show the variety of muddled ideas that surrounded this disease. William Hunter appears to have been alone in saying what others may have thought privately—that nothing was of any use. 'Of those attacked by this disease,' said Hunter in one of his lectures, 'treat them in any manner you will, at least three out of four will die . . . We tried various methods (bleeding, refrigerants, stimulants, mithridate) but everything failed.'[40] Hunter may have been right, but therapeutic nihilism, however honest, is unpalatable. What was needed was firm evidence of the cause of the disease that could point the way to prevention and treatment. This is what Alexander Gordon of Aberdeen appeared to provide, and we come to him next.

[40] As far as I can discover, Hunter never published these views, but they are reported by several authors as having been given in his lectures; e.g. Gooch, *An Account of Some of the Most Important Diseases Peculiar to Women*, 9.

3

Gordon of Aberdeen

In 1795 Alexander Gordon of Aberdeen (1752–99) published an account of an epidemic of puerperal fever. It is one of the most comprehensive accounts of an epidemic of puerperal fever ever written and a masterpiece of early epidemiology.[1] Gordon was the son of a tenant farmer in Aberdeenshire; he studied medicine at Marischal College in Aberdeen, and then in Edinburgh and possibly in Leyden. After serving as a surgeon in the Royal Navy, he spent just under a year in London studying midwifery before returning to Aberdeen towards the end of 1785 at the age of 33.[2]

He may well have been the only person in the far north of Scotland with an extensive knowledge of midwifery and the world of the London accoucheurs. He certainly knew, and probably owned, copies of the treatises we discussed in the last chapter. Soon after his return to Aberdeen, Gordon founded a dispensary for the poor and provided courses of instruction for the midwives of Aberdeen. Through the dispensary he established himself as the sole accoucheur to the poor, working closely with the midwives of the town. He also established a successful private practice.

Gordon would have been a worthy but unknown physician were it not for an epidemic of puerperal fever that began in Aberdeen in December 1789 and lasted until March 1792. The people of Aberdeen, knowing nothing of puerperal fever, believed it to be an epidemic of an ephemeral fever called the 'Weed', which was usually brief and seldom fatal, and for which, it was said, bleeding should never be employed. From his experience in London, however, Gordon could see at once that this was not the 'Weed' but puerperal fever. After the first few cases had occurred he began keeping careful notes . Because the epidemic occurred in a town as opposed to a lying-in hospital, Gordon was able to make three vital observations:

1. that the disease was contagious and was transmitted from one case to another by doctors and midwives;

---

[1] Alexander Gordon, *A Treatise on the Epidemic Puerperal Fever of Aberdeen* (London, 1795).
[2] I. A. Porter, *Alexander Gordon of Aberdeen, 1752–1799* (Aberdeen University Studies No. 139; Edinburgh, 1958); G. P. Milne, 'The History of Midwifery in Aberdeen', *Aberdeen University Review*, 47 (1978), 293–303. C. J. Cullingworth, *Oliver Wendell Holmes and the Contagiousness of Puerperal Fever* (London, 1906), 33–5, app. II, 'Biographical Sketch of Dr Alexander Gordon of Aberdeen, 1752–99'.

2. that there was a close relationship between puerperal fever and erysipelas;
3. (and here of course I am taking his conclusions at face value) that early and copious bleeding was the only hope of curing the disease.

Gordon's Treatise

The treatise opens with a description of the character of the epidemic, which was

not confined to the town of Aberdeen but extended to the suburbs and contiguous country where it proved as fatal as in the heart of the city. It was not peculiar to any particular constitution, or temperament, but promiscuously seized women of all constitutions and temperaments; for the strong and the weak, the robust and the delicate, the old and the young, the married and the single, those who had easy, and those who had difficult labours, were all equally and indiscriminately affected. It prevailed principally among the lower classes of women, and on account of my public office, and extensive practice in Midwifery, most of the cases came under my care. But women in the higher walks of life were not exempted, when they happened to be delivered by a midwife, or physician, who had previously attended any patients labouring under the disease.[3]

He then turns to the orthodox view that puerperal fever was influenced by the epidemic constitution. He had kept 'an account of the weather and the state of the atmosphere', but he soon came to the conclusion that the epidemic constitution was irrelevant, 'because I discovered that the disease was occasioned by a cause very different from the sensible qualities, or constitution of the air'.[4] The key paragraph on which the whole of the first part of the treatise was based is as follows:

I plainly perceived the channel by which it [puerperal fever] was propagated; and I arrived at that certainty in the matter, that I could venture to foretell what women would be affected with the disease, upon hearing by what midwife they were to be delivered, or by what nurse they were to be attended during their lying-in: and, almost in every instance, my prediction was correct.[5]

It was the ability to forecast that was so convincing. He went further. While others had emphasized the variability of the symptoms of puerperal fever, Gordon was convinced 'there is scarce any disease more regular in its time and manner of attack, or more uniform in its appearance and symptoms'. Almost all his cases began very early on the second or third day after delivery, and Gordon was yet another who emphasized the constancy of the abdominal pain: 'In the Puerperal Fever the abdomen cannot be pressed upon without occasioning great pain. The pain was so excruciating that the miserable patients described their torture to be as great, or greater than what they suffered during labour.'[6]

---

[3] Gordon, *A Treatise on the Epidemic Puerperal Fever of Aberdeen*, 2–3.
[4] Ibid. 3.   [5] Ibid. 3.   [6] Ibid. 7.

Gordon's views were highly unorthodox in that he insisted that all the cases were due to a single cause. He dismissed the notions of epidemic influence and the suppression of the lochia (in none of his cases, he wrote, was the lochia suppressed; at worst it was slightly diminished), and he could see no evidence of individual predisposition.[7]

The originality of Gordon's observations has been stressed by many; but the extent to which he rejected the received wisdom of the day has not attracted the attention it deserves. To many of his contemporaries Gordon—the son of a tenant farmer working amongst the poor in the extreme and barren north of Scotland, who held no hospital or university appointment—must have seemed far too cocksure, too dogmatic, too provincial, and too unknown to command the respect he deserved.

The Link with Erysipelas

Gordon's second great contribution was the demonstration of the link between puerperal fever and erysipelas. From the evidence of autopsies, Gordon was convinced that puerperal fever was an inflammatory disease, leading to 'mortification or suppuration of the parts contained within the cavity of the abdomen'.[8] He continued: 'Having proved that the Puerperal Fever is an inflammatory disease, I shall next endeavour to investigate the specific nature of the inflammation, or inquire, whether it be of the nature of Phlegmon or Erysipelas.' His certainty that there was a link between the two diseases was based not so much on appearances during life or at post-mortem as on epidemiological observations:

That the Puerperal Fever is of the nature of erysipelas, was supposed by Pouteau forty years ago, and has been the opinion of Doctors Young and Home of Edinburgh, since that time. I will not venture positively to assert, that the Puerperal Fever and Erysipelas are precisely of the same specific nature; but that they are connected, that there is an analogy between them, and that they are concomitant epidemics, I have unquestionable proofs. For these two epidemics began in Aberdeen at the same time, and afterwards kept pace together; they both arrived at their *acmè* together, and they both ceased at the same time.[9]

Further, Gordon noted that, while the epidemics of puerperal fever and erysipelas raged together, almost every surgical case admitted with a wound to the [Aberdeen] hospital 'was soon after his admission seized with erysipelas in the vicinity of the wound'. Thereby Gordon established the link through

---

[7] Gordon, *A Treatise on the Epidemic Puerperal Fever of Aberdeen*, 10–11.   [8] Ibid. 53–4.

[9] Ibid. 55–6. While quoting Young and Home, Gordon failed to mention Denman's passing comment that 'There is a peculiarity in this fever which I believe has never been observed. It is an erysipelatous appearance, of a dusky red colour, on the knuckles, wrists, elbows, knees, or ankles . . . This is always a mortal sign.' Possibly he thought it too trivial, or possibly he missed it. See T. Denman, *Essay on the Puerperal Fever* (London, 1768; 2nd edn., 1773); repr. in Fleetwood Churchill (ed.), *Essays on the Puerperal Fever and Other Diseases Peculiar to Women* (London, 1849), 43–60, at 48.

erysipelas between surgical infection and puerperal fever, a link whose import-ance was not fully realized for many years.

Notice that Gordon was not, and did not claim to be, the first to suggest that puerperal fever and erysipelas were due to the same 'poison'. He was, however, the first to provide convincing evidence that would be confirmed by scores of authors over the next fifty and more years.

Treatment

The final and largest part of Gordon's treatise is devoted to treatment. Here, Gordon's supreme self-confidence expands into an almost aggressive dogmat-ism. He was convinced he had found the cure for puerperal fever. Every case should be treated by bleeding and purging, but the crucial element was bleed-ing, which must be done early in the disease and must be copious. To take ten ounces of blood (the standard quantity in the treatment of inflammatory fevers) was insufficient. It had to be twenty ounces at least, and preferably twenty-four. If recovery was not rapid, bleeding should be repeated. Other treatments might assist to a minor degree, but compared with copious bleeding they were useless.

Every case, he said, in which venesection was carried out *early and copiously* recovered, and sometimes the recovery was spectacular. He cited instances where he saw a patient with a high fever and abdominal pain one day, bled her copi-ously, and found her the next morning sitting up in bed, free from pain, and feeling well. Patients who died were, according to Gordon, those not bled at all, or those who were bled too late, or too timidly.

Gordon's evidence seems so convincing that, if it were a modern form of treat-ment that claimed to produce such results in a fatal disease, it would pass today's ethical committees and probably receive a grant for a randomized trial, for he insisted that in the cure of this disease he had been 'much more successful than any other practitioner'.[10] But his insistence on copious bleeding put his reputation at stake. His methods came under the floodlight of public opinion, and he was well aware of the dangers:

According to vulgar custom in this country the women came from all quarters to see the patient[s] and to offer their advice. Several ladies joined the crowd; and though they neither knew the nature, nor even the name of the disease, yet they gave their advice with great freedom. Some said it was wrong to bleed, others that it was improper to purge . . . supposing the disease was what they called a weed; and, seemingly actuated by other motives than the good of the patient, they proposed different practitioners, every one recommending her own favourite.[11]

In the case of John Low's wife in August 1790, Gordon was called in when puerperal fever was established. He bled her and purged her, but she died and

---

[10] Gordon, *A Treatise on the Epidemic Puerperal Fever of Aberdeen*, 73.   [11] Ibid. 27.

Gordon was bitterly criticized. Gordon believed that in this case, as in several others, he was called too late for bleeding to be effective. Unfortunately, he believed that in the end his success would speak for itself: 'In this manner [bleeding], at last, I fairly got the better of a prejudice, which I thought invincible . . . and thus I had the satisfaction to see the voice of clamour effectually silenced.'[12] In fact, as we will see, the clamour was not silenced. It reappeared when his treatise was published.

I suspect there are two reasons why Gordon was so certain that bleeding was effective. First, he was sure that bleeding had to be performed very early in the disease. If he bled the patient copiously and she still died, he assumed it was because the disease had already been too well established; if only he had been called earlier, she would have survived. It was a general feature of epidemics that, the earlier the onset, the more likely the patient would die. Thus it would be in such cases of very early onset that, by the time Gordon was called, he would feel that the disease was so far advanced that his treatment was too late. A similar argument was, incidentally, used in the twentieth century to justify radical mastectomy for cancer of the breast: if the patient appeared to be cured, it was due to the operation; if secondaries appeared, that was proof that the operation had not been performed early enough.

The second reason was that Gordon did not arrive at his conclusion about early and copious bleeding until the epidemic was already established and had been present for several months. It was the nature of all epidemics of puerperal fever that the fatality rate was always highest at the beginning of the epidemic, and declined after the epidemic had been established for some months. Thus most of the cases that Gordon bled copiously were cases late in the epidemic —the very cases most likely to recover in any case. As the epidemic progressed, Gordon was able to see the decline in the case fatality rate (see Fig. 3.1) and, attributing this to his treatment, was able to sustain his belief in venesection.

The Epidemic and the Treatise

Table 3.1 and Fig. 3.1 are based on a table published by Gordon in his treatise.[13] It lists only cases in which Gordon was involved, directly or indirectly. There is no information on the total number of cases in Aberdeen, and none on how many deliveries were not followed by puerperal fever. We do not know how many midwives were practising at the time. He listed seventeen midwives in his treatise, and also mentions Mrs Jefferies, who had 'all the practice of the old town of Aberdeen'. Although the old town was 'only a mile from the new town', it was never visited by puerperal fever because, says Gordon,

---

[12] Gordon, *A Treatise on the Epidemic Puerperal Fever of Aberdeen*, 80.
[13] In Gordon's table there were seventy-seven cases in all, arranged in chronological order. Case 77 was doubtful. It occurred six months after the epidemic had ceased, and was associated with the delivery of a macerated stillbirth. It probably had no connection with the epidemic.

TABLE 3.1. *Cases of puerperal fever recorded during the epidemic in Aberdeen, 1789–1792, by birth attendant*

Birth attendant	Cured	Died	Total	Fatality rate (%)
Dr Gordon	11	5	16	31
Mr Harvey (a young surgeon)	0	1	1	
Midwives				
Mrs Blake	7	4	11	
Mrs Elgin	2	5	7	
Mrs Philp	3	1	4	
Mrs Smith	1	1	2	
Mrs Chalmers	1	1	2	
Mrs Coutts	1	1	2	
Mrs Mitchell	1	1	2	
Mrs Irvine	0	1	1	
Mrs Ogilvie	2	1	3	
Mrs Clark	3	1	4	
Mrs Taylor	2	0	2	
Mrs Emslie	1	1	2	
Mrs Balfour	1	1	2	
Mrs Anderson	7	0	7	
Mrs Keith	3	2	5	
Mrs Davidson	2	0	2	
Mrs Henderson	0	1	1	
Total	37	22	59	38
Total	48	28	76	37

Note: This table is based on seventy-six cases. The final case, case 77 in October 1792, is excluded. It was not part of the epidemic but was due to a delivery associated with a macerated stillbirth.

Source: Alexander Gordon, *A Treatise on the Epidemic Puerperal Fever of Aberdeen* (London, 1795), 17–21, table.

Mrs Jefferies 'was so very fortunate as not to fall within the infection'.[14] With these reservations in mind, there are some interesting features in Fig. 3.1.

    The epidemic began in December 1789, reached a high peak in the last quarter of 1790, and then declined, ending in the spring of 1792. The fatality rate was significantly higher up to the end of 1790 than it was thereafter.[15] Of

---

[14] Gordon, *A Treatise on the Epidemic Puerperal Fever of Aberdeen*, 66.

[15] There were thirty-eight cases and nineteen deaths from December 1789 to the end of 1790. From the beginning of 1791 to the end of the epidemic there were thirty-eight cases and nine deaths. The difference is significant: $0.02 > P > 0.01$.

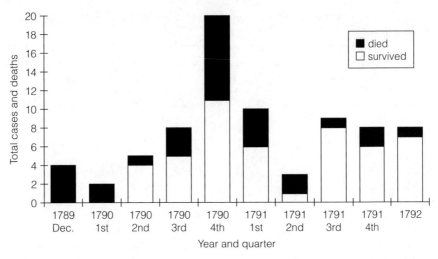

F IG. 3.1 Total cases of puerperal fever recorded every quarter during the epidemic in Aberdeen, 1789–1792

Source: Alexander Gordon, *A Treatise on the Epidemic Puerperal Fever of Aberdeen* (London, 1795), 17–21, table.

the twenty-eight fatal cases, twenty-four died on or before the seventh day, with the majority dying on the fifth post-natal day after a three-day illness, show-ing how rapidly this disease could kill.

It was only after the epidemic was well established that Gordon saw the way it was spreading, and suspected it was contagious or infectious (to Gordon the words were synonymous). His suspicion soon became a conviction:

That the cause of this disease was a specific contagion, or infection, I have unquestionable proof . . . [it] seized such women only, as were visited, or delivered, by a practitioner, or taken care of by a nurse, who had previously attended patients affected by the disease. In short I had evident proofs of its infectious nature, and that the infection was as read-ily communicated as that of the smallpox, or measles, and operated more speedily than any other infection, with which I am acquainted.[16]

Gordon admitted he did not understand the nature of the contagion, but he believed it was something that clung to the clothes and person of the birth attend-ants, in a similar way, perhaps, to the manner in which smoke from an autumn bonfire clings to one's clothes (my analogy, not his). He explained it thus:

With respect to the physical qualities of the infection, I have not been able to make any discovery; but I have evident proofs that every person, who had been with a patient in the Puerperal Fever, became charged with an atmosphere of infection, which was com-municated to every pregnant woman, who happened to come within its sphere . . .[17]

---

[16] Gordon, *A Treatise on the Epidemic Puerperal Fever of Aberdeen*, 63.   [17] Ibid. 63–4.

He also confessed, 'It is a disagreeable declaration for me to mention, that I myself was the means of carrying the infection to a great number of women.'[18]

When it came to writing his treatise, Gordon discussed preventive measures that might be applied in future epidemics, measures such as fumigation, which was already used widely in the attempt to control contagious diseases. Specifically, he recommended that 'The patient's apparel and bed-clothes ought, either to be burnt, or thoroughly purified; and the nurses and physicians, who have attended patients affected with the Puerperal Fever, ought carefully to wash themselves, and to get their apparel properly fumigated, before it be put on again.'[19] He foresaw the danger of broadcasting the names of practitioners and midwives who had been responsible for spreading the disease. It was a 'fatal secret', as he says in the following passage:

Those who propose to prevent the Puerperal Fever, must have two intentions in view. The one is, to prevent the infection from being communicated; and the other is, after the infection has been communicated, to prevent its action. My endeavours were entirely directed to this last purpose, for the Puerperal Fever had prevailed for some time, before I discovered that it was infectious: and after this discovery was made, I saw the danger of disclosing the fatal secret.[20]

In other words, he foresaw (correctly) the storm that could descend on himself and the midwives if everyone knew the names of those who, far from helping their patients, were inadvertently sending them to their graves. In retrospect it was foolish of Gordon to publish the names of the midwives who had spread the disease in his treatise, even though he openly confessed that he, too, had unwittingly transmitted it from one patient to another.

The midwives were furious. The women of Aberdeen, who had taken a keen interest in the outcome of the epidemic and had their own views, may well have pointed an accusing finger at Mrs Blake, the midwife who had had the greatest number of cases of puerperal fever—eleven in all. And it would not have escaped their attention that one midwife, Mrs Anderson, had had seven cases of puerperal fever but none of them had died, while another, Mrs Elgin, had also had seven cases but five of them had died. A little naïvely, perhaps, Gordon believed that his record of cures by copious bleeding would deflect criticism and earn him the gratitude of Aberdeen. But his critics persisted in the belief that the epidemic had been nothing more than the fever known as the 'Weed'. Far from praising Gordon, they blamed him for his insistence on copious bleeding and purging. It was this, they said, not this new disease called puerperal fever that no one had ever heard of, that was the cause of the high death rate.

Hurt by 'the ungenerous treatment which I met with from that very sex whose sufferings I was at so much pains to relieve', Gordon was forced to leave Aberdeen. He rejoined the Navy. But sadly he soon developed pulmonary

tuberculosis and returned to die at the age of 47 at his brother's farm, a disappointed man with a strong sense of the injustice of this world.[21]

The Reception of Gordon's Work

Gordon's legacy to medicine consisted of three propositions. First, that puerperal fever could be transmitted from one patient to another by the doctor or
nurse/midwife. Secondly, that there was a very intimate relationship between
puerperal fever and erysipelas. Thirdly, that copious bleeding performed very
early in puerperal fever was the only possible cure.

Today we would have no difficulty in ranking these propositions in the order
I have given. The first, on which his reputation rests, was of major importance,
because it unveiled the cause of puerperal fever and thereby pointed the way
to prevention. The second proposition was also an astute observation, but not
as fundamental from the practical point of view as the first. The third proposition is something of an embarrassment, for it makes us wonder how a man who
made such astute observations on two aspects of puerperal fever could go so
badly astray on the third. But these are judgements from a modern viewpoint.
They are totally different from the way Gordon's views were received at the
time. Indeed, Gordon is an example of a view cited by Oliver Sacks; namely,
'how odd, complex, contradictory, and irrational the process of scientific discovery can be. And yet, beyond the twists and anachronisms in the history
of science, beyond the vicissitudes and fortuities, perhaps there is an overall
pattern to be discerned.'[22]

Gordon's first proposition on the transmission of puerperal fever was not
so much rejected as apparently neglected and forgotten as if irrelevant. His
second proposition on the link with erysipelas was confirmed by others in the
early nineteenth century again and again, but Gordon was never given credit
for describing it. But his third proposition on the value of venesection was cited
frequently and always favourably. It was for this alone that Gordon retained a
toehold in the publications of the early and mid-nineteenth century.

Why was the first proposition so totally neglected? Some have suggested that
the very idea that doctors could be responsible for spreading pueperal fever was
accusatory, threatening, and repugnant to medical men. This was probably true
to a limted extent of Semmelweis, to whom we come later, but there is little
evidence that this was the prime reason as far as Gordon was concerned. I believe
that the explanation lies in the concept of prematurity.

In science, an idea may be rejected 'if its implications cannot be connected by
a series of simple logical steps to canonical, or generally accepted, knowledge'.[23]

[21] Porter, *Alexander Gordon of Aberdeen*, 51–2.
[22] O. Sacks, 'Scotomata: Forgetting and Neglect in Science', in R. B. Silvers (ed.), *Hidden Histories
of Science* (London, 1997), 141–88, at 141.   [23] Gunter Stent, cited in ibid. 158.

Unfortunately for Gordon, almost a century had passed before the bacterial basis of puerperal fever was beginning to be accepted. Only then could Gordon's first proposition be seen for what it was—a brilliantly original observation that could now, a century later, be connected by simple logical steps to the canonical knowledge of the late nineteenth century.

Thus we find in 1887 that Robert Lee chose the opportunity of the prestigious Goulstonian Lectures to praise Gordon in the warmest terms. He allowed that Gordon and Semmelweis were both 'possessed of powers of original thought', but he believed that Gordon had greater 'intellectual and moral superiority'. Lee remarked perceptively that Gordon's observations on contagion were unpopular because of the dominance of pathology. The pathological mind, said Lee, accepts only what it sees. Gordon's contemporaries knew of his concept of a 'specific poison' of contagion and they asked if specific poison could be seen. If not, it was of no importance.[24]

In the twentieth century, the slow revival of Gordon's reputation can be traced to C. J. Cullingworth in 1906, who added a brief appendix on Gordon at the end of his essay on the work of Oliver Wendell Holmes.[25] Nevertheless, the rehabilitation of Gordon was a slow process. In the 1929 edition of Garrison, although Gordon's name is mentioned in passing, nothing is said of his achievement.[26] Even at the end of the twentieth century he remains unknown to many who are conversant with the work on puerperal fever by Holmes and Semmelweis.

The reception of Gordon's third proposition on the effectiveness of bleeding was quite different. Medical practitioners in the eighteenth and first half of the nineteenth century were on the whole favourable to the idea that venesection was an appropriate treatment for at least some fevers, especially inflammatory fevers (which we discuss later), so they were in a frame of mind that was only too ready to accept and acknowledge Gordon's views on bleeding. Some fifty years after Gordon's death Charles Meigs, a well-known professor of obstetrics in Philadelphia in the mid-nineteenth century, urged his students to read Gordon's treatise, which he described in glowing terms as

a small unobtrusive book, written without arrogance or pretension. It is a plain unvarnished tale; being a history of his concern with the epidemic, and carries so convincing and truthful an air into every page and line, that I cannot imagine anything better fitted to impress the mind of the reader with the warm and intense convictions of the writer. Half a century has elapsed since it appeared . . . it never loses its good and solid reputation. Every medical practitioner, whether accoucheur or not, ought to read it with care . . . Gordon must ever be regarded as the reformer of our therapeutics on child-bed fever.[27]

[24] R. J. Lee, 'The Goulstonian Lectures on Puerperal Fever', British Medical Journal (1875), i. 267–70, 304–6, 337–9, 371–3, 408–9, 440–2, at 305–6.
[25] Cullingworth, Oliver Wendell Holmes, app. II.
[26] F. H. Garrison, An Introduction to the History of Medicine (4th edn., Philadelphia, 1929).
[27] C. D. Meigs, Females and their Diseases: A Series of Letters to his Class (Philadelphia, 1848), 591.

From this you would guess that Meigs was a firm supporter of the theory of contagion. Not a bit of it. He was totally scornful of even the remote possibility of contagion, dismissing in one short sentence all Gordon had to say on the matter as a minor flaw in an otherwise splendid treatise. And he dismissed the idea of a link between erysipelas and puerperal fever as rubbish. Erysipelas was a skin disease. How could you have erysipelas of the uterus? 'You might as well say that a woman has iritis of her pylorus, which would be absolute nonsense.'[28] Meigs, though widely read and no fool, was exceptionally forceful and opinionated. Most importantly, at a time when faith in the therapeutic importance of venesection was beginning to fade, he was utterly convinced of the importance of copious bleeding in puerperal fever, citing many cases in which he had saved lives by this form of treatment. This is why Meigs, while admiring Gordon for his literary style (Meigs was a bit of a stylist himself), succeeded, by a degree of wilful blindness that is astounding, to latch onto the third part of Gordon's treatise while ignoring the other two.[29]

And yet it would be wrong to see the rejection of Gordon's contagious proposition, and the acceptance of his doctrine of bleeding, as absolutes in black and white. Denman, who knew Gordon well, wrote a short passage on the contagiousness of puerperal fever in the second edition of his *Introduction to the Practice of Midwifery*.[30] He notes that the contagious nature of puerperal fever, 'long suspected' is now 'fully proved', but he failed to give credit where credit was due. Neither Gordon nor his treatise is mentioned.

And it was not only Denman. Throughout the first two-thirds of the nineteenth century (before, that is, the role of bacteria in infective disease was accepted), except as an advocate of copious bleeding, Gordon was rarely if ever cited, at least as far as contagion was concerned. Yet there were numerous reports that, in essence, confirmed Gordon's discovery that puerperal fever was contagious in the sense of being conveyed by birth attendants, that it was often limited to the practice of one or two practitioners or midwives, and that there was a clear link with erysipelas and other septic conditions. We come to examples in the following chapters. And we will then find our suspicion grows that Gordon had more influence than appears at first sight. His work was not cited because it smelt of unorthodoxy, because it lay outside the accepted canon of knowledge. Yet the traces of his influence were there below the surface.

Gordon's treatise was the first substantial account of an epidemic of puerperal fever in a town. We now come to other town epidemics of puerperal fever, and the way they show gradual changes in the understanding of the disease.

---

[28] C. D. Meigs, *Females and their Diseases: A Series of Letters to his Class* (Philadelphia, 1848), 612.

[29] Meigs had always believed in venesection. Referring to the time when he had visited lying-in hospitals in France, he said on the question of venesection, 'All that I saw on those occasions and all that I have myself witnessed before and since, confirm me in my admiration of Gordon's precepts [on venesection]; and I adhere to, and adopt, and I desire, as your Professor of Midwifery, to lead you also to adopt Gordon's views' (ibid. 634–5).

[30] T. Denman, *An Introduction to the Practice of Midwifery* (2 vols.; London, 1795; 2nd edn., 1801).

4

Epidemic Puerperal Fever in Towns

During the late eighteenth and nineteenth centuries, when families were often large, a substantial number of babies, ranging on average from a sixth to a third, died before their first birthday. In most years, however, the ratio of deaths from pregnancy-related causes (in other words, maternal deaths) to births was only about 1 to 200 or 250. In a market town of around 5,000 to 7,000 inhabitants during the early nineteenth century, the people would, on average, expect to witness the burial of an infant six or more times a year. But years might pass with only an occasional maternal death and even longer without a death from puerperal fever. Compared with the death of an infant, or the death of a young person from tuberculosis, a maternal death was a relatively uncommon event.

Every now and again, however, a village, town, or city might be struck by an epidemic of puerperal fever, similar to the epidemic in Aberdeen in 1789–92 described in the previous chapter. Epidemics of puerperal fever in lying-in hospitals (which are the subject of the next chapter) are comparatively well known, but town epidemics seem to have escaped the attention of historians. This is odd, because they were terrible outbreaks that arrived suddenly and without warning, striking terror into women, their families, and their medical attendants. Sometimes they lasted for a few months, sometimes for two or three years, and when they ceased they did so gradually by a process of fading away and a decline in severity. Nearly always they began in winter or early spring, which is characteristic of streptococcal epidemics. And they usually arrived without warning, although an astute local medical practitioner might note in retrospect that the epidemic of puerperal fever had been preceded by an outbreak of sepsis in various forms, especially erysipelas.

As the epidemic took hold and spread to surrounding villages, three features were frequently reported. The first was the extremely high fatality rate, especially in the early weeks of the epidemic, when it could be as high as 80 per cent —a far higher fatality than occurred in most outbreaks of the plague or smallpox. The second was the frequent tendency for the epidemic to be limited to the patients of one or two medical practitioners or midwives, while their colleagues —working in precisely the same area and not necessarily more experienced, careful, or respected than those singled out as the carriers of the disease— might have no cases at all. The third was the observation that the disease could be transmitted to mothers not only by birth attendants who had attended cases of puerperal fever, but also by birth attendants who had attended cases of erysipelas or septic lesions. The reverse also occurred. Doctors and midwives attending women with puerperal fever sometimes developed erysipelas, usually on their arms, and some of them died. Also, 'the newborn infants of mothers with puerperal fever die of erysipelas in an unusually large ratio'.[1]

Epidemics of puerperal fever were indiscriminate. They were as likely to affect the older multiparous mothers as the young primipara; they struck especially women who had had prolonged or difficult labours, but also numerous women who had had easy short ones. They were as likely to strike the robust as the delicate, the well-to-do as the poor. In most historical accounts of puerperal fever, hospital epidemics have tended to eclipse the terrifying epidemics that swept through towns and villages. Yet it is the latter, the town epidemics, that revealed many of the features that were gradually incorporated into the growing body of knowledge on the cause and the nature of puerperal fever.

The Frequency of Town Epidemics

How common were epidemics of puerperal fever? Table 4.1 is a list of epidemics of puerperal fever in towns and lying-in hospitals between 1770 and 1849, compiled from various sources. Although it is impressive in length, it should be read with three provisos in mind.

1. It consists solely of epidemics that happened to be reported. There are good reasons for believing that many other epidemics occurred that were never reported, especially in the eighteenth century, when puerperal fever had only just been recognized as a distinct entity.[2]
2. The table shows an apparent increase in the number of epidemics in the first half of the nineteenth century. This is probably due in part to the growing recognition of the problem of puerperal fever, and even more to the rapid growth of medical periodicals in which obstetricians and also general practitioners (most of whom would never have dreamt of writing a treatise) could publish reports of local epidemics.
3. A few so-called epidemics may have been small local random variations in the endemic level, not meriting the description of an epidemic.[3]

---

[1] A. Hirsch, *Handbook of Geographical and Historical Pathology* (2nd edn., 1881), trans. C. Creighton (3 vols., London, 1883), ii. 469.

[2] Hirsch found records of town epidemics in Copenhagen in 1672, in Rouen and Caen in 1713, in Paris in 1736 and 1746, and in Lyons in 1750. It is probable that many other unrecorded epidemics of puerperal fever occurred (ibid. ii. 442).

[3] Hirsch, one of the main sources for Table 4.1, said that in one instance he used 'epidemic' when the mortality rate in the hospitals rose by more than 6% above the prevailing average; 6% seems a low figure for the definition of an epidemic.

TABLE 4.1. *A chronological list of reports of epidemics of puerperal fever in lying-in hospitals, towns, counties, and regions, UK and the Continent of Europe, 1770–1849*

Year	UK		Europe	
	Lying-in hospitals	Towns or counties	Lying-in hospitals	Towns or regions
1770	London	London	Vienna	Rotterdam
1771	London			
1772				
1773	Edinburgh			
1774	Dublin		Paris	Paris
1775		Derbyshire	Paris	Paris, Vienna
1776				
1777			Vienna, Stockholm	
1778	Dublin		Paris, Copenhagen	Copenhagen, Berlin
1779	Dublin			Berlin
1780			Paris	Berlin
1781			Paris, Cassel	
1782			Paris, Copenhagen	Copenhagen
1783	London			Gladenbach
1784				Gladenbach
1785			Vienna	
1786			Paris, Copenhagen	Lombardy
1787	London, Dublin	London		Lombardy, Poitiers
1788	London, Dublin	London		
1789		Aberdeen		
1790		Aberdeen		
1791		Aberdeen	Copenhagen	
1792		Aberdeen	Copenhagen, Vienna	
1793			Vienna, Stockholm, Rouen, Amsterdam	
1794			Stockholm	
1795			Vienna	
1796			Vienna	
1797				
1798				Créteil
1799				Grenoble
1800				Grenoble, Trier
1801				Trier
1802				
1803	Dublin			
1804				
1805				Rostock
1806				
1807				
1808		Barnsley, Sunderland, Doncaster		
1809		Leeds		

TABLE 4.1. (*cont'd*)

Year	UK		Europe	
	Lying-in hospitals	Towns or counties	Lying-in hospitals	Towns or regions
1810	Dublin	Leeds	Stockholm, Milan	Landsberg
1811	Dublin	Leeds Yorkshire (W. Riding)	Stockholm, Heidelberg	Landsberg
1812	Dublin	Leeds, Durham	Heidelberg	
1813	Dublin	London, Abingdon, Dumfries		
1814	London, Edinburgh	Abingdon	Prague	
1815	Edinburgh, Dublin			
1816			Paris	
1817			Wurzberg	
1818	London		Paris, Lyons	Prague
1819	Dublin	Glasgow, Stirling	Stockholm, Vienna, Prague, Lyons, Wurzberg	Prague
1820	Dublin	Glasgow, Stirling	Stockholm, Kiel, Dresden, Wurzberg	Bavaria
1821		Edinburgh, Glasgow, Stirling	Lyons	
1822		Edinburgh, Glasgow, Stirling	Vienna, Marburg	
1823	London, Dublin		Vienna, Marburg	
1824	London		Munich	
1825	London, Edinburgh		Berlin, Hanover, Munich, Prague, Stockholm	Berlin
1826	Edinburgh, Dublin	Birmingham	Paris, Berlin, Stockholm	Nassau
1827	London			Bentheim
1828	London, Dublin	Birmingham, Dublin	Amsterdam	Bentheim
1829	London, Dublin	Birmingham	Paris, Vienna, Hanover, Amsterdam, Copenhagen	
1830		Birmingham, Manchester	Paris, Vienna, Prague, Giessen, Kiel	Toulouse
1831		Plymouth, Manchester, Aylesbury	Paris, Geissen, Stockholm	Nassau
1832			Munich, Bonn	Bonn
1833	Birmingham	Edinburgh	Vienna, Prague	Nassau

TABLE 4.1. (cont'd)

Year	UK		Europe	
	Lying-in hospitals	Towns or counties	Lying-in hospitals	Towns or regions
1834	Dublin, Birmingham		Paris, Vienna, Gratz, Prague, Kiel	
1835	London, Birmingham		Kiel, Prague, Bamberg	Bamberg Loire inférieur
1836	London, Dublin, Birmingham		Vienna	Nassau
1837	Dublin		Copenhagen, Dresden, Griefswald	Griefswald
1838	London, Edinburgh		Griefswald, Paris	Griefswald
1839			Copenhagen, Dresden, Wangen	
1840			Paris, Berlin, Copenhagen, Stockholm, Prague, Halle	Dulmen
1841		Doncaster	Paris, Berlin, Stockholm, Halle	
1842	London		Paris, Gratz, Rennes	Peitz
1843			Paris, Rouen, Dorpat	Paris
1844			Paris, Rouen, Rennes, Stockholm	Girresheim Aalborg
1845	Dublin		Copenhagen, Lyons	Greenland
1846			Paris, Lyons, Rouen, St Petersburg, Gronigen, Berlin, Wurzberg, Toulouse	
1847			Stuttgart, Kiel	
1848			St Petersburg, Kiel	Bornholm
1849			Stockholm, Stuttgart, Berlin, Tubingen, Stuttgart	Stuttgart

Note: Where the name of a town, county, or hospital appears for two or more sucessive years (as in the case of Aberdeen), this indicates one epidemic lasting two or more years not two or more separate epidemics. However, as it is the exception rather than the rule to find data on the length of an epidemic, many that appear as a single entry may well have lasted for more than a year.

Sources: A. Hirsch, *Handbook of Geographical and Historical Pathology* (2nd edn., 1881), trans. C. Creighton (3 vols.; London, 1883), i. 422–31; Fleetwood Churchill, 'An Historical Sketch of the Epidemics of Puerperal Fever', in Churchill (ed.), *Essays on the Puerperal Fever and Other Diseases Peculiar to Women* (London, 1849), 31; R. Gooch, *An Account of Some of the Most Important Diseases Peculiar to Women* (London, 1831; 2nd edn., 1838); Alexander Gordon, *A Treatise on the Epidemic Puerperal Fever of Aberdeen* (London, 1795); L. Le Fort, *Des maternités: Études sur les maternités et les institutions charitables d'accouchement à domicile dans les principaux états de l'Europe* (Paris, 1866). A few accounts of epidemics were culled from other occasional sources.

That epidemics of puerperal fever were common before 1850 seems beyond doubt, but, for reasons that are far from clear, it seems that the incidence of epidemics decreased steeply during the final third of the nineteenth century, and by the early years of the twentieth century they had become rare.[4]

The Abingdon Epidemic

Abingdon, a market town about six miles south of Oxford, with a population of 4801 in 1811, is an example. There had not been a case of puerperal fever in the town within living memory until it suffered a severe epidemic that was described by one of the local general practitioners, Mr Thomas West, in a short report that embraced all the characteristic features of a town epidemic due to what must have been a highly virulent strain of the Group A streptococcus.[5]

The epidemic began in the spring of 1813 with several cases of 'mortification in the leg' in a nearby village. Other cases of the same nature appeared in Abingdon, where Mr West was forced to amputate both legs of a 'healthy robust lad' aged 12 who had a similar condition (the boy survived). In July 1813 a few cases of erysipelas and two cases of puerperal fever occurred in Abingdon, and by the end of 1813 large numbers of people with trifling wounds, such as punctures by thorns or slight skin abrasions, developed erysipelas.

By the spring of 1814 both diseases (erysipelas and puerperal fever) rose to epidemic proportions. There were two fatal cases of what West referred to as *erysipelas gangrenosa* but that might now be described as necrotizing fasciitis, and many more cases of puerperal fever—twenty in all—of whom nearly all died. In these cases the onset of puerperal fever was rapid, and in only one case was the onset delayed to the sixth day; most occurred sooner. The last case of puerperal fever was in June 1814, there were a few minor cases of erysipelas in the summer, and the epidemic ceased in September 1814, approximately eighteen months after it had begun.

During the epidemic, many of the nurses attending on the lying-in women, as well as washer-women, were attacked with erysipelas in one or both arms, without any sores on the hand or fingers. One baby died of erysipelas. Although in some of the surrounding villages there were many cases of both diseases, 'other villages adjoining were totally free from either disease'. There was never a case of puerperal fever in a village where there was not also a case of erysipelas.[6]

[4] As far as hospital epidemics were concerned, this could be attributed at least in part to the use of antisepsis after 1880; but hospital deaths were always a very small proportion of total puerperal-fever mortality, and the introduction of antisepsis is not a plausible explanation for the disappearance of town epidemics.

[5] T. West, 'Observations on some Diseases, Particularly Puerperal Fever, which Occurred in Abingdon and its Vicinity in 1813 and 1814', *London Medical Repository and Review*, 3 (1815), 103–5.

[6] It is worth noting for future reference that West does not mention any cases of scarlet fever during the epidemic.

Other Epidemics

The similarity between the Abingdon epidemic and the Aberdeen one of 1789–92 is striking. One recalls Gordon's description of the way puerperal fever and erysipelas appeared together, 'reached their acmè' together, and disappeared simultaneously. What is especially interesting is that the Abingdon epidemic seems to have been part of a widespread epidemic in and around the second decade of the nineteenth century in various parts of Britain. Dr Bradley reported an outbreak of puerperal fever in the West Riding of Yorkshire in 1811, in which, on its first appearance, none survived.[7] Dr Armstrong described a similar epidemic in Sunderland in 1813 and said it had also appeared in epidemic form in Newcastle upon Tyne and in various parts of Northumberland and Durham.[8]

Armstrong, like so many authors, described the extraordinary rapidity of epidemic puerperal fever, the intense abdominal pain, the sunken countenance, the high mortality, and the occasional cases where the pain disappeared completely, convincing the patient and her family that recovery was at hand just before her inevitable death. Armstrong also noted the concurrence of erysipelas. Sunderland, with a population of 12,289 in 1811, was considerably larger than Abingdon. There were several practitioners in the town, but forty out of the fifty cases occurred in the practice of one surgeon and his assistant. Armstrong was unusual in citing Gordon and believing that Gordon was right: puerperal fever was a contagious disease.

An epidemic also occurred in Leeds (whose population at the time was about 62,000) between 1809 and 1812. It was the subject of a treatise by William Hey Jr. that reveals his wide knowledge of the subject.[9] Hey stated that the epidemic of puerperal fever first appeared in north-east England around 1808 in Barnsley and spread to Leeds in 1809. There were also epidemics in Scotland in 1813–14, suggesting that there was in this period a pandemic of puerperal fever (and erysipelas) in Britain, which followed a period when such epidemics had been rare. The epidemics in the north of Britain were seen as a new phenomenon. When the outbreak occurred in Leeds in 1809, although puerperal fever was known as a sporadic disease, no epidemic had occurred in the town within living memory.

The characteristics of the Leeds epidemic were the large number of cases and the much greater severity, rapidity, and fatality of the disease in epidemic rather than sporadic form. The clinical features of the disease were exactly as described by Armstrong and others—the sudden onset with a rigor, fever, headache, and the extreme abdominal pain and tenderness—and the very high

---

[7] Dr Bradley, 'On an Epidemic of Puerperal Fever', *Medical and Physical Journal*, 28 (1811), 193–201.

[8] J. Armstrong, *Facts and Observations Relative to the Fever Commonly Called Puerperal* (London, 1814).

[9] William Hey, *A Treatise on the Puerperal Fever Illustrated by Cases which Occurred in Leeds and its Vicinity in the Years 1809–1812* (London, 1815).

fatality, especially at the onset of the epidemic. As elsewhere, puerperal fever was closely accompanied by an epidemic of erysipelas that was also more fatal than usual.

The social-class distribution is interesting. In many epidemic diseases, especially gastrointestinal diseases, it was usual for the incidence and the fatality to be higher in the lower social classes than the upper. If anything, the opposite was true of epidemics of puerperal fever. In Leeds, when the epidemic of puerperal fever began, it was noticed that it attacked a higher proportion of the upper than the lower classes. Later it seemed to be equally distributed between all parts of the population.

Hey of Leeds, like Gordon of Aberdeen, was a fervent believer in early and copious bleeding as the only effective remedy. Although he was less dogmatic than Gordon, who had claimed that early and copious bleeding invariably cured, Hey took venesection further. Where Gordon had recommended that 20 to 24 ounces of blood should be taken away when others had suggested 10 ounces, Hey always removed at least 20 ounces, often took away 40 ounces, on two occasions bled 52 ounces, and once achieved 70 ounces. Hey did not claim, like Gordon, a success rate of 100 per cent, but he believed it was axiomatic that a measure that cures a disease must also be capable of preventing it.[10] The one major difference between Hey and Gordon was that Hey kept an open mind on the question of contagion. He had not seen enough evidence of contagion with his own eyes, but he was sufficiently impressed by other people's evidence to follow what was already becoming a golden rule amongst the better-informed practitioners. Whenever he attended a case of puerperal fever or erysipelas, he always washed thoroughly, and changed all his garments before attending another midwifery case.

Some twenty years after the Leeds epidemic, an epidemic occurred in Manchester (population 98,500 in 1811). It was described by John Roberton, a well-known and highly respected physician who was an honorary accoucheur to the Manchester Lying-in Charity.[11] This was one of many outpatient charities that trained and employed midwives under the general supervision of honorary accoucheurs to deliver the poor in their homes. The epidemic began in the practice of 'Mrs A. B., a midwife in great practice among the patients of the Charity', who had, on 4 December 1830, delivered a poor woman who had died of puerperal fever.

From this date to the 4th January 1831 inclusive—exactly one month—this midwife delivered thirty women residing in different parts of an extensive suburb, of which number sixteen caught the disease, and all of them ultimately died. These were the only cases of puerperal fever which had for a considerable time occurred in Manchester. The

---

[10] Nevertheless, he was scornful of the suggestion that, if a woman lost a copious quantity of blood during delivery—as if, in effect, she had performed venesection on herself—she should be protected against puerperal fever. He described this idea as 'specious', and said he had seen women who had lost much more blood in a delivery than would be taken by venesection who later developed puerperal fever.

[11] J. Roberton, 'Is Puerperal Fever Infectious?', *London Medical Gazette*, 9 (1831–2), 503–5.

midwives, commonly twenty-five in number, deliver on average, ninety women per week, which is about three hundred and eighty in a month. Now of this number delivered during the month in question, none had puerperal fever except the patients of Mrs A. B. Yet all this time this woman was crossing the other midwives in every direction, scores of patients of the Charity being delivered by them in the very same quarters where her cases of fever were happening.[12]

As Roberton realized, this was an astonishing story. Mrs A. B. was an efficient and respected midwife. No one could accuse her of ignorance or improper practice. Yet, through no fault of her own and for reasons she could not begin to understand, she had been singled out as a 'harbinger of death'. There must have been women who, seeing her pass on her rounds through the streets, pointed an accusing finger and vowed not to have her in their house. Mrs A. B. was advised by the Charity to cease practice for a short period and 'go to the country'.

Puerperal fever soon occurred all over Manchester and in the practice of many midwives instead of just one. Roberton concluded:

The fact that sixteen cases of puerperal fever occurred in one month in the practice of a single midwife, while the patients of the other midwives were exempted from the disease, leads naturally to the conclusion that this midwife was the medium of communicating (I take not upon myself to say in what manner) the malady from one woman to another.[13]

This was not the only instance of a midwife suffering a series of cases. Hirsch mentions that most of the cases of puerperal fever that occurred in the small Saxon town of Landsberg in 1810–11 happened in the practice of one midwife; 'after this woman ceased to attend midwifery cases, nothing more was seen of the disease'. Similarly, in Aarhaus in Denmark in 1850, nine cases of puerperal fever occurred in rapid succession, all in the practice of one midwife when the only other midwife in the town had none. The story was repeated in an epidemic of puerperal fever (fourteen cases in thirty-four successive confinements) that occurred in Schwenigen in 1879. There were two midwives in the town, but all the cases were confined to the practice of one midwife.[14]

When Roberton surveyed the evidence he had collected in Manchester, it seemed to him, as it did to most people, that, although there was cast-iron evidence that contagious transfer could and often did occur, that alone could not explain the whole cause of the disease. Roberton concluded that, as well as being infectious, 'this disease is propagated by some cause of a more general kind, probably existing in the atmosphere, after the fever has prevailed for some time in a locality . . . Numerous cases occurred during the late epidemic in Manchester, the origin of which could not, I apprehend, have been traced to

[12] Ibid. 503. Note that the number of deliveries per month by this charity exceeded the annual number of deliveries in nearly all the British and Continental lying-in hospitals in the 1830s. The lying-in hospitals have attracted so much attention it is easy to forget that a much larger as well as a much safer service was provided through outpatient charities. [13] Ibid. 504.
[14] Hirsch, *Handbook of Geographical and Historical Pathology*, ii. 456, 458, 459.

infection properly so called.' In a later publication Roberton made the important and unexpected observation that, in contrast with most epidemics, which seemed to single out the poor, deaths from sporadic puerperal fever seemed to be more numerous amongst the middle classes in the suburbs who were delivered by doctors, than amongst the poor in the slums who were delivered by midwives.[15]

Epidemics Spread by Doctors and Midwives

Similar stories continued to appear throughout the nineteenth century. At an inquest on a maternal death in Wigan it appeared that between 1 September and November 1882 there were 'from ten to twelve' maternal deaths in Wigan of which eight were due to puerperal fever and all had been delivered by the same midwife. She was persuaded to cease practice.[16] By the second half of the century it was felt that midwives (but not doctors) who had a series of cases of puerperal fever in their practice should cease practising midwifery, and some believed that this should be enforced by the law.

In 1874–5 there was a small outbreak of puerperal fever in Coventry. A series of cases of puerperal fever, most of which ended fatally, was traced to a Coventry midwife, Mrs Ingrams, and later to another midwife.[17] News of the outbreak got to the ears of the coroner, who 'sent a police-officer to warn her not to continue her occupation until two medical men had given her permission to do so'. She was, however, allowed to attend births provided she did not examine the patient or undertake the delivery, and she was told to notify a general practitioner, Dr Brown, who would undertake the delivery. This arrangement was successful in one case; but in the next Dr Brown was called by this midwife when he was occupied in delivering one of his own patients. He sent a message saying he was unable to come; and, since the midwife was already there, she had better undertake the delivery. She did, and the patient died. Mrs Ingrams was charged with manslaughter and tried at the Warwick Assizes.

This raised, as the *British Medical Journal* put it, 'several points of interest'. Did the coroner have the power to impose such an order? 'Coroners, unfortunately, were not always medical men.' In this case the coroner was a lawyer, and there was a danger that 'public opinion might report to him an embolic case as puerperal fever'. Mrs Ingrams was a 'useful, well-intentioned but ignorant midwife', who protested that she had 'never had a woman done badly before' and did not even know of the existence of puerperal fever until Dr Brown had

---

[15] J. Roberton, *Essays and Notes on the Physiology and Diseases of Women* (London, 1851). This work has a memorable account of the life of working-class women in Manchester and shows that Roberton, after a full day's work, would go on a round of the charity patients to see how they were and enquire after their welfare.   [16] *Lancet* (1882), ii. 862.

[17] The story of this and other incidents can be found in the correspondence columns of the *British Medical Journal* (1875), i. 185, 208, 313, 317, 331, 351, 356, 451–2.

told her about it. Partly because it was felt the coroner might have exceeded his powers, but mainly because Dr Brown had failed to attend the second case after the coroner's order (so that he, rather than Mrs Ingrams, was to blame for the death of the patient), the judge directed the jury to enter a verdict of not guilty. But this was soon followed by another case involving a midwife, Elizabeth Marsden. This took place in Manchester, where Mrs Marsden was ordered repeatedly to cease practice by a surgeon, but failed to do so. She was tried, convicted, and sentenced to six months' imprisonment. The conviction and the sentence were generally applauded by the medical press, but all of this raised the worrying possibility that, if midwives could be prosecuted, why not doctors?

The author of the leading article in the *British Medical Journal* found this potentially alarming. There should be, he wrote, a 'legal method for staying the death-dealing career' of any doctor who wilfully exposed his patient to danger by 'conducting a labour shortly after being in attendance upon a woman suffering from a contagious fever'.[18] But would it stop there? If medical practitioners were to be accused of 'manslaughter by infection', they would have to tread very warily. Otherwise:

Down comes the policeman to Sir William Jenner, to tell him to see no more cases of croup for three months, at his peril, as the coroner has heard he has been attending some fatal cases; to Sir William Gull, to give up practice for two months, as he hears he has been attending some fatal cases of scarlatina; to Dr Farre, to give up practice, because he has been in repeated consultation in a fatal puerperal case. The vista opened up by such prosecutions leads a long way, and is lost in a rather obscure shade.[19]

This, however, is to jump ahead. By the 1870s few obstetricians doubted that puerperal fever was contagious in the sense that it could be transferred from one midwifery case to another by a doctor or midwife, and few disagreed in principle that failure to take steps against such an occurrence was little short of murder, even though, as we will see, they disagreed on the mechanism of contagion. In the 1820s, it was different.

William Campbell of Edinburgh published a treatise on puerperal fever in 1822 in which, although he included Gordon's treatise as an appendix, he refuted the idea of contagion.[20] By 1831, however, he had changed his mind. In a passage that speaks volumes about notions of cleanliness of hands and clothes, he allowed that contagion could occur after 'the dissection of the bodies' of women who had died of puerperal fever:

In October 1821, I assisted at the dissection of a woman who died of the disease, after an abortion in the early months; the pelvic viscera, with the external coats, were removed, and *I carried them in my pocket to the classroom*. The same evening, without changing my clothes, I attended the delivery of a poor woman in the Canongate; she

---

[18] Ibid. 313.   [19] Ibid. 351.
[20] W. Campbell, *A Treatise of the Epidemic Puerperal Fever as it Prevailed in Edinburgh in 1821–22* (Edinburgh, 1822).

died; next morning, I went, in the same clothes, to assist some of my pupils, who were engaged with a woman in Bridewell, whom I delivered with forceps; she died; and of many others, who were seized with the disease, within a few weeks, three others shared the same fate in succession. (emphasis added)[21]

Campbell had heard of others who had infected women after attending a post-mortem, and 'for the last two years [that is, since 1829] I have scrupulously avoided by actual contact assisting at such post-mortem examinations', which he always left to 'gentlemen who were not likely to be engaged with women in child-bed'.[22]

There was a steady accumulation of similar evidence. During an epidemic of puerperal fever in Aylesbury (Buckinghamshire) in 1831 it was noted that 'Wounds of all kinds, contusions, simple abrasions, and common attritions of the cuticle' turned septic and the contagiousness of puerperal fever was 'as palpable to us as smallpox'. He added, 'The more severe and protracted the labour, the greater the probability—nay, the certainty—of an early and severe attack.'[23]

In Birmingham, Dr Elkington received an urgent summons to a midwifery case while attending a case of erysipelas. He had no time to wash or change, for it was, as he suspected, a case of placenta praevia, which he 'turned and delivered'. The woman survived the delivery but died of puerperal fever five days later.[24]

Eighteen cases of puerperal fever occurred in quick succession in the practice of one accoucheur, most of which were fatal, during an epidemic of puerperal fever in Plymouth in 1845. The origin of the initial series of cases seems to have been a case of erysipelas. For the first few weeks of the epidemic no one else had any cases; then, as in the Leeds and Manchester epidemics, it spread to the patients of other practitioners. The author of the report in which this was described concluded: 'That it [puerperal fever] is contagious is beyond dispute.' But he also believed that it was due to atmospheric influence.[25]

Robert Lee, one of the most distinguished obstetricians in London during the early- to mid-nineteenth century, was persuaded of the link between puerperal fever and erysipelas. He was less certain that contagion was involved in every case. He noted that Hulme in London and Tonnellé in Paris, both rated highly as authorities on puerperal fever, had witnessed drastic epidemics

---

[21] W. Campbell, 'On Puerperal Fever', *London Medical Gazette*, 9 (1831–2), 353–4. The odd thing is that this episode occurred before Campbell published his treatise in 1822. But it was not until 1831 that he realized, or decided to admit, what he had done.   [22] Ibid. 354.

[23] R. Ceely, 'Account of a Contagious Epidemic Puerperal Fever which Prevailed in Aylesbury and its Vicinity, in the Autumn of 1831', *Lancet* (1834–5), i. 813–18.

[24] F. Elkington, 'Observations on the Contagiousness of Puerperal Fever', *Provincial Medical Journal*, 7 (1844), 287–8. The phrase 'turn and deliver' refers to the standard procedure for placenta praevia, which required the practitioner to plunge his hand through the placenta, turn the baby in utero, grasp the baby's foot and deliver it as a breech.

[25] E. Blackmore, 'Observations on Puerperal Fever', *Provincial Medical Journal*, 9 (1845), 173–8, 210–13, 228–30, 242–5, 321–4, 338–41, 353–5, 369–71, 387–90, 399–401, 638–9.

in hospitals, but neither believed that puerperal fever was contagious. Gordon of Aberdeen had been convinced of contagiousness, but Hey of Leeds and Armstrong of Sunderland were undecided. Lee concluded:

It is difficult to reconcile this conflicting evidence; and the facts I have observed, though they have led me to believe the disease is sometimes communicable by contagion, yet they have not perhaps been sufficiently numerous, and of so decisive a character, as to dispel every doubt on the subject of its contagious or non-contagious nature. It is but proper to state that it has occurred in many cases, in the most destructive form, where contagion could not possibly be supposed to have operated as the cause.[26]

Charles Sidey, an Edinburgh surgeon, remarked in 1839 that

we notice puerperal fever giving rise to erysipelas under certain circumstance; and erysipelas on the other hand giving rise to puerperal fever . . . but whatever treatment was pursued, I scarcely saw any recover except one; and I am confident that a great many cases reported as recoveries have not been puerperal fever in its pure form, but common acute inflammatory cases.[27]

Epidemics of puerperal fever were commonplace in Scotland. In Dumfries and neighbourhood in 1813, just at the time when so many outbreaks occurred throughout England, 'twenty-seven individuals in the better ranks died from this affection in about six weeks, and only one recovered'. In 1823 Dr Kellie in Leith attended sixteen midwifery cases in succession, all of whom died of puerperal fever. Dr Hamilton saw one of Dr Kellie's cases in consultation, following which a series of cases he attended all developed puerperal fever and died. Later, a pupil of Dr Hamilton wrote to him to say he had visited Ireland, where he had volunteered to deliver the poor gratuitously. The third case he attended developed puerperal fever 'and from that time not one escaped it who came under my care'. The disease even followed him out of Ireland, for it developed in one woman he attended after his return to London, and in another he attended soon afterwards during a voyage to New South Wales. He had given the woman (there being nothing else available on the ship) 'some old sheets and a piece of garment which had been packed in one of my trunks at the time I was attending the puerperal fever case in London'; she also died of puerperal fever.

It was remarked by Dr Hamilton that 'when puerperal fever prevailed in the lying-in wards of the Royal Infirmary, all the sores in the surgeon's ward which was on the same floor, were in a very bad condition; and erysipelas followed every operation . . .'. It was also noticed that several of the pupils of the hospital 'had a succession of cases in various quarters of the town; while other

---

[26] R. Lee, *Researches on the Pathology and Treatment of Some of the Most Important Diseases of Women* (London, 1833). Nevertheless it was in this book that Lee suggested that serious consideration should be given 'on the grounds of humanity, [to] whether Lying-in Hospitals should not be altogether abolished' (p. 114).
[27] C. Sidey, 'Cases of Puerperal Fever', *Edinburgh Medical and Surgical Journal*, 51 (1839), 91–9, at 95.

pupils, as extensively engaged at the same time in midwifery practice, and in the same localities, had none'.[28]

There were similar stories from the Continent. In Belgium M. Grisar reported that he had attended a case of prolonged labour in 1842 in which the woman was delivered of a dead baby by forceps. Two days later she died of puerperal fever. Between 2 December and 19 March, M. Grisar delivered sixty-four women, of whom sixteen developed puerperal fever and eleven died. None of his colleagues in the same town had a single case of the disease. M. Grisar concluded that he was responsible for transmitting the disease, took all the usual precautions such as changing all his clothes and repeatedly washing himself, and the outbreak ceased.[29]

It was very alarming that experienced, careful, and skilful practitioners could find their reputation torn to shreds if they suffered a series of puerperal-fever deaths in their practice. Gooch (a noted London obstetrician) recalled that 'In the winter of the year 1824, puerperal fever was prevalent in London and its neighbourhood', and he told the following story:

A general practitioner in large midwifery practice lost so many patients from puerperal fever, that he determined to deliver no more for some time, but that his partner should attend in his place. This plan was pursued for one month, during which not a case of the disease occurred in the practice. The elder practitioner, being then sufficiently recovered, returned to his practice. But the first patient he attended was attacked by the disease and died. A physician who met him in consultation soon afterwards about a case of a different kind, asked him whether puerperal fever was at all prevalent in his neighbourhood, on which he burst into tears, and related the above circumstances.[30]

These histories of epidemics are only a small selection of the total.[31] The common features that recur are the close link between puerperal fever and erysipelas, the high fatality rate in epidemic as opposed to sporadic puerperal fever, the tendency for cases to be confined to one or two birth attendants when others were not affected, and the consequent effect on the practices of medical practitioners and midwives. Most authors concluded that puerperal fever

---

[28] All these reports from Scotland can be found in a discussion on puerperal fever in Edinburgh, published in the *London and Edinburgh Monthly Journal of Medical Science*, 13 (1851), 70–1. Although not stated, it is my guess that all the women 'in the better ranks' were delivered by a doctor or doctors, while the poor were delivered by midwives. This social-class differential is discussed in Chapter 12.

[29] Léon Le Fort, *Des maternités: Études sur les maternités et les institutions charitables d'accouchement à domicile dans les principaux états de l'Europe* (Paris, 1866), 113.

[30] R. Gooch, *An Account of some of the Most Important Diseases Peculiar to Women* (London, 1831; 2nd edn., 1838), 71–2.

[31] For the interested reader, there are three easily available and comprehensive sources. First, O. W. Holmes, *Puerperal Fever as a Private Pestilence* (Boston, 1855), including his 'additional references and cases' at the end of the pamphlet. Secondly, Hirsch, *Handbook of Geographical and Historical Pathology*, ii. 471–5, 'List of Writers on Puerperal Fever'. Thirdly, the useful list of references at the end of the pamphlet by C. J. Cullingworth, *Oliver Wendell Holmes and the Contagiousness of Puerperal Fever* (London, 1906), 37–41. Taken together they cover a reasonable proportion of the main nineteenth-century publications on epidemics of puerperal fever.

was sometimes contagious, but few believed that contagion occurred in every case, especially the sporadic cases that provided the strongest argument against a unitary theory of contagion.

Erysipelas and Puerperal Fever in the USA

How much were medical practitioners in Western countries aware of what was going on abroad? In the nineteenth century there was a greater mutual awareness of other practitioners' work between Britain and Germany than between Britain and France. As Robert Ferguson, a London surgeon, remarked in 1859: 'Content to remain within the pale of their own genial activities and rich literature, the French, unlike the Germans, rarely glance at the labours of foreigners; hence I cannot but accept the coincidence of opinions common to them and me as confirmations of results arrived at by independent workers in a common field.'[32] But the closest links between practitioners were, for the obvious reason of a common tongue, between Britain and the USA. Editors frequently reprinted each other's articles, in summary or in whole, in their medical periodicals with no apparent worries about copyright.[33] Certainly, American physicians knew about many of the British and European publications on puerperal fever and erysipelas. But there is one event (or series of events) that seems to have been relatively little known outside the USA at the time, and seems not to be well known to historians. This was an epidemic of erysipelas in mid-nineteenth-century America of quite astonishing ferocity, accompanied by high mortality from puerperal fever.

According to Daniel Drake, sporadic erysipelas had always been well known as a serious but usually limited infection, usually of the face. Epidemic erysipelas, however, was unknown within living memory in the 1820s. There was a slight epidemic in 1826, but the main outbreak began in the 1840s and lasted on and off to the 1860s.[34] During this period it spread in a south-westerly

---

[32] R. Ferguson (ed.), *Gooch on Some of the Most Important Diseases of Women* (London, 1859), p. xii.

[33] The *British and Foreign Medico-Chirurgical Review*, founded in 1848, was devoted to reprinting British and foreign papers on medicine, and in the USA the *American Journal of the Medical Sciences* reprinted many papers and reports published in British and European journals.

[34] D. Drake, *Systematic Treatise on the Principal Diseases of the Interior Valley of N. America*, 2nd edn., ed. S. H. Smith and F. G. Smith (Philadelphia, 1854), 622. See also E. Bennett, 'On the Identity of Erysipelas and a Certain Form of Puerperal Fever, and its Contagiousness', *American Journal of the Medical Sciences*, 19 (1850), 376–83; C. Hall and G. Dexter, 'Account of the Erysipelatous Fever, as it appeared in the Northern Section of Vermont and New Hampshire, in the Years 1842–43', *American Journal of the Medical Sciences*, 7 (1844), 2–27; D. Leasure, 'The Erysipelatous Disease of Lying-in Women', *American Journal of the Medical Sciences*, 31 (1856), 45–9; J. F. Peebles, 'Facts in Relation to Epidemic Erysipelas, as it Prevailed in Petersburg, Virginia, during the Winter and Spring, 1844–45', *American Journal of the Medical Sciences*, 11 (1846), 23–44; R. T. P. Ridley, 'Cases of Erysipelas which Occurred in Platte County, Missouri, in which there were Marked Evidences of Propagation of the Disease by Contagion', *New York Journal of Medicine*, 10 (1853), 41–8; Report of the Medical Society of Montgomery County, *Transactions of the Medical Society of the State of Pennsylvania*, 2 (1852), 128–9.

direction from New England to Mississippi and Louisiana, but the main outbreak seems to have been greatest in the north-east.[35]

It was, incidentally, an extraordinary and inexplicable feature of this epidemic
that it appeared to be a rural phenomenon. It occurred in small towns, villages, and settlements, but missed cities such as 'Buffalo, Pittsburg, Cleveland,
Cincinnati, Louisville, St. Louis and New Orleans, where it was scarcely known,
even as a sub-epidemic, except in their hospitals, and there it never prevailed
with a violence approaching that which it displayed in the country'.[36]

Unlike sporadic erysipelas, the epidemic form often produced gangrene
and the 'submucous and subcutaneous areolar tissue was ravaged by disease in
almost every violent case'.[37] The epidemic form was not confined to skin and
subcutaneous tissue, but often spread down from the mouth, tongue, and throat
to the larynx and lungs.[38] Whether such extension of the disease could still be
called erysipelas is doubtful, but there is no doubt that erysipelas of the skin
was accompanied by infection elsewhere.

In 1844 Dr Hall and Dr Dexter reported their experience of this epidemic
in Burlington, Vermont, and Lancaster, New Hampshire, during the years
1842–3.[39] It started in the spring of 1842. In a community of only 1,500–1,600
people, it had killed seventy people in six months.[40] There were numerous
fatal cases in which there was extremely rapid dissolution of skin, muscles, and
even bones in a manner strongly suggestive of necrotizing fasciitis. As the disease progressed, usually with remarkable rapidity, suppuration and dissolution
of tissue spread to huge areas of the body. In one case it rapidly covered the
whole of the trunk from the pelvis to the chin. In another it covered the whole
of one side of the chest, and spread in hours rather than days round beneath
the armpit to the muscles of the back and the shoulder. The disease tended to
produce a fluid exudate rather than pus, and when such areas or blisters were
opened to let the fluid out physicians found 'long strips of the cellular membrane protruded, resembling pieces of wet rotten linen, which could be drawn
out by the forceps'. Unlikely though it sounds, Hall and Dexter claimed that
the fluid exudate was capable of attacking the metal blade of a scalpel as if it
was nitric acid.[41]

The disease often began in the arm, where

the point of the attack was observed to be a little raised . . . and after a lapse of a few
hours, to present a jet black appearance the size of a large pin head. In all cases of this
kind the patients were somewhat advanced in years and died in five or six days with
extensive sloughing of the whole arm . . . No language can give an adequate description of the revolting aspects of this form of the epidemic. In many individuals . . . the
flesh would drop from the limb, or the whole member present the disgusting spectacle
of a livid mass of putrefaction.[42]

[35] Drake, *Systematic Treatise*, 623.   [36] Ibid. 625.   [37] Ibid. 633–4.
[38] Ibid., and also especially Peebles, 'Facts in Relation to Epidemic Erysipelas'.
[39] Hall and Dexter, 'Account of the Erysipelatous Fever'.   [40] Ibid. 14.
[41] Ibid. 17.   [42] Ibid. 18–19.

In 1852 a New England physician reported a case of erysipelas of the head that led to the whole of the scalp sloughing off the head, followed by suppuration with 'necrosis and separation of the entire bones of the area of the skull'. Astonishingly there was 'no sign of any disorder of the cerebral system', although the brain, 'covered by integument', was exposed to the air and 'the movements of elevation and depression of the brain were perceptible'.[43] In a similar case 'a large portion of the external table of the skull was removed through the incised scalp'.[44] In another case, reported in 1865, the skin and underlying tissue of the penis and scrotum were completely eaten away by erysipelas. Against expectations, the patient did not die, but, by frequent dressings and stretching the skin on the inner side of the thigh the genitals were decently covered with healthy skin in a period of four weeks—a result of which a modern plastic surgeon might well be proud.[45]

During this epidemic there were numerous instances of the transfer of erysipelas to puerperal fever and vice versa. A physician described how, when he was treating a judge for erysipelas, he was called to a remote mountain settlement to attend a woman who had a quick normal labour. The settlement had not seen a single case of erysipelas or puerperal fever, but the woman died of puerperal fever. In a town in Vermont affected by epidemic erysipelas, thirty cases of puerperal fever occurred of which only one recovered. In a town of 1,500 inhabitants in New Hampshire, twenty mothers died of puerperal fever and about forty people died of erysipelas.[46] Physicians themselves were at great risk, and, when two young physicians died of erysipelas after carrying out post-mortems, their colleagues decided it was wise to cease from 'prosecuting the inquiry on the dead subject'.[47]

A doctor from Western Missouri reported that, while he was attending an epidemic series of cases of erysipelas, 'I acted as accoucheur to three ladies within the space of a week. The labor of each was without difficulty [and] all were safely delivered,' but all three died of puerperal fever, 'not one surviving four days from the invasion of the disease'.[48] At least one physician at this time believed that puerperal peritonitis was simply erysipelas of the womb, and remarked in passing that epidemics of erysipelas 'have frequently made a hospital of a whole neighbourhood'.[49] When one reads the accounts of the violence inflicted on skin, subcutaneous tissue, and muscle by this variant of the streptococcus, what it must have done to the uterus, pelvis, and peritoneum of lying-in women does not bear thinking about.

[43] M. Larrey, 'Report', *American Journal of the Medical Sciences*, 23 (1852), 254.

[44] Hall and Dexter, 'Account of the Erysipelatous Fever', 17.

[45] A. W. King, 'Case of Gangrenous Erysipelas of Penis and Scrotum', *American Journal of the Medical Sciences*, 44 (1865), 274.   [46] Leasure, 'The Erysipelatous Disease of Lying-in Women', 47.

[47] Ibid. 48.

[48] T. P. Ridley, 'Cases of Erysipelas which Occurred in Platte County, Missouri, in which there were Marked Evidences of Propagation of the Disease by Contagion', *New York Journal of Medicine*, 10 (1853), 41–8.

[49] R. S. Holmes 'On Erysipelas', *Transactions of the American Medical Association*, 7 (1854), 143–66, at 147, 153.

At all events, the link between the two diseases was beyond doubt. A physician who worked in Newcastle, Pennsylvania, and gave his paper the title 'The Erysipelatous Disease of Lying-in Women', mentioned the case of a baby that died of erysipelas after its mother had died of puerperal fever. Furthermore, the mother was attended by an 'old lady who washed and dressed her for the grave [and] took erysipelas within five days of the time she [the mother] died and was the most hideous case of that foul disease I ever met'.[50]

What remained obscure was the mechanism by which the diseases were transferred from patient to patient. Hall and Dexter cited Dr Calvin Jewett's observations:

I do not believe the disease [erysipelas] contagious like smallpox or measles, it approaches more nearly epidemic typhus. I speak of the disease generally, not of puerperal cases, for these are unquestionably communicated by individuals, whether physician or nurse, who have been much with the disease, to women, at or immediately after childbirth. I believe the clothing, not the hand of the physician communicates the disease. *I wish I were mistaken on this point.* (emphasis in original)[51]

Likewise, the physician Ezra Bennet of Connecticut recognized that puerperal fever could be the result of indirect contact with erysipelas, so he took care when he had just attended a case of erysipelas to wash his 'whole person with soap and water and then with a solution of chloride of lime' before attending a midwifery case. But he believed other factors played an important part in causing puerperal fever—for instance, vitiation of the atmosphere, and especially anaemia. Few cases of puerperal fever, he thought, occurred in healthy red-faced women who were florid and did not flood, while the pale and weak, who were prone to flooding, were much more susceptible. Other factors included the 'Peculiar condition of the system induced by labour, exposure to cold, [or] abuse of stimulating drinks'.[52]

Hirsch, who reported this epidemic in detail, believed that erysipelas, puerperal fever, and hospital gangrene 'are in their origin dependent on the existence of some breach of continuity in the external and internal surfaces of the body' and that, although most cases were transmitted by contagion 'through contact with surgical instruments, bandages or other things used by patients . . . in the majority of cases . . . one is rather driven to think that the reproduction of the morbid poison really takes place outside the human body and that the virus is for the most part carried by currents of air'.[53] We return to the question of contagion in Chapter 6.

Was the USA unique in suffering such terrible epidemics of erysipelas? I have been unable so far to find reports of such terrifying epidemics of erysipelas

[50] Leasure, 'The Erysipelatous Disease of Lying-in Women', 48.

[51] Hall and Dexter, 'Account of the Erysipelatous Fever', 19.

[52] E. Bennett, 'On the Identity of Erysipelas and a Certain Form of Puerperal Fever, and its Contagiousness', *American Journal of the Medical Sciences*, 19 (1850), 376–83, at 382.

[53] Hirsch, *Handbook of Geographical and Historical Pathology*, ii. 389, 415. For the use of the word 'virus' in the nineteenth century, see Ch. 6 below.

from Britain or Continental Europe in spite of searching for them, and August Hirsch, in his magnificent *Handbook of Geographical and Historical Pathology*, does not mention similar epidemics in other countries. Of course, they may have occurred and not been reported, or the reports may have escaped notice. I suspect at least some similar outbreaks occurred. In most of the standard texts and surgical dictionaries of the nineteenth century, under the heading of erysipelas, the 'gangrenous' form is mentioned in passing, but usually receives little attention. However, the reader may recall that, in the account of the Abingdon epidemic of puerperal fever, the outbreak began with several cases of erysipelas, including the unfortunate boy who had both legs amputated for infective gangrene, and the two cases described as *erysipelas gangrenosa*. What would be described today as erysipelas and necrotizing fasciitis seem to have occurred together in the American epidemic and may well have occurred elsewhere. It was, however, as a result of these utterly horrifying epidemics of puerperal fever and erysipelas in the USA that one of the most famous accounts of puerperal fever came to be written by Oliver Wendell Homes.

Oliver Wendell Holmes and Puerperal Fever

It was just as the outbreak of erysipelas was beginning in New England, in May 1842, that there was a meeting of the College of Physicians of Philadelphia. At this meeting:

Dr Condie begged leave, as there appeared to be no other written communications to be presented, to call the attention of the College to a subject of very great interest to the medical profession . . . He alluded, he remarked, to the prevalence, at the present time, of puerperal fever of a peculiarly insidious and malignant character . . . The remarks he was about to offer, were founded upon cases that had occurred in the southern sections of the city . . . In the practice of one gentleman, extensively engaged as an obstetrician, nearly every female he has attended in confinement, during several weeks past within the above limits, had been attacked by the fever . . . The disease has been found to occur alike in the young and the middle aged—the robust and delicate—in those surrounded by every comfort and afforded every attention demanded by their situation, as in the poor and destitute . . . and as well after the most rapid and easy labours, as after those that were protracted and difficult.[54]

In the subsequent discussion numerous instances of the same kind were mentioned. Dr Jackson of Northumberland County, Pennsylvania, for example, had recently suffered seven successive cases of puerperal fever in his practice, although there were no other cases of puerperal fever within a radius of fifty miles. Two of his cases recovered, five died. During this time erysipelas was

---

[54] College of Physicians of Philadelphia, 'Discussion', *Transactions of the College of Physicians of Philadelphia*, 1 (1841–6), 50–62, at 50–1. The 'one gentleman, extensively engaged as an obstetrician', was Dr Rutter.

unusually prevalent and severe, and the first of Dr Jackson's cases followed the treatment of 'a limb extensively mortified from erysipelas'. He went straight from this case to a woman in labour 'with my clothes and the unfortunate gloves most thoroughly embued with the effluvia of that sphacelation'. Dr Jackson soon found that 'Women who had expected of me to attend upon them, now becoming alarmed, removed out of my reach, and others sent for a physician residing several miles distant. These women, as well as those attended by mid-wives, all did well . . .'.[55]

The case most frequently cited was that of Dr Rutter of Philadelphia, who had a large obstetric practice. He was not a specialist obstetrician but a respected general practitioner who had been a pupil of Professor Charles Meigs. During the 1840s Rutter suddenly found that almost every midwifery case he attended developed puerperal fever. Nothing remotely like this had happened to him before. During a period of twelve months in 1841–2 he had no less than seventy cases of the disease in his practice. The number that died is not recorded, but very few of the women he delivered escaped the disease.

The effect on Dr Rutter's reputation can be imagined, because his colleagues, no more careful, experienced, or competent than himself, had only sporadic cases in their practices or none at all. No one could explain why Dr Rutter alone had such a devastating series of cases. Greatly distressed, Rutter ceased practice and quarantined himself for several weeks. He washed frequently and thoroughly. His head and face were shaved. He changed all his clothing and all the equipment he carried about with him even to the pencil he carried for taking notes. In spite of these measures, when he resumed practice puerperal fever still followed him wherever he went, until, worn out and disappointed, he was forced to leave Philadelphia.[56]

As it happened, at about the same time that puerperal fever was discussed in Philadelphia, it also cropped up at a meeting of the Boston Society for Medical Improvement. One of those present was Oliver Wendell Holmes (1809–94), better known today as a poet than a physician. This is how Holmes described the meeting:

It happened, some years ago, that a discussion arose in a Medical Society, of which I was a member, involving the subject of a certain supposed cause of disease, about which something was known, a good deal suspected, and not a little feared. The discussion was suggested by a case, reported at the preceding meeting, of a physician who

[55] College of Physicians of Philadelphia, 'Discussion', *Transactions of the College of Physicians of Philadelphia*, 1 (1841–6), 60.

[56] Ibid. A description of this incident can also be found in J. S. Parry, 'Description of a Form of Puerperal Fever which Occurred at the Philadelphia Hospital Characterized by Diphtheritic Deposits of Wounds of the Genital Passages and by other Peculiar Phenomena', *American Journal of Medical Sciences*, 69 (1875), 46–76. See also correspondence between C. Meigs and D. Rutter in *Medical Examiner*, 6 (1843), 3. In 1889 an American obstetrician, Harold C. Ernst, said, without giving any authority for the assertion, that Rutter had 'an oezena on his hand', and that this was the source of infection (H. C. Ernst, 'The Etiology of Puerperal Fever', in B. C. Hirst (ed.), *A System of Obstetrics by American Authors* (2 vols., Edinburgh, 1889), ii. 401–59).

made an examination of the body of a patient who had died with puerperal fever, and who himself died in less than a week, apparently in consequence of a wound received at the examination, having attended several women in confinement in the mean time, all of whom, as alleged, were attacked with puerperal fever. Whatever apprehensions and beliefs were entertained, it was plain that a fuller knowledge of the facts relating to the subject would be acceptable to all present. I therefore felt that it would be doing a good service to look into the best records I could find, and inquire of the most trust-worthy practitioners I knew, to learn what experience had to teach in the matter, and arrived at the results contained in the following pages.[57]

Holmes first presented the results of his investigations to the Boston Society for Medical Improvement on 13 February 1843. He was still a relatively obscure young physician, aged 33. It was not until 1847 that he was appointed to the Parkman Professorship of Anatomy and Physiology in the Medical School of Harvard University. With the encouragement of the Society, the paper was published in April 1843 in the *New England Quarterly Journal of Medicine*, which had a very restricted circulation and ceased publication in 1844. Few knew of Holmes's work until he republished the paper as a pamphlet with the title *Puerperal Fever as a Private Pestilence* twelve years later in 1855.

Holmes began his paper by disputing the view that 'the facts are too generally known and acknowledged to require any formal argument or exposition, that there is nothing new advanced, and no need of laying additional statements before the profession'. He pointed out that in the two leading midwifery text-books in the 1840s one ignored the evidence of contagion and the other flatly denied that puerperal fever was ever under any circumstances a contagious disease.[58] As for the negative evidence produced by physicians who protested they had attended cases of puerperal fever without transmitting the disease to other patients, Holmes replied that 'children that walk in calico before open fires are not always burnt to death', but no one would use this as 'an argument against woollen frocks and high fenders'. Holmes then presented the evidence of contagion based on an extremely thorough search of everything he could find that had been published on the subject.[59]

The greatest part of the paper consists of a review of the reports we have already discussed in this and the previous chapter with some additional sources, mostly American. The fame of Holmes's paper rests on its clarity, force, and style. In the most memorable and readable account of puerperal fever that has ever been published, he sets out an unanswerable case for the contagiousness of puerperal fever. It is the work of a man who loved writing, who was old enough to marshall his material skilfully, but young enough to be passionate

---

[57] Holmes, *Puerperal Fever as a Private Pestilence*. See also Cullingworth, *Oliver Wendell Holmes*.
[58] Holmes, *Puerperal Fever as a Private Pestilence*, 27.
[59] It is salutary for the modern historian, with all the facilities of computerized catalogues and indices and numerous secondary sources, to discover the thoroughness of Holmes's research. Apart from sources quoted in the text, he added an appendix containing a list of 'additional references and cases', and there is very little in the way of publications on puerperal fever before 1850 that he missed.

and angry and to let these qualities show. His main thesis was (with the original emphasis):

The disease known as puerperal fever is so far contagious as to be frequently carried from patient to patient by physicians and nurses.

He admitted that he had no idea whether the contagion was carried on the hands of the birth attendant or whether it consisted of some kind of miasm or atmospheric infection. Nor could he provide an explanation for the most puzzling of all the characteristics of the disease—the tendency for one physician or midwife to be singled out as the carrier of the disease while his or her colleagues escaped such a fate. But it was something that happened so often that it was impossible to dismiss it as an occasional chance event:

In the view of these facts, it does appear a singular coincidence that one man or woman should have ten, twenty, thirty, or seventy cases of this rare disease, following their footsteps like a beagle through the streets and lanes of a crowded city, while the scores that cross the same paths on the same errands know it only by name.[60]

He argued correctly that one did not need to know the mechanism of contagion in order to prove that it occurred, and he found that the evidence of contagion was overwhelming. He ended his paper with a list of recommendations to the effect that anyone who attended an autopsy, a case of puerperal fever, or a case of erysipelas should take precautions against conveying puerperal fever to a midwifery case. No physician 'who held himself in readiness to attend cases of midwifery' should ever attend an autopsy on a case of puerperal fever. And every physician who had 'three or more closely connected cases of puerperal fever should regard it as prima facie evidence that he is the vehicle of contagion'. His final conclusion, from which he took the title for his pamphlet, was:

The time has come when the existence of a private pestilence in the sphere of a single physician should be looked upon not as a misfortune but a crime; and in the knowledge of such occurrences, the duties of the practitioner in his profession, should give way to his paramount obligations to society.[61]

It has often been said that Holmes was the first to discover the contagiousness of puerperal fever. Holmes never made such a claim, and it is, of course, manifest nonsense. His contribution was to assemble, like a skilled lawyer, all the published evidence he could find and weld it into a coherent and unanswerable case. Who, then, could fail to be convinced? As he said, fifty years later, 'I thought I had laid down the rules which promised to ensure the safety of the lying-in woman from disease and death carried to her unconsciously by her professional attendant.'[62]

It may have been the use of the word 'crime' ('not as a misfortune but a crime') that upset some of his colleagues; or he may have seemed too young,

---

[60] Holmes, *Puerperal Fever as a Private Pestilence*, 7–8.
[61] Ibid. 57.   [62] Cullingworth, *Oliver Wendell Holmes*, 20.

too inexperienced, to be so sure of himself. But he certainly upset some estab-lished obstetricians, such as the two professors in Philadelphia: Charles Meigs, who held the chair of midwifery and the diseases of women at Jefferson Col-lege, and Professor Hodge, who held the chair of obstetrics at the University of Pennsylvania. Hodge disagreed courteously with Holmes. Meigs, on the other hand, attacked Holmes with an unseemly ferocity, dismissing the paper as offen-sive nonsense, the 'maunderings of a sophomore', the work of an obscure, young, upstart physician. As a man who often boasted about his extensive experience, he was scornful of a paper written by someone with a limited practical know-ledge of obstetrics.

Holmes declined to take offence. 'No man', he said, 'makes a quarrel with me over the counterpane that covers a mother, with her new-born infant at her breast.'[63] Instead, he answered the objections of his critics with quiet reason. To critics who objected that there were many occasions when they had attended cases of puerperal fever without transmitting the disease, Holmes replied with a memorable passage from Watson's *Lectures on the Practice of Physic*:

A man might say, 'I was in the battle of Waterloo, and saw many men around me fall and die, and it was said that they were struck down by musket-balls; but I know bet-ter than that, for I was there at the time, and so were many of my friends, and we were never hit by any musket-balls. Musket-balls, therefore, could not have been the cause of the deaths we witnessed.'[64]

But the opposition was formidable, especially from Professor Charles Meigs, who was 51 when the essay was published. Meigs (as we saw in Chapter 3 on Alexander Gordon) possessed an extraordinary ability to blind himself to un-palatable facts. He dismissed the seventy cases of puerperal fever in Dr Rutter's practice when others had none (together with all the other examples of this kind) as nothing more than pure chance.[65] Meigs was a highly successful obstet-rician with a large private practice, a popular and persuasive teacher, and the author of a widely read text on the practice of midwifery; as such, his opinion carried weight. To his dying day he denied the possibility that puerperal fever was a contagious disease, and for doing so he was ultimately ridiculed and his reputation was damaged—not so much for his denial of contagion (honest dif-ferences of opinion were acceptable) as for the offensiveness of his attacks on Holmes, whose fame as a poet and physician grew with the passage of time.

---

[63] Ibid. 17.   [64] Ibid.
[65] C. D. Meigs, *Females and their Diseases: A Series of Letters to his Class* (Philadelphia, 1848).

5

Puerperal Fever and the Lying-in Hospitals

There was an extraordinarily rapid growth of hospitals in the eighteenth century. In London the Westminster Hospital was founded in 1720, Guy's in 1724, St George's in 1733, the London in 1740, and the Middlesex in 1745. In addition, thirty-two hospitals were established in provincial England by 1799, starting with Winchester and Bristol in 1736, followed by York (1740), Exeter (1741), and Bath (1742). Although historians have argued whether these hospitals did more harm than good, they were seen at the time not just as symbols of the philanthropic impulse, but as genuinely helpful and humane institutions providing medical care for the poor. They also formed a nucleus for the teaching of medicine, and in that respect proved to be remarkably robust. Although many have had to move from their original sites, every one of the eighteenth-century voluntary hospitals in England still exists in name as a National Health Service hospital, and often as a teaching hospital.

When they were founded, strict rules were devised (but not always kept) to exclude undesirable patients such as those suffering from smallpox or other contagious diseases including 'the itch' (scabies), patients with venereal disease, and children except those who needed 'cutting for stone'. They also excluded 'women big with child', and this was perhaps the most glaring exclusion. It was only natural, therefore, that philanthropists decided to establish separate hospitals, known for many years as 'lying-in' hospitals, for the delivery of poor women.

The Establishment of Lying-in (Maternity) Hospitals

The lying-in hospitals were closely modelled on the larger general hospitals.[1] In the UK they were voluntary institutions in the sense of depending on the voluntary contributions of the public, and they appointed honorary obstetricians, although they were known at the time as 'accoucheurs'.[2] The early lying-in

---

[1] At this early stage, maternity wards within general hospitals were rare. There were maternity wards in the Edinburgh Infirmary, and the Middlesex Hospital opened a maternity ward before the century was out. But they were the exceptions.

[2] It is difficult to put a precise date on the use of the modern term 'obstetrician', but it gradually became more popular during the nineteenth century. It may come as a surprise that right up to the end of the nineteenth century accoucheurs were much more likely to be physicians than surgeons. Obstetrics was shunned by hospital surgeons as a low-status occupation associated with general practice,

hospitals were the British Lying-in Hospital, founded in 1749, the City of London Lying-in Hospital in 1750, Queen Charlotte's Hospital in 1752, and the Westminster Lying-in Hospital in 1765. The Dublin Lying-in Hospital, later known colloquially as the Rotunda, was founded in 1757. Many lying-in hospitals were likewise founded on the Continent. There was an obstetric ward in the Hôtel Dieu in Paris as early as 1664, and lying-in hospitals were founded in the eighteenth century in many European cities including Paris, Berlin, Vienna, and Göttingen. Almost always, such hospitals on the Continent were funded by local or national government.[3]

In the history of maternal care in the UK, before the lying-in hospitals were founded the only resource for the poor in childbirth had been the untrained midwife, with a very occasional visit by a surgeon in an obstetric emergency. The lying-in hospitals provided what was perceived as skilled maternal care in the form of trained midwives backed up by accoucheurs, as well as the warmth, shelter, a week or two's rest, and adequate food that were highly valued by the patients. They also played an important role in training midwives and medical students and became centres for the investigation and treatment of the complications of pregnancy, labour, and the post-natal period. In short, they promised to be useful, charitable, institutions. From the accoucheurs' point of view they raised the status of man-midwifery, and also, through enhanced reputation, the incomes of those lucky enough to be appointed as honorary accoucheurs and who depended on private practice for their living.

Although intended to bring skill and comfort to the poor in childbirth, and save them from the perceived ignorance of untrained midwives, the lying-in hospitals were from the early years plagued by recurrent epidemics of puerperal fever with appalling mortality rates. By choosing delivery in a lying-in hospital, women (although they seldom knew it) were exposing themselves to a risk of dying that was many times higher than if they had stayed at home in the worst of slums and been attended in their birth by no one except family and an untrained midwife. The lying-in hospitals were such a disaster that, in retrospect, it would have been better if they had never been established before the introduction of antisepsis in the 1880s.[4] As John Burns remarked in his

---

until the late-nineteenth- and early twentieth-century growth in operative gynaecology moved (after a great struggle) away from general surgery and linked up with obstetrics, which thereby became a branch of surgery rather than medicine.

[3] Léon Le Fort, *Des maternités: Études sur les maternités et les institutions charitables d'accouchement à domicile dans les principaux états de l'Europe* (Paris, 1866). Oddly, although provincial towns in England were falling over each other in the rush to build voluntary general hospitals, none, as far as I can discover, established a lying-in hospital in the eighteenth century.

[4] There were occasional exceptions. Fleetwood Churchill wrote in 1849: 'Perhaps I may be allowed to mention as a curious exemption from this disease [puerperal fever], that during the whole time the Western Lying-in Hospital in this city has been open for the poor, we have never had puerperal fever prevailing there. A single case of uterine inflammation has occurred occasionally . . . but it has never been followed by a second soon after. I do not pretend to account for this; I am far from supposing that the credit is due to better management' (Fleetwood Churchill, 'An Historical Sketch of the Epidemics of Puerperal Fever', in Churchill (ed.), *Essays on the Puerperal Fever and Other Diseases Peculiar to Women* (London, 1849), 3–42, at 28.

widely read textbook on midwifery in the 1830s: 'The Puerperal fever is most frequent and most fatal, in hospitals. In private practice, it is less malignant, though still very dangerous. In hospitals, it has conspicuously appeared as a contagious disease.'[5] In 1872, William Farr, the Compiler of Abstracts at the General Register Office, was more forceful:

Seeing how destitute of comforts, means, and medical appliances many women are, the thought occurred to some benevolent persons that they might be received and delivered in hospitals. It was the extension of the hospital system to midwifery cases, which have some analogy with wounds and injuries for which hospitals had been used since the date of their foundation. Contrary to expectations, the advantages these institutions offered were over-balanced by one dread drawback; the mortality of mothers was not diminished; nay, it became in some instances excessive; in other instances appalling.[6]

As we will see, there had been for more than a century, ample reason for such worries.

Death in the Lying-in Hospitals

Table 5.1 shows the number of maternal deaths per 10,000 deliveries in certain UK and Continental lying-in hospitals in the late eighteenth and early nineteenth centuries. Bearing in mind that the average maternal mortality rate in the UK and on the Continent, where the large majority of deliveries were attended by midwives or general practitioners, was in the region of 40 to 50 per 10,000 deliveries (of which approximately half were due to puerperal fever), this table is a vivid illustration of the danger of these institutions. It was not just the epidemics, when the mortality could be twenty or more times the rate in home deliveries; the endemic rate was usually considerably greater (by a factor of three or four) than the mortality rate of home deliveries (see Table 5.3).[7] Further, in certain hospitals on the Continent (Paris and Vienna, for example) some of the sick maternity cases were removed in the early stages of puerperal fever from the maternity wards to general wards. If these patients died, their deaths were recorded in the lists of deaths on the medical wards. Semmelweis, to whose work we come later, emphasized that for this reason the published mortality rates, already alarmingly high, were sometimes an understatement of the true level of mortality.[8]

The danger of the lying-in hospitals was thrown into stark contrast by the other form of charitable maternal care: the lying-in dispensaries and hospital schemes for providing maternal care on an outpatient basis, which were more

[5] J. Burns, *The Principles of Midwifery* (9th edn., London, 1837), 601–2.
[6] *Report of the Registrar General for England and Wales for 1870* (1872), 407.
[7] Léon Le Fort showed that some of the deaths in Parisian maternity hospitals were due to incidental diseases such as typhus, typhoid, and phthisis, and some were certainly due to other puerperal causes; but the large majority were due to puerperal fever (Le Fort, *Des maternités*, 35–7).   [8] Ibid.

TABLE 5.1. *Deliveries and maternal mortality rates in certain lying-in hospitals in the UK and on the Continent of Europe during the late eighteenth and first half of the nineteenth century*

Lying-in hospital and period	Average annual no. of		Maternal mortality rate		
	Deliveries	Deaths	Average for period	Highest annual rate	Lowest annual rate
London Lying-in Hospital					
1770–1779	564	13	*230*	398	67
1780–1789	555	9	*162*	—	—
1791–1799	591	2	*34*	—	—
1833–1842	170	10	*587*	—	—
Dublin Lying-in Hospital					
1790–1799	1,604	13	*81*	156	50
1800–1809	2,218	20	*91*	216	47
1810–1819	2,968	40	*134*	294	51
1815–1833	2,691	35	*130*	n.a.	n.a.
1833–1840	1,881	32	*172*	n.a.	n.a.
Vienna Maternity Hospital					
1790–1799	1,757	17	*97*	261	25
1800–1809	1,777	14	*79*	198	49
1810–1819	2,061	40	*194*	498	50
1820–1829	2,830	120	*424*	745	85
Paris Maternité					
1810–1814	2,192	107	*488*	686	301
1820–1824	2,423	114	*474*	633	215
1830–1834	2,648	145	*547*	880	371
1840–1844	3,516	163	*463*	697	255
Paris Hôtel Dieu					
1802–1821	85	4	*123*	—	—
Dresden Maternity Hospital					
1825–1834	263	8	*304*	—	—
Leipzig Maternity Hospital					
1810–1829	81	1	*123*	—	—
Average mortality rates in home deliveries in Britain and on the Continent			*40–50*		

Notes: Maternal mortality rates are expressed as maternal deaths per 10,000 deliveries.
   The most important data are italicized.
   Average numbers of deliveries and deaths, and maternal mortality rates, are shown to the nearest whole number. The highest and lowest annual rates of mortality are not shown where the average number of maternal deaths per year was less than 10.
   n.a. = not available.

Sources: William Heberden, *Observations on the Increase and Decrease of different Diseases* (London, 1801); L. Le Fort, *Des maternités: Études sur les maternités et les institutions charitables d'accouchement à domicile dans les principaux états de l'Europe* (Paris, 1866); T. D. O'Donel Browne, *The Rotunda Hospital, 1745–1945* (London, 1947).

TABLE 5.2. *Maternal mortality rates due to puerperal fever, General Lying-in Hospital, London, 1835–1859*

Periods	No. of deliveries	No. of deaths due to puerperal fever	Maternal mortality rate due to puerperal fever
Five-year periods			
1835–39	835	52	623
1840–44	819	53	639
1845–49	1,241	8	64
1850–54	1,113	29	260
1855–59	1,262	26	206
Total period			
1835–59	5,270	168	319
England and Wales			
1835–59			17

Note: Maternal mortality rates are expressed as the number of maternal deaths per 10,000 deliveries.

Source: W. T. Fox, 'Puerperal Fever', *Transactions of the Obstetrical Society of London*, 3 (1862), 368–71.

common in the UK (and later in the USA) than on the Continent of Europe. These charities also provided trained midwives, backed up by consultant accoucheurs, but they delivered poor women in their own homes and achieved very low rates of maternal mortality.[9] Just how successful they were, compared with the lying-in hospitals, can be seen in Tables 5.3 and 5.4. Table 5.3 shows the maternal mortality rates in home deliveries in various countries, and Table 5.4 shows the records of the Royal Maternity Charity—a charity that served the East End of London and worked amongst the most deprived section of the poor.

The low mortality achieved by such outpatient charities as the Royal Maternity Charity and the Westminster General Dispensary in London was in part due to the skill of the midwives and obstetricians (although these were available in the lying-in hospitals) but much more to the striking difference in cases of puerperal fever. Thus, in the period 1831–43, the mortality due to puerperal fever amongst the patients of the Royal Maternity Charity was 10 per 10,000 births, while the corresponding figure for the General Lying-in Hospital in the same period was over 600 (Tables 5.2 and 5.4).

The strikingly lower rates of puerperal fever in the Royal Maternity Charity were associated with low rates of interference in normal labours, and to the fact

---

[9] The best-known example was the Royal Maternity Charity in London, founded in 1757, and we saw an example in Manchester when discussing the views of Roberton in the previous chapter.

TABLE 5.3. *Maternal mortality rates of home deliveries in various towns, for various indicated periods*

Town and period	No. of deliveries	Maternal mortality rate
Paris, 12th Arrondissement (1856)	3,222	31
Paris, Bureau de Bienfaisance (1861–2)	12,634	55
City of Paris (1861–2)	87,277	51
Leipzig Polyclinique (1849–59)	1,203	108
Berlin Polyclinique (1864)	500	140
Munich Polyclinique (1859–63)	1,911	84
City of St Petersburg (1845–52)	209,612	67
London, all home deliveries (1860–4)	562,623	39
Edinburgh, all home deliveries (1858)	5,486	50
London, Westminster General Dispensary (1818–28)	7,717	22
Total deliveries and average maternal mortality rate of all home deliveries investigated by Le Fort	934,781	47

Note: Maternal mortality rates are expressed as maternal deaths per 10,000 deliveries.

Source: Le Fort, *Des maternités*, 32–3.

TABLE 5.4. *Deliveries and maternal deaths, Eastern Division of the Royal Maternity Charity, London, 1831–1843*

Births and deaths	No. of births or deaths	Percentage of deaths in each group	Maternal mortality rate
Total number of live births	33,868		
Total maternal deaths	166	100	49.0
Direct maternal deaths	126	75.9	37.2
Haemorrhage	56	33.7	16.6
Puerperal fever	34	20.4	10.0
Other	36	21.6	10.6
Indirect maternal deaths	40	24.0	11.8
Phthisis	15	9.0	4.4
Pneumonia	6	3.6	1.8
Typhus	6	3.6	1.8
Other	13	7.8	3.8

Notes: Maternal mortality rates are expressed as maternal deaths per 10,000 live births.

For comparison with the maternal mortality rates in Continental lying-in hospitals such as those in Paris, the correct comparison is with total maternal deaths, that is with direct maternal deaths + indirect maternal deaths.

Source: F. H. Ramsbotham, 'The Eastern District of the Royal Maternity Charity', *London Medical Gazette*, NS 2 (1843–4), 619–25.

that the patients were delivered separately in their homes and not crowded together in a hospital where cross infection was inevitable, especially when one remembers that post-mortem examinations were routinely performed in many lying-in hospitals. With hindsight it is easy to condemn the lying-in hospitals and their staff for not closing these lethal institutions. But we will see later why they were allowed to continue.

Descriptions of Hospital Epidemics

In the lying-in hospitals the striking feature of puerperal fever was its periodicity. In their earliest days, from about 1740 to 1780, there were many severe epidemics in which the fatality rates were the highest ever recorded. There was one in the Hôtel Dieu in Paris in 1746 and another in Edinburgh in which it was said that every woman who contracted the disease died of it and 'whole wards were swept away'. The years 1770 and 1771 were said to be particularly bad. In his *Practical Essays on the Arrangement of Pregnancy and Labour*, first published in 1793, John Clarke said: 'In the year 1770 this [puerperal] fever raged violently in several of the London Hospitals. In the Westminster Hospital between November 1769 and May 1770, of sixty-three women delivered, nineteen had the fever and fourteen died; which is nearly every fourth woman.'[10]

But there were some periods of several years when there was scarcely a case of the disease, and the staff would be lulled into a state of false security. From about 1785 to 1810 mortality in most lying-in hospitals was low and there were few reports of town epidemics.[11] The fact that this was a period in which scarlet fever was said to be particularly severe is a matter whose significance is discussed in Chapter 12. From about 1810, however, severe epidemics returned, and for the next seventy years the mortality in lying-in hospitals not only failed to improve, but got worse. Desperate attempts were made to prevent the series of increasingly severe epidemics, with little or no effect. Once again, however, periods of awful mortality alternated with periods of calm. This was vividly described by one of the most noted of the London obstetricians in the first half of the nineteenth century, Robert Gooch:

[10] John Clarke, *Practical Essays on the Arrangement of Pregnancy and Labour and on the Inflammatory and Febrile Diseases of Lying-in Women* (London, 1793; 2nd edn., 1806).
[11] DeLacy has argued that hospital delivery was only slightly more dangerous than delivery at home, basing her view on a comparison between the mortality rates of the London lying-in hospitals at the end of the eighteenth century and calculations of mortality rates of home deliveries taken from the London Bills of Mortality. Her finding of low hospital mortality is likely to be due to the fact that the period she chose happens to have been a period in which hospital mortality rates were much lower than they were either before or afterwards. She also suggests that there may have been selection of high-risk cases for hospital delivery, but there is clear evidence that selection on clinical grounds was rare in the lying-in hospitals before the late nineteenth century (M. DeLacy, 'Puerperal Fever in Eighteenth-Century Britain', *Bulletin of the History of Medicine*, 63 (1989), 521–56).

I was appointed physician to the Westminster Lying-in Hospital in the year 1812, and as the elder physician, Dr Thynne, was aged and infirm, the whole task devolved upon me for several years, to attend both the in and the out-patients in their difficult labours, and their illnesses . . . My situation gave me ample opportunities of observing the diseases of lying-in women among the poor of London and its neighbourhood.

I had not been physician to the hospital long before I remarked how much more healthy it was at one time than at another; sometimes, for many months, there was no sickness among the patients; as soon as the labour was over they were well; they required nothing but an opiate for their after-pains, and a few doses of aperient medicine, and the medical part of my office was almost a sinecure. At other times, cases of illness were perpetually occurring; as soon as one was over another began; often I had several at the same time under my care; this would go on for several months, and then cease, leaving the hospital healthy for a long time.

The cases which were so numerous in these unhealthy seasons had the common symptoms and course of puerperal fever . . . The disease generally began very suddenly. After being quite well, feeling no sense of illness, or at least making no complaint, the patient was seized at once with chilliness, or shivering, and pain in the belly, and the pulse rose to 120 or 130 . . . I soon found that I had to deal with a very fatal disease. When I saw the patients after it had been going on two or three days or even longer (which was no unusual circumstance among the *out* patients) I seldom or never saved them; the sunk countenance, the small weak pulse of 140 or 160, the tympanitic belly, the short breathing, and sometimes the clammy sweat, all indicated a fatal disease, past the reach of depletion, even if it had ever been fit for it.[12]

Here, when Gooch is writing about 'saving' patients, he means bleeding. In this, the age of 'heroic therapy', Gooch, citing Gordon and Denman as his authorities, was a firm believer in 'depletion' or venesection. He insisted, like Gordon, that to be effective it had to be carried out in the very early stages of the disease, when the patient's pulse was full and strong:

A vein was opened in the arm, with a wide orifice, so that the blood flowed in a full stream, and it was allowed to flow until the patient felt faint; the arm was then tied up, and her head was raised so as to encourage the faintness for many minutes . . . When the patient had thoroughly recovered from her faintness, from ten to twenty leeches were applied to the painful and tender parts of the abdomen . . . when the leeches had fallen off, a bag, long enough and broad enough to cover the whole abdomen, was stuffed with hot poultice which was spread so as to form a cushion nearly an inch thick; this was laid hot over the whole abdomen, and renewed so often as to keep up heat and moisture.[13]

---

[12] Robert Gooch, *An Account of Some of the Most Important Diseases Peculiar to Women* (London, 1831; 2nd edn., 1838), 38–42. Robert Gooch (1784–1830) MD LRCP, began medical practice as a general practitioner in Croydon. He soon moved to London and became lecturer on midwifery at St Bartholomew's Hospital and Honorary Consultant Accoucheur to the Westminster Lying-in Hospital in 1812 at the age of 28. He quickly had a large practice in midwifery, but was later forced to abandon most of his work because of becoming increasingly feeble and emaciated, and he turned to the writing for which he had had no time as a busy accoucheur. He died of consumption in 1830 at the age of 45. (*Dictionary of National Biography*). [13] Ibid. 44–5.

Unfortunately, however, Gooch found that the disease was already too advanced for depletion by the time he arrived at the patient's bedside. Delay could occur for various reasons, as he explains.

Within the hospital I used to see it [puerperal fever] earlier, sometimes within a few hours of its commencement, although even here this was not always the case . . . the patients of a lying-in hospital are slow to confess themselves ill; they look upon pain in the belly as nothing but after-pains, and dread the active remedies which a confession of illness brings upon them; even after the confession, the nurses are often dilatory in communicating it [or] the patient would go to bed complaining of nothing and be waked . . . by pain in the belly or chilliness, but the night-nurse thought it unnecessary to disturb anybody, and I lived two miles from the hospital.[14]

Gooch found similar problems of being called late amongst his outpatient cases, but, whenever he felt that bleeding was indicated, if he was not satisfied with the results of the initial bleeding, venesection was performed again, once more to the point of fainting.

There were similar epidemics of puerperal fever at the Rotunda (the Dublin Lying-in Hospital) that are especially instructive because it was an institution in which there was a large number of births, and that kept meticulous records throughout the nineteenth century. Table 5.5 and Fig. 5.1 show the annual rates of mortality in this hospital between 1781 and 1868.

In the thirty years 1770–99, when (in round numbers) there were about 1,200 deliveries a year, the average maternal mortality was 97 per 10,000 births. During the next forty years, 1800–39, when there were close to 3,000 deliveries a year, mortality rose to 134. But it was after 1840 that maternal mortality rose spectacularly, reaching a peak of 714 in 1862. During the nineteen years 1840–68, when the annual number of deliveries was about 2,500, the average maternal mortality rose to 216. This was more than twice the mortality in the late eighteenth century and four times the average maternal mortality in England and Wales between 1847 and 1868 (national vital statistics for Ireland were not available for this period). Here is an account by the Master of the Rotunda, Dr Labatt, of the terrible Dublin epidemic of 1819.

During the years 1815–16–17 the hospital was very healthy; of nearly 10,000 women admitted sixty-six died . . . The epidemic which is the immediate object of this statement, commenced in a most insidious way, so as to excite but little alarm. During the months of June, July and August last we continued healthy, and without a single case of fever. On the 8th of September, however, two women were attacked, and on the following day, one; on the 20th one; on the 28th one; and on the 4th of October, one; all in different wards.

No new cases occurring for several days after this last attack, I was in hopes that I should be relieved of all anxiety; but on the 15th of October, I was much alarmed on finding seven women complaining, and from this time until the beginning of December, there was scarce a day that two or more were not attacked.

[14] Robert Gooch, *An Account of Some of the Most Important Diseases Peculiar to Women* (London, 1831; 2nd edn., 1838), 42–3.

TABLE 5.5. *Annual maternal mortality rates, Dublin Lying-in Hospital, 1781–1868*

Year	No. of deliveries	No. of deaths	Maternal mortality rate	Year	No. of deliveries	No. of deaths	Maternal mortality rate	Year	No. of deliveries	No. of deaths	Maternal mortality rate
1781	1,027	6	5.8	1811	2,561	24	9.4	1841	2,025	23	11.3
1782	990	6	6.0	1812	2,766	43	15.5	1842	2,171	21	10.0
1783	1,167	15	12.8	1813	2,484	62	24.9	1843	2,188	22	10.0
1784	1,261	11	8.7	1814	2,508	25	10.0	1844	2,176	14	6.4
1785	1,292	8	6.2	1815	3,075	17	5.5	1845	1,411	35	24.8
1786	1,351	8	5.9	1816	3,276	18	5.5	1846	2,025	17	8.4
1787	1,347	10	7.4	1817	3,473	32	9.2	1847	1,703	47	27.5
1788	1,469	23	15.6	1818	3,539	56	15.8	1848	1,816	35	19.2
1789	1,435	25	17.4	1819	3,197	94	29.4	1849	2,063	38	18.4
1790	1,546	12	7.7	1820	2,458	70	28.4	1850	1,980	15	7.5
1791	1,602	25	15.6	1821	2,849	22	7.7	1851	2,070	14	6.8
1792	1,631	10	6.1	1822	2,675	12	4.5	1852	1,963	11	5.6
1793	1,757	19	10.8	1823	2,584	59	22.8	1853	1,906	17	8.9
1794	1,543	20	12.9	1824	2,446	20	8.2	1854	1,943	37	19.0
1795	1,503	7	4.6	1825	2,746	26	9.5	1855	1,060	35	33.0
1796	1,621	10	6.2	1826	2,440	81	33.2	1856	1,600	25	15.6
1797	1,712	13	7.6	1827	2,550	33	12.9	1857	1,509	33	21.9
1798	1,604	8	5.0	1828	2,856	43	15.0	1858	1,084	30	27.6
1799	1,537	10	6.5	1829	2,141	34	15.9	1859	1,389	21	15.1
1800	1,337	18	13.4	1830	2,288	12	5.2	1860	1,404	26	18.5
1801	1,725	30	17.4	1831	2,176	12	5.5	1861	1,135	59	52.0
1802	1,985	26	13.0	1832	2,242	12	5.3	1862	800	58	72.5
1803	2,028	44	21.6	1833	2,138	12	5.6	1863	1,228	32	26.0
1804	1,915	16	8.3	1834	2,024	34	16.8	1864	1,184	26	21.9
1805	2,220	12	5.4	1835	1,902	34	17.9	1865	1,332	30	22.5
1806	2,406	23	9.5	1836	1,810	36	19.9	1866	1,074	40	37.2
1807	2,511	12	4.8	1837	1,833	24	13.1	1867	1,146	40	35.0
1808	2,665	13	4.9	1838	2,126	45	21.1	1868	1,022	39	38.2
1809	2,889	21	7.3	1839	1,951	25	12.8	TOTAL	170,972	2,373	13.9
1810	2,854	29	10.2	1840	1,521	26	17.1				

Note: Maternal mortality rates are expressed as maternal deaths per 1,000 deliveries.

Source: E. Kennedy, 'Zymotic Diseases, as More Especially Illustrated by Puerperal Fever', *Dublin Quarterly Journal of Medical Sciences*, 47 (1869), 292–3.

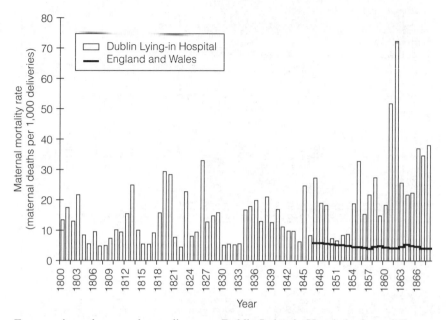

FIG. 5.1 Annual maternal mortality rates, Dublin Lying-in Hospital, 1800–1868, with the maternal mortality rates for England and Wales, 1847–1868, shown for comparison

Sources: E. Kennedy, 'Zymotic Diseases as More Especially Illustrated by Puerperal Fever', *Dublin Quarterly Journal of Medical Sciences*, 47 (1869), 292–3; *Annual Reports of the Registrar General for England and Wales.*

Early in December, with the concurrence of several medical governors, I sent notices of the unhealthy state of the hospital through the city, in order to prevent those from coming in who could provide themselves with accommodation at home, to whom, at the same time, I offered our gratuitous attendance at their residences. This had the effect of lessening our numbers; but many wretched creatures still continued to present themselves for admission at our gates, saying that they would rather run the risk of fever in the hospital where they would have food and attendance, than remain at home destitute of both.

From the 1st of Sept. to the 31st of Dec., of 1010 admitted, 129 took the fever, and sixty-one died [a mortality rate of 604 per 10,000 deliveries and a case fatality rate of just under 50 per cent] . . . from the 1st to the 31st of January, 1820, of 171 patients admitted, sixty three were attacked, and twenty five died [a mortality rate of 1,462 per 10,000].[15]

---

[15] This report was never published but was given directly to Fleetwood Churchill, who includes it in his introductory essay, 'An Historical Sketch', in his *Essays*, 17–20. See also accounts of earlier epidemics at the Rotunda in J. Brenan, *Thoughts on Puerperal Fever Illustrated by Cases in the Lying-in Hospital, Dublin* (London, 1814), which is a short work and much less informative.

This extract, incidentally, answers an important question. What did the poor of Dublin feel about such mortality? Why did women agree to admission to a hospital where the risk of dying was so much greater than in a home delivery? As Dr Labbatt explained, even in an epidemic so terrible that the hospital was closed, women still longed for the comforts of a hospital, the warmth, the food, and the attention. More importantly, their appreciation of the danger would be slight, for even in the worst years in the worst lying-in hospitals, the majority of women survived. A mortality as high as 500 per 10,000 (or 5 per cent) was terrible from the obstetrician's point of view, but it meant that 95 per cent of the women entered the hospital, had their babies, and in most cases returned home none the worse for a hospital delivery. Chatting amongst themselves, women would have known that far more of their neighbours were safely delivered than perished.

If women were reluctant to enter a hospital, it was usually because they feared methods of treatment, as Gooch hinted, or because the staff had a reputation of being unkind and treating them roughly. It is unlikely that working-class women would have appreciated the difference between a survival rate of 99.5 per cent (a mortality of 50 per 10,000 births) and one of 95 per cent (a mortality of 500 per 10,000).

The staff of the lying-in hospitals, of course, were only too aware of the reality of hospital delivery. Their fears might be lulled by a series of years in which there were only occasional maternal deaths, but sooner or later the hospital would be struck by an epidemic, with deaths occurring in rapid succession. Believing that the origin of epidemics lay in the fabric of the hospitals, the almost invariable response was to fumigate and sometimes to combine fumigation with closing the wards for a period of several weeks or even months. This often seemed to keep puerperal fever at bay, but not for long.

In a survey of Parisian lying-in hospitals, published in 1830 in the *Edinburgh Medical and Surgical Journal*, the author noted that French obstetricians were convinced that outbreaks of puerperal fever originated from disease that was lodged in the walls of the hospitals. He also noted that the French completely rejected ideas of contagion 'to which so much importance is attached by many obstetricians in Britain', and he drew attention to the fact that the new lying-in hospital in Paris, the Maternité, had just suffered a large epidemic.[16]

The Maternité in Paris was one of the most famous institutions of its day. It was deliberately built on high ground in an open district to reduce the risk of miasmatic influences. It was considered a model of what a lying-in hospital should be, designed to prevent puerperal fever. It was clean, tidy, and well equipped, and the food and care were excellent. Patients were delivered in a labour ward containing twelve beds, and after delivery they were carried to a long gallery divided into single rooms. If any signs of sickness appeared, the

[16] Anon., 'Critical Analysis: Puerperal Fever', *Edinburgh Medical and Surgical Journal*, 34 (1830), 328–49.

patient was promptly removed to a separate sick-ward. 'The whole medical service of the hospital is confessedly one of the most complete in Europe.'[17]

And so it was, for it seemed that everything that should be done had been done in the way of siting, design, isolation of feverish patients, avoidance of overcrowding, and general administration. If anywhere was safe to have a baby, it should have been the Maternité. Yet this hospital, for all its modern structure and organization, was plagued by epidemics of puerperal fever as frequently and with as high a rate of mortality as those that occurred in old, dirty, and overcrowded lying-in hospitals of the city. In 1829 there were 2,735 deliveries and 252 deaths, a rate of 921 deaths per 10,000 births, almost all due to puerperal fever.[18]

In 1866 Léon Le Fort, whose large and impressive work *Des maternités* was the standard work on lying-in hospitals, discussed the cause of puerperal fever in hospitals. He allowed that contagion could on occasions play some part, but the main reason was, in his view, simple. In every maternity hospital, he said, the walls, the bedding, and the furniture were saturated with the noxious influence that caused the disease. For this reason—and in spite of the unhappy example of the Maternité—he believed that new hospitals were safer than old ones, pointing to the high mortality of old dilapidated hospitals, the apparent benefits of repainting and fumigating after an epidemic, and the fact that when a new maternity hospital was built it usually escaped outbreaks of puerperal fever for a number of years.[19] In fact, the Parisian maternity hospitals were, from the point of view of mortality, amongst the worst in the world; and Parisian doctors were aware of it. In the 1850s they were close to despair. It is said that, when an elderly accoucheur was leaving his lying-in hospital, he met a poor woman in labour on her way to the entrance. He stopped the woman and tried to turn her away, saying, 'Do not come in here unless you wish to die.'[20]

The first to throw some light on the problem was a French doctor, Étienne Stéphane Tarnier (1828–97), who became one of the leading accoucheurs and the leading authority on puerperal fever in Paris in the second half of the nineteenth century.[21] At the beginning of his career he showed that maternal mortality in all the prestigious Parisian lying-in hospitals was much higher than the mortality of home deliveries in the city. The mortality in the Maternité, for example, was seventeen times greater than the mortality in the surrounding district. When Tarnier presented his findings in his inaugural thesis, his seniors at the Maternité were not impressed. Indeed, they were deeply offended at this

[17] Anon., 'Critical Analysis: Puerperal Fever', *Edinburgh Medical and Surgical Journal*, 34 (1830), 328–49.   [18] Le Fort, *Des maternités*, 24.

[19] Ibid.

[20] C. J. Cullingworth, 'Biographical Note on Étienne Stéphane Tarnier', *Transactions of the Obstetrical Society of London*, 40 (1898), 78–89.

[21] Tarnier was born near Dijon, where his father, who was a country doctor, was often assisted by his son in the latter's student days. Tarnier was educated first at Dijon and then in Paris, where he went to study medicine. He gradually became interested in the science of obstetrics and was appointed as a resident in the Maternité in 1856 (ibid. 80).

slur on their establishment, and their reaction was initially so hostile that Tarnier nearly abandoned medicine. However:

A discussion on the nature of puerperal fever took place at the Académie de Médecine, which extended over four months of the year 1858. The thesis of Tarnier was constantly quoted. Dubois [Director of the Maternité] became interested, and promised Tarnier that he would install him as *chef de clinique*; whereupon Tarnier set to work with renewed ardour, and wrote a fresh monograph on puerperal fever as observed at the Maternité. This was published at the end of 1858. When he presented himself to the publisher with his manuscript, M. J. B. Baillière, glancing from the title to his unknown visitor, exclaimed, 'I know only one man, sir, in Paris, who is competent to deal with such a subject.' 'Who is that?' 'Dr Tarnier.' 'I am Dr Tarnier.'[22]

Soon, this feature of Parisian maternity institutions became widely known in a city where they were not especially interested in what had been the experience in other countries. Léon Le Fort, however, investigated rates of puerperal fever in several European countries and showed that what was found in Paris was found everywhere else. Even in the poorest and most deprived areas of European cities, home deliveries were much safer than hospital deliveries (see Table 5.3).[23]

The Cause of Hospital Epidemics

In the next chapter, ideas on fever, contagion, and epidemics will be discussed in depth. It is appropriate, however, to end this chapter by a summary of the views of hospital accoucheurs in the first half of the nineteenth century on the causes of the high hospital mortality and the recurrent epidemics that were suffered by all of them. 'Causes' was the operative word, for everyone believed the high mortality was due to a number of causes, which differed in relative importance in different places at different times.

Most believed that epidemic influence was an important factor in precipitating epidemics. The high endemic level was usually explained in the same terms as those given by Le Fort in 1866—namely, that the walls, the bedding, and the furniture of lying-in hospitals became saturated with the noxious influence that caused the disease, as a result of the crowding-together of so many parturient women under one roof. Sometimes puerperal fever was attributed to defective drainage, especially if there were open drains or sewers in the vicinity; and sometimes the old theory of telluric (meaning 'of the earth' or 'of the soil') influence was held to be a prime cause, if it was felt that a lying-in hospital had been established in an unhealthy area.

[22] Ibid.
[23] Gabriel-Paul Ancelet, *Essai historique et critique sur le création et la transformation des maternités à Paris* (Paris, 1896), and Le Fort, *Des maternités*.

What is surprising is the scant attention paid to contagion, especially in France. Although the role of contagion in town epidemics was well established in the UK during the first half of the nineteenth century, it was mentioned comparatively rarely in connection with hospital epidemics. The Dublin accoucheur Dr Douglas, while believing that hospital epidemics were due to multiple factors such as epidemic influence, miasmas and atmospheric pollution, overcrowding, and so forth, allowed that occasionally puerperal fever could be contagious:

I am rather apprehensive that such contagion may be conveyed by persons much engaged in hospital duty, at a time when the atmosphere is heavily loaded with this peculiar effluvium. I have been informed of the circumstance of a pupil in midwifery having remarked, at the period of an epidemic, that several patients successively, upon who he waited during labour, were seized with this disease, and died . . . the young gentleman became so apprehensive that he himself had been the medium of the conveyance, that he resolved not to attend upon any other patient during the prevalence of the epidemic.[24]

Evory Kennedy recalled a similar episode with a foreign student:

I recollect being very much struck with the evidence afforded of this fact [contagion by the 'medical attendant or nurse-tender'] in the case of a most assiduous and indefatigable physician who was sent over by his Government from the North of Europe to study under me at the Lying-in Hospital. He was with me during one of the earlier outbursts of puerperal fever, when it became necessary to partially close the hospital and attend patients at their own homes. This gentleman was not remarkably attentive in exercising that virtue which is said to be second only to Godliness. He never appeared to change linen or woollen habilaments, and absolutely lived in a shaggy pilot coat by night and by day. He was so unceasing in his duties that he attended two patients for every other pupil's one; but the unhappy part of it was that I traced him through his rounds of duty like the pale horse of the Apocalypse, and the fatality attending his steps was such that I was obliged to request him to desist from visiting patients at their homes, when the proportion of cases sensibly diminished.[25]

What seems so remarkable is the difference between home and hospital practice in this respect. Most practitioners in the 1830s and 1840s who practised home midwifery had learnt that they themselves could be the vehicle of contagion. They knew, in theory at any rate, that, if they were called to a midwifery case following an attendance on a case of puerperal fever or erysipelas or a post-mortem examination, they must change their clothes and wash thoroughly. The same rules do not appear to have been followed in lying-in hospitals. There is no evidence in the first half of the nineteenth century that hospital obstetricians washed or changed their clothes after performing a hospital post-mortem examination and before attending a patient on the wards. Indeed, the possibility that hospital epidemics might be in whole or even in part due to the

---

[24] J. C. Douglas, 'On Puerperal Fever', *Dublin Hospital Reports and Communications*, 3 (1822), 141–60, at 145. This interesting paper consists unusually of a series of questions put to Douglas by the Board of Health and his answers to them.

[25] E. Kennedy, 'Zymotic Diseases, as More Especially Illustrated by Puerperal Fever', *Dublin Quarterly Journal of Medical Science*, 47 (1869), 269–307, at 272, 297.

process of contagious transfer by birth attendants was rarely mentioned. It was as if the causes of hospital epidemics were not the same as those outside the hospitals. And they held these views in spite of the fact that the link between puerperal fever and erysipelas (which was one of the components of the theory of contagion) was also recognized in hospitals.

Indeed, as we saw in the previous chapter, some believed that puerperal fever was neither more nor less than erysipelas in lying-in women. Epidemics in the Dublin Lying-in Hospital in 1835–7 and again in 1845 were accompanied by an outbreak of erysipelas in surgical hospitals, and in the 1845 epidemic some of the babies died of erysipelas.[26] Dr Rigby reported that, in one epidemic in the General Lying-in Hospital, the child of every woman who died of puerperal fever 'perished of erysipelas, which ran its course in a few hours'.[27] It was the abundance of such evidence that led Fleetwood Churchill to conclude that it was probable that erysipelas and puerperal fever were, 'as it has been asserted by many, and with great probability, essentially the same disease'.[28]

There were other ideas of relatively minor importance. Dr Collins, Master of the Rotunda, considered, but dismissed the possibility, that puerperal fever was associated with 'long lingering labours'; it was, he said, no more common in long and lingering labours in which intervention had often proved necessary than in short and normal ones. His colleague, Dr Cusack, however, was quick to point out the fallacy of his reasoning. There were 15,084 short labours (95 per cent of the total) and 748 (5 per cent) prolonged labours. Seventy-one cases of puerperal fever in 15,084 short labours 'comes to about 1 in 212' [or 47 per 10,000], while 13 cases in 784 prolonged labours come to '1 in 58' [or 172 per 10,000].[29] Nevertheless, these data show that the high rate of puerperal fever cannot be attributed solely to a high rate of interference in normal labours in such hospitals as the Rotunda. Certainly the risk of developing puerperal fever

---

[26] Churchill, 'An Historical Sketch', in Churchill (ed.), *Essays*.

[27] The evidence of Rigby is quoted in J. Copland, *Dictionary of Practical Medicine* (3 vols.; London, 1858), iii. 507–8, a rich source that also includes the memorable report of M. Dugés in Paris, who said that, during the epidemic of 1819, several cats 'who frequented the wards of the Maternité . . . were attacked by painful distension of the abdomen' and proved at post-mortem to have signs of peritonitis (iii. 505). I have not as yet found any other reports to support this startling observation.

[28] Churchill, 'An Historical Sketch', in Churchill (ed.), *Essays*, 28–36. There were many other references to erysipelas and puerperal fever in hospitals, including R. Yates Ackerley, 'Remarks on the Nature and Treatment of Puerperal Fever', *London Medical Gazette* (1837–8), ii. 462–6; G. B. Clarke, 'Observations on Malignant Puerperal Fever', *London Medical Gazette*, NS 5 (1847), 331–4; C. Sidey, 'Cases of Puerperal Fever', *Edinburgh Medical and Surgical Journal*, 51 (1839), 91–9, R. Storrs, 'Puerperal Fever', *London Medical Gazette* (1845), i. 1087–8; and J. Cross, 'Sketches of the Medical Schools of Paris', *London Medical and Physical Journal*, 34 (1815), 478–87. G. H. Weatherhead, in *An Essay on the Diagnosis between Erysipelas, Phlegmon and Erythema, with an Appendix Touching on the Probable Nature of Puerperal Fever* (London, 1819), was a rare example of an author who did not believe in this linkage. He tried to inoculate himself with erysipelas by abrading his arm and wrapping the abraded area in dressings from a man with erysipelas. The foolhardy experiment failed, in the sense that Weatherhead suffered no symptoms and the author assumed that erysipelas could not be transmitted from one individual to another.

[29] S. Cusack, 'On Puerperal Fever', *Dublin Journal of Medical Science*, 9 (1836), 162–5. The difference is highly significant: $P < 0.001$.

was higher following prolonged labours (about 50 per cent), but such difficult labours were themselves a small proportion of all deliveries (less than 5 per cent), so the majority of cases of puerperal fever (over 95 per cent) followed the far more numerous normal deliveries.[30]

Finally, there was the question of the relationship between town epidemics of puerperal fever and epidemics in hospitals. Opinion was divided. Some saw town epidemics as the source of hospital ones, some believed the link was in the other direction, and some believed there was no connection. If one examines town and hospital epidemics for the period 1770–1850, there is a moderately close correspondence. Thus, the period 1790–1810 was relatively free of town and hospital epidemics. In the next two decades, however, that is 1810–30, there was a large number of both town and hospital epidemics, but from 1830 to 1840, when there was a surge of hospital epidemics, few town epidemics were reported.

Once again, it is interesting to note for future reference that scarlet fever was a deadly disease between about 1795 and 1802, when epidemics of puerperal fever were rare, but scarlet fever became a mild disease between 1802 and 1835, when some of the worst epidemics of puerperal fever occurred. And when scarlet fever once more became deadly after 1835, with high peaks of mortality in 1840 and 1848, there were few reports of town epidemics of puerperal fever and comparatively few hospital epidemics. We will return to scarlet fever in Chapter 12.

---

[30] There were a few lying-in hospitals where a high rate of interference was the rule. For example, Osiander in Göttingen was famous in the early nineteenth century for an exceptionally high rate of forceps deliveries in the lying-in hospital. The reason was that he applied forceps on every possible occasion, even in normal labours, to teach the students (J. F. Oznan, *Histoire médicale, générale et particulière des maladies contagieuses et épizootiques* (Lyons, 1835), and Ulrich Tröhler, *Tracing Emotions, Concepts and Realities in History: The Göttingen Collection of Perinatal Medicine* (Florence, 1993)).

6

Puerperal Fever: Causes and Contagion

In the previous chapters we have dealt mainly with descriptions of puerperal fever and erysipelas, both sporadic and epidemic. Before we come to the central figure of Semmelweis, it will be helpful to discuss the views of mid-nineteenth-century authorities on the nature and causes of puerperal fever and whether or not it merited the description of a contagious disease. I shall do so within the wider context of ideas about other diseases, epidemics, and contagion in general.

Changing Definitions of Fevers

To understand ideas on causation and disease nomenclature, it is important to recognize that, broadly speaking, the classification and definition of fevers were based on symptoms, signs, and external appearances for most of the eighteenth century; on morbid anatomy (post-mortem findings) from the late eighteenth to the late nineteenth centuries; and on specific microbiological causes from the late nineteenth century to the end of the twentieth century.[1] During the nineteenth century, the post-mortem had become the final court of appeal to such an extent that the essence of hospital medicine was the clinico-pathological correlation—that is, the correlation between the diagnosis made by a physician on the basis of clinical observation and examination, and the evidence revealed by the 'opening' of the body. Opening the body was seen as the way to the truth. As Bichat, one of the founders of morbid anatomy, said in a memorable passage:

For twenty years from morning to night, you have taken notes at patients' bedsides on affections of the heart, the lungs, and the gastric viscera, and all is confusion for you in the symptoms which, refusing to yield up their meaning, offer you a succession of incoherent phenomena. Open up a few corpses: you will dissipate at once the darkness that observation alone could not dispel.[2]

---

[1] 'Eighteenth-century medicine was primarily one of symptoms, not lesions, of patients, not their organs' (W. F. Bynum, *Science and the Practice of Medicine in the Nineteenth Century* (Cambridge, 1994), 30).

[2] Quoted in ibid. 33, and by K. Codell Carter, 'The Development of Pasteur's Concept of Disease Causation and the Emergence of Specific Causes in Nineteenth-Century Medicine', *Bulletin of the History of Medicine*, 65 (1991), 528–48, at 543. Marie-François-Xavier Bichat (1771–1802) is described by Garrison as 'the creator of descriptive anatomy' (F. H. Garrison, *An Introduction to the History of Medicine* (4th edn., Philadelphia, 1929), 444–5.

Post-mortem examinations were, of course, carried out in the eighteenth century, but the new emphasis on gross pathology represented a major shift in the way doctors thought about diseases. In the case of puerperal fever it led to such questions as whether it was a disease of the uterus, the peritoneum, the pelvic veins, the lymphatics, or the blood, because all such organs revealed signs of disease in some cases on some occasions. Denman believed puerperal fever was a disease of the uterus. Robert Gooch classified puerperal fever as a form of peritonitis, and he renamed it 'puerperal peritonitis'[3]—a name that appears frequently throughout the nineteenth century. Because signs of disease were found in so many organs, puerperal fever rapidly acquired a host of new names that we discussed in Chapter 1.

The terminological confusion that resulted tended to foster a suspicion that puerperal fever might be not one, but several different diseases. If that was so, did they all belong to the same group of fevers? Was puerperal fever in its various forms an inflammatory or erysipelatous fever, or a low, nervous and, asthenic type of fever? This was not a frivolous or academic question. The answer had a profound bearing on treatment, for bleeding was indicated for inflammatory fevers, but never for low nervous fevers. And if that difficult question could be resolved, another question remained. Was puerperal fever a specific fever, running true to form like measles or smallpox, or was it a fever that arose from, and conversely could give rise to, other diseases such as erysipelas, scarlet fever, typhus, diphtheria, and so forth?

Confusion was worsened by the question of contagion. If it was contagious, it was conspicuously different from other contagious diseases such as smallpox or measles, which were transmitted directly from one patient to another. Puerperal fever, if contagious at all, was transmitted *indirectly* from one patient to another by a doctor or nurse/midwife. That was the crucial difference that separated puerperal fever from other contagious diseases, and partly explains why even the most eminent obstetricians were often deeply divided on the contagiousness of puerperal fever.

Contagionism, Anticontagionism, and Puerperal Fever

Before the work of Gordon of Aberdeen (1795) no one believed puerperal fever was contagious.[4] Denman was initially sceptical, but came round to the view

---

[3] R. Gooch, *An Account of Some of the Most Important Diseases Peculiar to Women* (London, 1831; 2nd edn., 1838).

[4] The only possible exceptions were when Professor Young described an outbreak of puerperal fever in 1773 in Edinburgh Infirmary as 'a local infection' (Alexander Gordon, *A Treatise on the Epidemic Puerperal Fever of Aberdeen* (London, 1795), 55. Also Joseph Clarke, Master of the Dublin Lying-in Hospital, wrote in 1790 that it was 'probable that this [puerperal] fever derived its origin from local contagion' (Joseph Clarke, 'Observations on the Puerperal Fever etc.', *Edinburgh Medical Commentaries*, 15 (1790), repr. in Fleetwood Churchill (ed.), *Essays on the Puerperal Fever and Other Diseases Peculiar to Women* (London, 1849), 351–62, at 353. Both remarks were very tentative, but both pre-date Gordon's description of contagion.

that it was sometimes contagious. In 1833 Robert Lee of London wrote a review of past and current opinion.[5] Quoting Tonnellé and Dugés of Paris, he noted that the French were totally against the idea of contagion, and for the most part remained sceptical until well into the second half of the century. Indeed, the concept of puerperal fever as a contagious disease found so little support on the Continent in the first half of the nineteenth century that it was often described on the Continent as the English theory. Lee himself was inclined to agree with the French, but he kept an open mind on the subject.[6] Hey of Leeds, as we saw in Chapter 4, thought that puerperal fever was contagious only to a 'very inferior degree'. Armstrong of Sunderland, however, was sure it was often, if not always, a contagious disease, while Roberton of Manchester was convinced it could be contagious on some occasions, but not on others (see Chapter 4).

Clearly, ideas on the contagiousness of puerperal fever were influenced by ideas on contagion in other diseases, and it so happens that there was a well-known and prolonged debate between the contagionists and the anticontagionists in the first half of the nineteenth century, which has attracted the attention of many historians.[7] Few historians, however, have taken any interest in puerperal fever. At first sight, this omission is curious, for it raises the obvious question of how much this famous debate on contagionism and anticontagionism (which I will call the 'main debate') affected, and how much it was affected by, the arguments about the contagiousness of puerperal fever? The quick answer is very little, and the reason is simple.

The main debate on contagion was concerned not with infectious ('zymotic') diseases as a whole, and least of all with puerperal fever, but rather with a limited number of diseases of particular importance to the public health—namely, cholera, typhus, and especially in the USA yellow fever.[8] From the modern point of view it is tempting to see the contagionists as the pioneers, the men of vision, because they were proved right in the end. We might, therefore, assume that the anticontagionists were the enemies of progress, clinging desperately to outdated views. This is virtually the exact opposite of how the two opposing camps were seen at the time, because contagion was far from being a new concept. It was, in fact, so ancient—dating back as it did to the plague and the idea of

[5] R. Lee, *Researches on the Pathology and Treatment of Some of the Most Important Diseases of Women* (London, 1833). [6] Ibid. 92.

[7] It would be inappropriate to try to survey all the major publications on this subject. Those which I have found most useful are E. H. Ackernecht, 'Anticontagionism between 1821 and 1867', *Bulletin of the History of Medicine*, 22 (1948), 562–93; M. Pelling, *Cholera, Fever and English Medicine* (Oxford, 1978), and 'Contagion/Germ Theory/Specificity', in W. F. Bynum and Roy Porter (eds.), *Companion Encyclopedia of the History of Medicine* (London, 1993), i. 309–34; J. M. Eyler, *Victorian Social Medicine: The Ideas and Methods of William Farr* (Baltimore, 1979); C. Rosenberg, *Explaining Epidemics and Other Studies in the History of Medicine* (Cambridge, 1992), ch. 14, 293–304; and C. Hamlin, 'Predisposing Causes and Public Health in Early Nineteenth-Century Medical Thought', *Social History of Medicine*, 5/1 (1992), 43–70.

[8] Rosenberg feels that the debate was more polarized earlier in the nineteenth century, more confrontational in regard to yellow fever than to cholera, and more marked in cholera than in typhus (Rosenberg, *Explaining Epidemics*, 299 n. 10).

quarantine—that it was looking distinctly threadbare by the mid-nineteenth century.

Before the ultimate triumph of the contagionists at the end of the century, it was anticontagionism that 'reached its highest peak of elaboration, acceptance, and scientific respectability' in the first half of the nineteenth century.[9] The anticontagionists were the optimists, the forward-looking pioneers. They believed that something could be done by looking for the causes, prevention, and cure of epidemics in social and political terms, thereby laying the groundwork for nineteenth-century public health. Conversely, the contagionists have been described as the pessimists whose only remedy for epidemics was isolation and quarantine, measures that involved government control, and interference with trade and with the liberty of the individual, and thus with the political and economic affairs of a country.[10] In an era of *laissez-faire*, contagionism went against the grain of public and private prosperity and the policies of political parties.

Now consider puerperal fever. Questions of isolation, quarantine, loss of liberty, and interference with trade were totally irrelevant to a disease confined to lying-in women. Likewise, considerations of public health, hygiene, and social policies (the anticontagionist issues) had no apparent relevance to puerperal fever. In the main debate, neither side could call on the evidence of puerperal fever to support their stance. And there was more to it than that. In the case of puerperal fever it was the contagionists who were often seen as the radical and forward-thinking men, because they could at least suggest preventive measures such as changing clothes and washing themselves after attending a septic case. But the anticontagionists in the field of puerperal fever had nothing to offer except cleaning out drains and worrying about miasmas.

Thus the two debates—the main debate and the one over the contagiousness of puerperal fever—were like two arguments taking place on the opposite sides of a wall. Each side could hear the other indistinctly, but the two never met, never shared ideas. Thus, what appears to be a paradox—that the gradual acceptance of the contagiousness of puerperal fever occurred at the very time when the main contagion/anticontagion debate was swinging towards the anticontagionist position—was no paradox at all. There was no conflict. A man could believe puerperal fever was contagious while holding ferociously anticontagionist views in the main debate (or vice versa) without being in the least inconsistent.

Contagions, Infections, and Miasmas

Further, the arguments about contagion were much more complicated than appears at first sight. There was never an iron curtain between the anticonta-

---

[9] Ackerknecht, 'Anticontagionism', 565.

[10] J. C. Riley, *The Eighteenth Century Campaign to Avoid Disease* (London, 1987), quoted in Hamlin, 'Predisposing Causes and Public Health'.

gionists and their opponents. In the mid-nineteenth century, even the most rabid anticontagionist accepted that certain diseases such as syphilis, gonorrhea, smallpox, measles, and 'the itch' were contagious. Likewise, Hamlin has shown that, although miasmatic theory has been seen as the foundation of the anti-contagionist position, and although miasmatic theory and contagion are usually presented as opposite poles, the 'contagionist and anticontagionist miasmatic explanations were neither mutually exclusive nor essentially in opposition'.[11] Miasms (or miasmas) were, in Hamlin's words, un-isolatable and (according to some) inodorous materials in the air emanating from vegetable decomposition. They differed, on the one hand, from vitiated air lacking some essential ingredient such as oxygen, and, on the other (although practitioners often appeared to forget it), bad smells. Bad smells and miasmas were not the same thing.[12] The 'poison' or 'miasma' of a fever could be produced by putrefaction, but transmitted by contagion. This is certainly a view that would have appealed to Alexander Gordon, who thought that the epidemic of puerperal fever in Aberdeen was both miasmatic and contagious, providing an example of what Hamlin calls 'the miasm of contagion, or of contagion produced by miasm'.[13]

An example of further potential confusion is the use of the word 'virus' in the early nineteenth century. 'Virus' did not, of course, mean what it means at the end of the twentieth century—an infectious micro-organism, smaller than a bacterium, and usually beyond the resolution of the light microscope. It indicated, vaguely rather than precisely, the agent or agents by which fevers could occur, as when in 1846 Dr Peddie of Edinburgh suggested that puerperal fever was due to a 'specific virus of an animal nature' that frequently originated from erysipelatous inflammations.[14] For 'virus' we could substitute the word 'poison', which is all that the word 'virus' means in Latin. In the *Edinburgh Medical and Physical Dictionary*, published in 1807, 'Virus' is defined as 'a synonyme [*sic*] of poison or contagion'. Miasma is defined as 'a particle of poison in a volatile state, borne on the wings of the atmosphere, and capable of attaching itself to an animal body so as to produce disease . . . as in the case of CONTAGION'. Under 'Contagion' the entry reads 'The same as *Effluvia, Miasma, Virus, or Lues*' (emphasis in original).[15]

Parsons has explored this muddled area as far as it affected puerperal fever and the question of contagion in the USA between 1840 and 1860.[16] She suggests that the anticontagionists were not a homogeneous group. There were the 'iatro-anticontagionists', who believed that, where puerperal fever was transmitted by a doctor to a lying-in woman from a case of erysipelas, it must be by miasmatic *infection*, not contagion. The others were the 'environmental-anticontagionists', who, holding that puerperal fever was never transmitted,

---

[11] Hamlin, 'Predisposing Causes and Public Health', 47.   [12] Ibid. 55.   [13] Ibid. 48.
[14] Dr Peddie, 'On the Contagiousness of Puerperal Fever', *London Medical Gazette* (1846), ii. 835–7.
[15] R. Morris and J. Kendrick, *Edinburgh Medical and Physical Dictionary* (2 vols.; Edinburgh, 1807).
[16] G. P. Parsons, 'Puerperal Fever, Anticontagionists, and Miasmatic Infection, 1840–1860: Toward a New History of Puerperal Fever in America', *Journal of the History of Medicine*, 52 (1997), 424–52.

thereby absolved doctors (and midwives) from ever transmitting puerperal fever; this group preferred to 'locate the pathogen in the environment to which women were exposed'.[17]

Parsons stresses that physicians distinguished between 'infection' and 'contagion'. The words do, of course, imply an obvious difference: contagion being the transmission of disease between people by direct physicial contact (because *tangio* means touch), while infection was transmission through the air. Parsons, however, asserts that in the period 1840–60 it was believed that one of the key features of contagious disease was that it always 'bred true' in the sense that smallpox caused smallpox and nothing else. If puerperal fever was always contagious, how could there be sporadic cases, and how could it apparently arise from contact with a separate disease, erysipelas? An infection, he says, need not 'breed true' and could arise in isolation because a 'confluence of personal and environmental factors had compromised the victim's resistance to infection'. When the first or solitary case had occurred, however, the disease could spread to a healthy woman by contagion.[18]

Certainly both words were used, but careful distinctions between infections and contagions were, I believe, rarely important. Most medical writers were happy to use 'contagions' to cover 'infections' as well. Dr Samuel Kneeland of Boston wrote about this very issue with clarity in 1846.

Very nice distinctions are to be found in various authors between contagion and infection, which need not be insisted on in treating of an affection where both probably operate; in fact, contagion is used by many as including infection. Dr Elliotson remarks that 'the word "contagious" is used in the same way as the term "horse"'. The latter is used to include both a horse and a mare; but it is frequently applied to the male only; and so these diseases are all continually spoken of as contagious; but the word is also employed in a limited sense to signify those diseases which are communicated by actual contact; or by touching something which the patient has touched; or something which has palpably proceeded from him . . . Some diseases are communicable by contagion alone; others by infection alone; others by both contagion and infection: as instances of the three may be mentioned syphilis, hooping cough, and smallpox—in the latter case we would place puerperal fever.[19]

We have seen more than enough of the variety of opinions on the contagiousness of puerperal fever, but it is notable that, whatever views they held, the majority of medical men in the 1840s who were involved in the practice of midwifery knew it was sensible to deflect criticism by following certain well-known rules such as changing clothes and washing thoroughly if called to a midwifery case after attending a case of puerperal fever or erysipelas. That was

[17] G. P. Parsons, 'Puerperal Fever, Anticontagionists, and Miasmatic Infection, 1840–1860: Toward a New History of Puerperal Fever in America', *Journal of the History of Medicine*, 52 (1997), 424–52.

[18] Ibid. 434.

[19] S. Kneeland, 'On the Contagiousness of Puerperal Fever', *American Journal of the Medical Sciences*, 11 (1846), 45–63, at 47. This is an interesting, well-written paper, which appeared three years after Oliver Wendell Holmes's famous paper, on which it was closely modelled.

what most teachers told their students, as Watson did in 1850, when he issued a grim warning: 'The hand which is relied upon for succor in the painful and perilous hour of childbirth . . . may literally become the innocent cause of [the mother's] destruction; innocent no longer, however, if, after warning and knowledge of the risk, suitable means are not used to avert a catastrophe so shocking.'[20]

Kneeland produced a list of nine propositions about puerperal fever, which I have paraphrased as follows:

1. From the confinement of cases to the practice of single physicians and nurses in populous cities; from the fatal results attending post-mortem examinations; from its ravages in hospitals it is definite that puerperal fever is contagious. It may have other means of propagation depending on the atmosphere, but contagion is proved by the way it is conveyed by practitioners.
2. Puerperal fever can be conveyed not only from other cases of the disease, but also from 'effluvia' arising from the dead, the sick, hospitals, clothes, bedding, and so on.
3. Epidemics are the *effects* not the *causes* of contagion.
4. Although poverty and misery seem to predispose to it, communication of puerperal fever is none the less fatal to the higher classes.
5. A mild case may communicate a severe disease, and vice versa.
6. Immunity provides nothing against contagion. (I think this means that a woman could suffer two or more attacks of puerperal fever.)
7. It is contagious at its commencement and after death.
8. Physicians should not make, nor be present at, an autopsy, but if they attend an autopsy they should wash and change their clothes before attending a woman in labour. They should do the same after attending a case of puerperal fever; and people who have washed the clothes or bedding soiled by a case of puerperal fever 'should not approach, much less nurse, a woman after a delivery'.
9. When the disease is prevalent, contact with a physician who has attended cases of puerperal fever should be avoided, and 'a strict attention to ventilation, cleanliness, quiet, proper food &c., are the dictates of a reasonable fear'.[21]

Explaining Epidemics of Puerperal Fever

How can we fit these ideas about epidemic puerperal fever into the ideas about epidemics in general in the mid-nineteenth century, where the main emphasis

---

[20] T. Watson, *Lectures on the Principles and Practice of Physic* (London, 1843; 4th edn., 1857), ii, Lecture LXV, 384. Watson was firmly entrenched in the contagionist camp, especially as far as typhus was concerned.   [21] Kneeland, 'On the Contagiousness of Puerperal Fever', 62–3.

was on the relative importance of predisposing causes, on the one hand, and exciting causes in the form of some contagion, specific poison, or miasm, on the other.

Predisposing causes included exposure to cold, breathing vitiated air, over-crowding, mental depression, malnutrition or its opposite (gluttony), and so on. There were, broadly, two views on the relative importance of predisposing and exciting causes. According to one view, predisposing causes could be sufficient *per se* to produce a fever or epidemic. According to a later view, associated espe-cially with Southwood Smith, the exciting cause was the essential cause.[22]

Southwood Smith held that a predisposing cause could never on its own produce a fever or epidemic. It could only modify the form taken by the dis-ease in different individuals. An exciting cause, on the other hand, would affect anyone exposed to it. His ideas predated bacteriology, and it is important to recognize that he was not thinking in modern terms of specific 'poisons' related to specific diseases. Indeed, the characteristic feature of all ideas on the cause of fevers was their non-specificity. Nevertheless the emphasis on exciting causes was an important step towards the radical change in concepts of causa-tion that took place during the second half of the nineteenth century and was associated with the discoveries of bacteriology. To jump ahead, the essence of the change at the end of the century was the recognition of specific, single, and necessary causes as opposed to non-specific, multiple, and unrelated causes. The specific causes—micro-organisms—became the sole means of identifying, separating, and naming fevers.

Configuration, Contamination, and Predisposition

In his essay 'Explaining Epidemics', Rosenberg provides a useful framework of ideas.[23] 'Before physicians had any knowledge of specific infectious agents,' he writes, 'medical explanations of epidemic disease tended to be holistic and inclusive . . . a disturbance in a "normal" . . . arrangement of climate, environ-ment, and communal life'. This, which he calls the *configuration* view, lived in 'relatively peaceful, if not always logical coexistence' with what he calls the *contamination* view. The most obvious component of contamination was person-to-person contagion by the transmission of some morbid material from one individual to another; but it also included 'any event that might subvert a health-maintaining configuration'. A third element is *predisposition*, which was simply the attempt to explain why some succumb to epidemics while others escape. 'In most historical instances, of course, all three elements—configurational, contamination, and predisposition—were brought to bear in creating culturally appropriate explanatory frameworks'. But, he adds later, 'It

---

[22] Hamlin, 'Predisposing Causes and Public Health', 43–70. I can give only a summary version of a long and complex debate, which is fully described by Hamlin in his paper.

[23] Rosenberg, *Explaining Epidemics*, 293–304.

is fair to say that the emphasis in epidemiological thought from the eighteenth through the mid-nineteenth century was on configurational—that is, environmental, additive and aggregate—models of health and disease.'[24]

For puerperal fever in the first half of the nineteenth century, the *configuration* view keeps appearing in remarks about epidemic influence (which appeared to be confirmed by the seasonal tendency of the disease) and the believed importance of telluric influence, which we might translate as environmental factors.[25] The contamination element was also prominent in hospital epidemics, not just in the sense of contagion, but rather in Rosenberg's sense of 'any event that might subvert a health-maintaining configuration' such as overcrowding and the way the fabric of the hospitals was believed to be soaked with and contaminated by noxious influences. Predisposition was also mentioned frequently as a factor in puerperal fever.

It was thoughts like these that governed the plans on which the Paris Maternité, mentioned in the previous chapter, was built. It was erected on high, open, and supposedly healthy ground for configurational reasons, and provided with well-ventilated, spacious, and separate rooms for patients, because of the danger of contamination from the fabric of the hospital. As we have seen, the French, who spurned the idea of contagion, thought it would be the healthiest lying-in hospital in Europe, but its puerperal mortality was as high as that in any other European maternity hospital.

In Britain and the USA during the mid-nineteenth century the emphasis, as far as puerperal fever was concerned, on the three factors—environment, contagion, and predisposition—was changing. There seems to have been a tendency between 1800 and 1850 to play down the importance of environmental factors, especially epidemic influence. The importance attached to predisposition, however, was increasing and would continue to occupy an important place right up to and beyond the discovery of the role of bacteria. The role of contagion (in the broad sense of strict contagion and infection) was certainly becoming more prominent but never to the exclusion of the other factors. We will trace these intellectual changes in Chapter 8.

Clarity and Confusion

What we are trying to do in discussions such as this is to get under the skin (or into the minds) of past practitioners as they struggled to make sense of the vagaries of fevers and epidemics. Most historians do so by constructing models or frameworks. Rosenberg's now famous essay 'Explaining Epidemics'

---

[24] Ibid. 295–8.

[25] 'Telluric', which means 'of the soil', was used in the broad sense of the place, the district, and the environment, and was based on the idea that there were healthy or salubrious and unhealthy or insalubrious areas. It was an idea that received support from nineteenth-century observations of differentials in morbidity and mortality in rural and industrial areas.

is not, of course, an explanation of epidemics in the light of modern knowledge, but an attempt to explain how medical practitioners in any given period
tried to explain epidemics in the light of contemporary knowledge and beliefs.
One of the pitfalls of constructing such historical models is the inevitable
temptation to make them internally consistent and all-embracing. We assume
that practitioners in, say, the 1840s possessed a clear and agreed system of
beliefs that it is our job as historians to interpret and understand. One has only
to spell out such an assumption to see that it leaves no room for plain, ordinary, muddle and confusion, which, I strongly suspect, was, in many instances,
the prevailing state of mind.

Consider what it must have been like in New England during the epidemic
of erysipelas and puerperal fever in the 1840s described in Chapter 4. Experienced country physicians would have been familiar with sporadic cases of both
diseases and would have had no difficulty in accommodating such cases within
their limited knowledge and framework of thought about disease. When the
epidemic arrived, however, they suddenly found themselves in the middle of
a situation where numerous patients were suddenly subjected to a terrible
disease, agonizing pain, and horrendous mortality. Nothing remotely like it
had occurred within living memory. They would have had no explanation, no
guidance from past experience, no concepts of germs or anything else to guide
them. And it cannot have made them feel any better to know that they themselves were at risk.

Physicians such as Oliver Wendell Holmes and Samuel Kneeland—educated
men with access to what were clearly excellent libraries in cities such as Boston
and Philadelphia—may have been able to construct a framework of understanding that included such concepts as the influence of the environment and
weather, the role of contagion, and the importance of predisposition. But they
were a small minority. The average country doctor, who would have had little
access to books or medical journals, must have been confused when it came to
explaining epidemics.

In 1845 J. Waddy, Physician to the Birmingham (England) Lying-in Infirmary, seeing the muddle that surrounded puerperal fever, tried to reconcile
conflicting views. He concluded there was not one, but many forms of puerperal fever, the sporadic, the epidemic, the inflammatory, the typhoid, the
gastrobilious. If anything, his ideas simply added to the prevailing confusion.
But he made one interesting suggestion, which might, in view of much later
knowledge of the role of the carriers of the streptococcus, be described as a
lucky guess. When dealing with the problem of doctors and nurses who had
a series of cases in their practice, he suggested that healthy birth-attendants
might carry something in the blood which they exhaled through their breath
and which infected the patient with puerperal fever. It was not, however, an
idea that caught on.[26]

[26] J. Waddy, 'Puerperal Fever', *Lancet* (1845), i. 671–5; (1845), ii. 531–2, 671–2; (1846), i. 38–9, 697–700.

What I have tried to do in this chapter is explain the evolution of ideas on the nature of fevers and epidemics in general and of puerperal fever in particular before we come to Semmelweis. What was lacking most of all in the pre-Semmelweis era was an explanation of the *mechanism* of contagion. For this reason, I want to introduce at this point a little-known paper by James Young Simpson. The paper was published in 1850. Semmelweis's observations were made in 1847. Simpson, however, had formulated his ideas over a period of more than ten years and knew nothing about Semmelweis when he wrote his paper, putting forward ideas that were remarkably similar to those of Semmelweis. Likewise, Semmelweis was unaware of Simpson's views until long after he had formulated his theories. New ideas in medicine seldom come completely out of the blue. They arise with a certain inevitability out of the slow accumulation of knowledge. It is, therefore, a banal commonplace that two or more doctors and scientists often make independent but simultaneous announcements of certain theories or discoveries. This is a case in point.

James Young Simpson and Puerperal Fever

Simpson, who is famous for having introduced chloroform anaesthesia for childbirth, took a keen interest in puerperal fever. In 1850 he summarized his views in a paper on the analogy between surgical fever and puerperal fever.[27] His main conclusions were as follows:

I shall content myself with observing here (what I have taught for the last ten years) that there exists, I believe, on record, a series of facts amply sufficient to prove this at least, that patients during labour have been and may be locally inoculated with a materies morbi capable of exciting puerperal fever; that this materies morbi is liable to be inoculated into the dilated and abraded lining membrane of the maternal passages during delivery, *by the fingers of the attendant*; that thus in transferring it from one patient to another, *the fingers of the attendant act, as it were, like the ivory points formerly used by some of the early vaccinators*; that the materies morbi most capable of being thus inoculated and generating the disease in a new individual seems to be the inflammatory products effected upon the serous or mucous membranes of females who are suffering under puerperal fever, or who have died from it; and lastly, that other inflammatory effusions, when in the same way transferred and inoculated into the puerperal female, appear to have sometimes the same effect, such as the effusions into tissues, that are the seat of an asthenic, erysipelatous, or gangrenous type of inflammation. (emphasis added)[28]

Simpson was, I believe, the first (in Britain at any rate) to suggest that puerperal fever was transmitted to the patient by the fingers of the birth attendant, and to underline that view by the memorable analogy of the ivory points used

---

[27] James Young Simpson, 'Some Notes on the Analogy between Puerperal Fever and Surgical Fever', *Monthly Journal of Medical Science* (Nov. 1850), 414–29.   [28] Ibid. 428.

in vaccination. He had identified the *mechanism* of contagion. A year later he repeated his view by saying that the material carried by nurses and doctors from one subject to another 'was an inflammatory secretion just as the inoculable matter of small-pox, cowpox, syphilis etc. was an inflammatory secretion'.[29] By this time, two words were becoming commonplace—septicaemia and pyaemia. Septicaemia was the presence of a toxin or poison in the blood (hence the still common phrase, 'blood-poisoning'). Pyaemia was pus in the blood, which was liable to be carried by the circulation to various parts of the body and set up septic foci or abscesses.

Simpson explained the link between puerperal fever and erysipelas in terms of the analogy between puerperal and surgical fever. In both there was a 'solution of continuity', an abrasion or loss of the surface or lining of an organ. The surface might be a surgical incision, a wound in the skin (often so small as to be virtually invisible), or the raw surface of the uterus after childbirth. In all instances, septicaemia could result from the entry of the infection into the blood through the exposed mouths of veins and arteries:

In the surgical patient, we have a wound or solution of continuity of the external part of the body, made by the knife of the surgeon; this wound has, opening upon its free surface, the mouths of numerous arteries and veins . . . In the puerperal patient, we have a wound or solution of continuity on the whole internal surface of the womb made by the separation of the placenta, and the exfoliation of the decidua or mucous membrane of the uterus; this wound has, opening upon its free surface, and specially at the former site of the placenta, the mouths of numerous arteries and veins . . .[30]

The mechanism was clear. Puerperal fever, like surgical fever, was caused by the introduction of a 'materies morbi' in the form of inflammatory effusions. Simpson cited the case of a surgeon who had a series of cases of puerperal fever while holding a surgical post at a hospital:

A gentleman, who was formerly surgeon to a very large hospital, and also an extensive practitioner in midwifery, informs me that during the period of his superintendence of the hospital, when consequently often touching the discharges from all kinds of wounds and breaches of surface, puerperal fever was, from time to time, common in his private obstetric practice—and at the same period he saw many of his surgical patients die with similar symptoms. Since giving up the surgical charge of the hospital, the occurrence of puerperal fever has ceased in his private practice.[31]

Simpson was cautious to this extent. He did not claim that all cases of puerperal fever were contagious; only that many were the result of contagion, and as far as these were concerned he provided the first clear description of the mechanism of contagion. Inflammatory exudate was introduced into the genital

[29] James Young Simpson, 'Discussion of Arneth's Paper Read to the Edinburgh Medico-Chirurgical Society, April 16, 1851', *Monthly Journal of Medical Science*, 13 (1851), 72–80, at 75.   [30] Ibid.
[31] J. Y. Simpson, 'The Analogy between Puerperal Fever and Surgical Fever', *Monthly Journal of Medical Science* (Nov. 1850), 414–29, at 429.

tract on the fingers of attendants. Septicaemic puerperal fever resulted from the exudate entering the open mouths of the blood vessels on the raw internal surface of the post-partum womb. These were the views of Simpson at the very time that Semmelweis was independently formulating closely similar views in Vienna.

7

Semmelweis

For many people, the history of puerperal or childbed fever is virtually synonymous with Ignaz Philipp Semmelweis (1818–65), probably the most famous figure in the history of obstetrics.[1] His treatise, *Etiology, Concept, and Prophylaxis of Childbed Fever* (1860–1), has been described as one of the greatest medical treatises of the nineteenth century. It is commonly believed that he was the first to state that puerperal fever is contagious and to introduce a way of preventing the disease, thereby abolishing, or at least greatly reducing, the mortality rate from puerperal fever. He is often described as a misunderstood martyr, driven insane by the united, stupid, and implacable opposition of his contemporaries, who refused to accept or implement his doctrines. This picture of Semmelweis began to be constructed some twenty-five years after his death, and in a short time he was glamorized and presented as genius and hero. In fact, many of the above attributions turn out to be untrue, and the real story of Semmelweis is much more interesting than the traditional hagiographic version.

Semmelweis Arrives in Vienna

Semmelweis, the son of a well-to-do grocer, was born in Taban (now part of Budapest) in 1818. Initially he intended to study law but changed to medicine, receiving his doctorate and degree of Master of Midwifery in the University of Vienna in 1844. A brief chronology of his life and work is shown in the appendix to this chapter. In February 1846 he was appointed as an assistant in the lying-in hospital that was part of the Vienna Allgemeines Krankenhaus (the Vienna General Hospital).

---

[1] Amongst the main sources for this account of the life and work of Semmelweis are, Sir William Sinclair, *Semmelweis, his Life and his Doctrine* (Manchester, 1909); I. P. Semmelweis, 'The Etiology, the Concept and the Prophylaxis of Childbed Fever', trans. with an introduction by F. P. Murphy, *Medical Classics*, 5/5 (1941), 339–478, 481–589, 591–715, 719–73; F. P. Murphy, 'Ignaz Philipp Semmelweis: An Annotated Biobibliography', *Bulletin of the History of Medicine*, 20 (1946), 653–707; I. P. Semmelweis, *The Etiology, Concept, and Prophylaxis of Childbed Fever*, trans. and ed. with an introduction by K. Codell Carter (Wisconsin, 1983); Iván Kápolnai, 'An Overview of University Education in Obstetrics and Gynaecology in Hungary', in Zoltan Papp, (ed.), *Past and Present of the First Department of Obstetrics and Gynaecology of Semmelweis University Medical School* (Ignaz Semmelweis Foundation; Budapest, 1996), 11–16.

At the time Semmelweis was appointed, this was the largest lying-in hospital in the world. In the 1850s there were about 7,000 deliveries a year compared (in round figures) with 3,000 in the largest lying-in hospital in Paris and about 2,000 each in the Prague and the Moscow maternity hospitals and in the largest lying-in hospital in the UK, the Rotunda in Dublin. In the lying-in hospitals in London, Edinburgh, Stockholm, and Boston, Massachusetts, the annual number of deliveries was only about 200–300, and about 500 in the New York Lying-in Hospital.[2] With the possible exception of the Rotunda in Dublin, no lying-in hospital had as high a reputation as Vienna for teaching obstetrics, not only to Viennese medical students, but also to 'foreigners [who] come to Vienna in order to complete a medical education already obtained in other universities'.[3]

The Vienna Lying-in Hospital was a part of the General Hospital from the time it was opened in 1784. The maternity wards soon became so overcrowded that separate wards were built in 1833. From then onwards the lying-in hospital was divided into two clinics, the first and the second clinics.[4] Patients were admitted to the first and second clinic on alternate days. The arrangements and facilities were identical in the two clinics and male and female students were taught in both clinics until 1839.[5] From 1839, however, it was decided to allocate the teaching of male medical students and visiting doctors to the first clinic and the training of female midwives to the second. The consequences of this change were described by Arneth, a colleague of Semmelweis, as follows:

Medical students were, almost without exception, in the daily practice of assisting at autopsies, of which eight or ten took place in our large hospital almost every day. The dissections were sometimes executed by the students, or they handled at least the pathological preparations, and examined them carefully. Moreover, the assistant used to lecture on the obstetrical operations. These were performed on dead bodies, and, of course, sometimes repeatedly. Now, after such investigations and such practice, it was not rare to see the students going immediately to the wards of the lying-in hospital, and examining the pregnant and parturient women. It is scarcely necessary to state, that the pupils of the other [second] clinic, being midwives, did not take any share in the occupations just alluded to; nay, even the assistant of that clinic had comparatively seldom to deal with post-mortem examinations, as it was not a part of his duty to give instructions to the midwives in pathology or operative midwifery.[6]

All that needs to be added is that the male students neither washed their hands nor changed their clothes when they passed from the post-mortem room to the

---

[2] Leon Le Fort, *Des maternités: Études sur les maternités et les institutions charitables d'accouchement à domicile dans les principaux états de l'Europe* (Paris, 1866), 14–33.

[3] Semmelweis, 'Etiology', ed. Murphy, 407.

[4] There was also a small private clinic for paying patients, which delivered on average around 200 patients a year. In the ten years 1839–48 there were 2,839 births and 72 deaths, a fatality rate of 2.5%, roughly the same as the mortality in the second (midwives) clinic, which we describe below (ibid. 446).

[5] F. H. Arneth, 'Evidence of Puerperal Fever Depending upon the Contagious Inoculation of Morbid Matter', *Monthly Journal of Medical Science*, 12 (1851), 505–11, at 506. This paper was read before the Edinburgh Medico-Chirurgical Society on 16 April 1851. Arneth (1818–1907) was a colleague and supporter of Semmelweis.   [6] Ibid. 507–8.

wards of the first clinic, where they carried out repeated vaginal examinations of women in labour. On average, each maternity case in the first clinic was submitted to five vaginal examinations for the purpose of teaching medical students.[7]

The Two Clinics

As soon as the two clinics were separated, certain features became evident. Between 1833 and 1839 the mortality rate had been much the same in the two clinics. After 1839, when the first clinic was reserved for male students and the second for female, the mortality became much worse in the first clinic compared with the second. This can be seen in Tables 7.1–7.4. One can see that, before the separation of male and female students, there was little to choose between the maternal mortality rates in the two clinics. After the separation in 1840, however, the mortality rate was consistently higher in the first clinic and the difference was very large indeed. This was the cause of much concern. Why should women delivered by students and doctors, who were supposed to be better educated and more skilful, suffer a much higher mortality than women delivered by midwives?

There were other differences between the clinics that, before the observations of Semmelweis, seemed to defy explanation. In the first clinic the patients often became sick in rows, while in the second clinic the cases were scattered through the ward. As Semmelweis was to remark later, 'For the purposes of instruction, all the parturients, as they lay alongside one another, were examined along the rows . . .'.[8] Further, the mortality of women in premature labour was exceptionally low. It was noted that women in premature labour were never examined because 'the first requirement in premature births is to delay the birth if possible'.[9]

Another important observation was the very low mortality rate of the 'street-births' (*Gassengeburten*) who were admitted to the first clinic after delivery. They rarely developed puerperal fever. But why were they admitted at all when they had already given birth? The reason was usually simple. Women who were admitted to the Vienna Lying-in Hospital could arrange to have unwanted babies placed in the Foundling Hospital across the street, where they would be cared for by the state.[10] Well-to-do women with illegitimate pregnancies could also be admitted, but to the private ward of the Lying-in Hospital, where their anonymity would be preserved and their infants sent to the Foundling Hospital. Similar arrangements were made in some of the lying-in hospitals of

[7] F. H. Arneth, 'Evidence of Puerperal Fever Depending upon the Contagious Inoculation of Morbid Matter', *Monthly Journal of Medical Science*, 12 (1851), 508.

[8] Semmelweis, 'Etiology', ed. Murphy, 369, and P. M. Dawson, 'Semmelweis, an Interpretation', *Annals of Medical History*, 6 (1924), 258–79.   [9] Semmelweis, *Etiology*, ed. Carter, 101.

[10] Mothers who took advantage of this arrangement, however, were required to act as wet-nurses to the abandoned infants (ibid.; Sinclair, *Semmelweis*, 42–6).

other countries.[11] Some of the 'street-births' were genuine precipitate births. Others were women who wanted to part with their babies secretly, and therefore arranged to be delivered at home by a midwife and taken quickly by coach to the hospital, claiming they had given birth *en route*. They thereby avoided intrusive vaginal examinations and the consequent humiliation and danger.[12]

Semmelweis made another significant observation. From the opening of the Lying-in Hospital in 1784 until 1823, 'Vienna did without pathological studies'; in other words, no post-mortem examinations were carried out.[13] Although this was the period when, throughout Europe, morbid pathology came into fashion, the director of the Vienna Lying-in Hospital from 1789, Lucas Böer, refused to make use of the cadaver for teaching, although he was pressured to do so, because he foresaw the dangers of infection.

Lucas Böer's successor, Klein, took a different view when appointed director in 1823. He introduced the routine of teaching on post-mortem material as described above. The mortality rate in the hospital promptly rose, as one can see in Table 7.1. Before 1823 the average annual level of maternal mortality since the hospital had opened was in the region of 125 per 10,000 births. After 1823 it rose to about 500 per 10,000 births. This seemed to Semmelweis to be further evidence of a connection between puerperal fever and post-mortem examinations.

Before Semmelweis was appointed, however, the rise in mortality was investigated in 1846 by a commission of inquiry. Various explanations were offered. It was said the bedlinen was not washed with sufficient care, that the wards were unfavourably situated; that there were faults in the drains, that the outbreaks of puerperal fever were due to epidemic influences and miasmas, and so forth. None was convincing. In 1846 the commission suggested that the high mortality in the first clinic might be due to too many medical students carrying out too many examinations, and the number of foreign students was drastically reduced. At first it seemed that mortality was falling. But the mortality rate rose again in the early months of 1847, showing that 'the real cause of the fact occupying our attention had not then been discovered'.[14]

This was the state of affairs when Semmelweis was appointed assistant to the first clinic in July 1846. He was deeply shocked by the terrible mortality and determined to discover the cause. The initial clue came from the accidental death of one of the medical staff, Professor Kolletschka, a forensic pathologist and pupil of Rokitansky, who died of blood poisoning following an accidental injury during an autopsy. The post-mortem examination of Kolletschka's body showed pathological lesions that Semmelweis recognized as similar to those found in women who had died of childbed fever.[15]

---

[11] I. Loudon, *Death in Childbirth: An International Study of Maternal Care and Maternal Mortality 1800–1950* (Oxford, 1992), 429.   [12] Semmelweis, 'Etiology', ed. Murphy, 435.
[13] Ibid.   [14] Arneth, 'Evidence of Puerperal Fever', 507.
[15] Semmelweis was not present at the post-mortem. He was on a brief holiday in Venice visiting art galleries and heard of Kolletschka's death and the post-mortem findings only on his return.

This observation was the basis of Semmelweis's core hypothesis. 'Suppose', he said, 'cadaverous particles adhering to the hands cause the same disease among maternity patients that cadaverous particles adhering to the knife caused in Kolletschka.' (The use of the word 'cadaverous' would, as we will see, turn out to be very important, and we should note that another phrase he used meaning exactly the same as 'cadaverous particles' was 'morbid matter'.) This hypothesis could explain not only the high mortality of the first clinic but also the odd features mentioned above, such as the relative immunity of premature births and the street-births—the two groups of patients who were not subjected to vaginal examinations by the students. Everything that Semmelweis proposed stemmed from these original observations.

The Introduction of Antisepsis

Once he had postulated that the high mortality of the first clinic was due to the transfer of cadaverous particles on the hands of the students, Semmelweis took the logical step of preventing puerperal fever by insisting that students washed their hands in a disinfectant solution of chlorine before examining patients. At first he used chlorina liquida, but he changed to chloride of lime because it was cheaper; fortunately it was also the more effective disinfectant.

Thus from May 1847 a bowl of chloride of lime was placed at the entrance of the lying-in ward. Once the student had disinfected his hands and entered the ward there was no further disinfection. 'Washing with chlorine water between patients was superfluous', because the patients were alive and therefore could not produce cadaverous particles. Chlorine had been recognized for many years as possessing disinfectant properties. Indeed, Semmelweis remarked in his treatise that he did not discover the disinfectant properties of chloride of lime; he only brought them into use.[16] Chloride of lime also had the ability to remove from the hands the clinging smell of decomposing bodies after an autopsy. Semmelweis saw this as evidence of the destruction of the cadaveric poison.[17]

The introduction of such a simple measure was highly effective. Mortality in the first clinic promptly declined by an amount that is statistically significant (see Tables 7.1–7.4). In fact, the fall in mortality after 1847 was even larger than

[16] In 1794 the French government had authorized its use in the treatment of sick sheep and horses and the disinfection of stables. In 1800 Guyton de Morveau had published a treatise on *Disinfecting the Air*; he recommended chlorinated lime in the second (1802) edition. In 1801 Rollo in London had recommended chlorine as a way of combating infection and destroying miasmata. Dr Labatt had used chlorine for puerperal fever at the Rotunda in 1814, as had Dr Peddie of Edinburgh in 1846 (J. Barker Smith, 'Semmelweis—Physician, Martyr, Pioneer', *Medical Times*, 52 (1924), 38–9, 51–3). In Chapter 4 we noted (note 52) that the American physician Ezra Bennett also used chloride of lime, but it is very doubtful that he had heard of Semmelweis. See also Oliver Wendell Holmes, *Puerperal Fever as a Private Pestilence* (Boston, 1855), 43.

[17] Semmelweis, 'Etiology', ed. Murphy, 369. The deodorant effect of chlorine and its significance is discussed by E. W. Murphy, 'Puerperal Fever', *Dublin Quarterly Journal of Medical Science*, 24 (1857), 1–31, at 28–9, where Murphy mentions Semmelweis's work favourably.

TABLE 7.1. *Maternal mortality rates, Lying-in Department of the Vienna Maternity Hospital, 1784–1859*

Period	Characteristics of the period	No. of deliveries	No. of maternal deaths	Maternal mortality rate
1784–1822	The years in which post-mortem examinations were not routinely carried out	71,395	897	125
1823–1832	The years in which post-mortem examinations were carried out routinely	28,429	1,509	530
1833–1838	Separation of the maternity hospital into two clinics with equal numbers of students and midwives in both			
	first clinic	23,509	1,505	640
	second clinic	13,097	731	558
1839–1847	Separate arrangement of the two clinics			
	first clinic, medical students	20,204	1,989	984
	second clinic, student midwives	17,791	691	388
1848–1859	Period following the introduction of chlorine washing in the first clinic			
	first clinic, medical students	47,938	1,712	357
	second clinic, student midwives	40,770	1,248	306
1784–1859	Total deliveries, deaths, and MMR during the period of 75 years	263,133	10,282	391

Note: Maternal mortality rates are expressed as the number of maternal deaths per 10,000 deliveries.

Source: based on I. P. Semmelweis, 'The Etiology, the Concept, and the Prophylaxis of Childbed Fever', trans. with an introduction by F. P. Murphy, *Medical Classics*, 5/5 (1941), 339–478, 481–589, 591–715, 719–73, at 460–2, table xxiv.

the statistics suggest, for it was the custom in the first clinic to remove some of the ill maternity patients to the general hospital during times of high mortality. Only those who could not be transferred because of the rapid course of their illness remained on the first clinic. The mortality of the first clinic between 1839 and 1846, high though it was, would have been even higher if the deaths of all the transferred patients had been included. In the second (midwives') clinic such transfers were never made.[18] Some modern critics have wondered whether the high mortality of the first clinic might have been due to a selective

[18] Semmelweis, *Etiology*, ed. Carter, 65.

TABLE 7.2. *Annual maternal mortality rates in the two clinics of the Vienna Maternity Hospital, before the introduction of Semmelweis's reforms, 1833–1839*

Year	First Clinic			Second Clinic		
	Births	Deaths	Maternal mortality rate	Births	Deaths	Maternal mortality rate
1833	3,737	197	*527*	353	8	*226*
1834	2,657	205	*771*	1,744	150	*860*
1835	2,573	143	*555*	1,682	84	*499*
1836	2,677	200	*747*	1,670	131	*784*
1837	2,765	251	*908*	1,784	124	*695*
1838	2,987	91	*304*	1,799	88	*489*
1839	2,781	151	*543*	2,010	91	*452*

Notes: During this period, 1833–9, medical students and student midwives were taught in both the first and the second clinics.

Maternal mortality rates (MMR) are expressed as the number of maternal deaths per 10,000 deliveries.

The most important data are italicized.

Source: Semmelweis, 'Etiology', ed. Murphy.

TABLE 7.3. *Annual maternal mortality rates in the two clinics of the Vienna Maternity Hospital before the introduction of Semmelweis's reforms, 1840–1846*

Year	First Clinic			Second Clinic		
	Births	Deaths	Maternal mortality rate	Births	Deaths	Maternal mortality rate
1840	2,889	267	*924*	2,073	55	*265*
1841	3,036	237	*780*	2,442	56	*229*
1842	3,287	518	*1,575*	2,659	202	*760*
1843	3,060	274	*895*	2,739	169	*617*
1844	3,157	260	*823*	2,956	68	*230*
1845	3,492	241	*601*	3,241	66	*204*
1846	4,010	459	*1,144*	3,754	105	*280*

Note: During this period, 1840–6, medical students were taught solely in the first clinic and student midwives in the second clinic.

Maternal mortality rates (MMR) are expressed as the number of maternal deaths per 10,000 deliveries.

Source: See Table 7.2.

TABLE 7.4. *Annual maternal mortality rates in the two clinics of the Vienna Maternity Hospital after the introduction of Semmelweis's reforms in 1847*

Year	First Clinic			Second Clinic		
	Births	Deaths	Maternal mortality rate	Births	Deaths	Maternal mortality rate
1847	3,490	176	*504*	3,306	32	*96*
1848	3,556	45	*127*	3,219	43	*133*
1849	3,858	103	*267*	3,371	87	*258*
1850	3,745	74	*197*	3,261	54	*165*
1851	4,194	75	*179*	3,395	121	*356*
1852	4,471	181	*405*	3,360	192	*571*

Note: During the period 1847–52 medical students were taught in the first clinic and student midwives in the second clinic. Chlorine washings were introduced by Semmelweis in the first clinic from May 1847.

Maternal mortality rates (MMR) are expressed as the number of maternal deaths per 10,000 deliveries.

Source: See Table 7.2.

policy of admission of complicated cases to the first clinic and their exclusion from the second. This was not so. Patients were admitted on a strictly random basis on alternate weekdays, and to the first clinic only at the weekends.

For all its success, the disinfection measures introduced by Semmelweis did not *abolish* puerperal fever in the Vienna Lying-in Hospital. Mortality decreased sharply, but was still at a very high level because there were many sources of infection in the hospital apart from the unwashed hands of students. There is evidence of a low standard of hygiene in such things as the bedlinen, dressings, instruments, and so forth. When James Young Simpson first heard of the rate of maternal mortality in Vienna, he failed to appreciate its significance and clearly had not heard of the theories or practice of Semmelweis, although he wrote in the following terms in June 1848, just over a year after Semmelweis's introduction of disinfection:

A few weeks ago I had a communication from Vienna telling me that formerly 70 in every 100 women delivered in the hospital died of puerperal disease. They delivered new patients in beds still hot and warm with the bodies of those just dead. The physician wrote to me to say they had now reduced last year the deaths to 10 per cent by using means against contagion. Formerly they refused to believe in contagion— that is to say, they sacrificed the lives of 70 per cent of the women delivered to their inhumane medical prejudices. Is it not a terrible illustration of the extent to which medical prejudices will carry men?[19]

[19] This quotation comes from a letter from Simpson to his friend, the London obstetrician, Francis Ramsbotham, dated 23 June 1848. National Library of Medicine, Bethesda, Manuscript Collection, correspondence between Francis Henry Ramsbotham and James Young Simpson, MC 22.

Semmelweis's Concepts of the Etiology of Puerperal Fever

For several months Semmelweis was convinced that the only cause of puerperal fever was the transfer of cadaveric particles from a corpse to a lying-in woman, and not necessarily a human corpse. Semmelweis believed that, if a veterinary surgeon performed a post-mortem on an animal and then examined a parturient woman, that woman would develop puerperal fever.[20] This was his first theory, the cadaveric theory. No corpse, no puerperal fever. Further, Semmelweis believed that all cases of puerperal fever, anywhere, at any time, were due to this cause. For reasons that will appear, this theory—the cadaveric theory—became firmly attached to the name of Semmelweis, and continued to be so attached for many years after Semmelweis himself had abandoned it. This was the cause of much confusion and was a major reason for the rejection of Semmelweis's hypothesis.

In fact, after much agonizing, Semmelweis changed his mind about six months after he had propounded the cadaveric theory, and he did so because of a sudden rise in the incidence of puerperal fever in the first clinic in spite of the continued routine of chlorine disinfection. The infection was soon traced to the admission of a woman with cancer of the uterus in October 1847. It is possible that this patient had cancer of the cervix secondarily infected with streptococci. By ill luck she was in the bed by the door at which the rounds always started. The students examined her and then proceeded up the row of beds along the ward, examining each patient in turn. Eleven of the twelve women in the beds next to the woman with cancer subsequently died of puerperal fever. A similar incident occurred in November 1847, when a woman was admitted to the ward with 'a discharging carious left knee'. Neither woman was a corpse. Yet each of them had appeared to produce the 'cadaveric particles' that Semmelweis had identified as the sole cause of puerperal fever.[21]

It had already become clear to his critics that the cadaveric theory as the explanation of all and every case of puerperal fever was untenable. In most cases of puerperal fever—in other hospitals, for instance, and above all in home deliveries—it was rare for the birth attendant to have come straight to the patient from performimg an autopsy. This was the major reason why Semmelweis's theory seemed wrong in general, even if it was correct under the special circumstances prevailing in the Vienna Lying-in Hospital. Semmelweis's first response was to postulate that the two cases mentioned above—the case with uterine cancer and the case with the carious knee—must have produced dead matter (cadaveric particles) as a result of their lesions. But he soon abandoned the view that all cases of puerperal fever were due to 'cadaveric particles' or 'morbid matter' and substituted the important new concept of '*decomposing animal organic matter*'.

---

[20] Semmelweis, *Etiology*, ed. Carter, 148.
[21] Semmelweis's own description of these incidents can be found in ibid. 93–4.

This was a much broader and more useful concept. It explained why puerperal fever was caused by the transfer of matter from the two cases on his ward, and it also allowed him to state that puerperal fever could be produced by any disease whatsoever, provided it produced decomposing animal organic matter. Further, if it was shown that puerperal fever followed indirect contact with any disease, the disease in question must have produced such decomposing matter. It was a nice example of a circular argument, which Semmelweis explained in a passage that is as clear as it is dogmatic:

I believe childbed fever, no single case excepted, to be a resorption fever, dependent upon the resorption of a decomposed animal organic matter, and the first result of this resorption is a disintegration of the blood, and after this, of the exudates . . . The decomposed animal-organic matter . . . is in the vast majority of cases conveyed to the individuals from the outside . . . In rare cases, the decomposed animal-organic matter . . . is produced within the limits of the affected organism, and these are the cases of auto-infection, and these cases cannot all be prevented.[22]

This allowed Semmelweis to explain the link between erysipelas and puerperal fever, a feature that was stressed by the British but scarcely noticed in Vienna. Erysipelas, he said, produced decomposing animal organic matter because:

The sources of the decomposed animal organic material which, conveyed to the individual from without, causes puerperal fever, are all diseases whatever the age and sex if only the disease in its progress produces a decomposed animal organic material, without regard to the fact whether the patient suffered from puerperal fever or not: only the decomposed animal organic material as a disease-product has to be taken into consideration.[23]

Animal organic matter could also be produced by 'physiologic blood or normal lochia . . . in as much as if they were left for a long time soaking the bed-linen and undergoing decomposition'. Furthermore, said Semmelweis, whatever its origin, 'the carrier of the decomposing animal organic material is the examining finger, the operating hand, the bedclothes, the atmospheric air, sponges, the hands of midwives and nurses which come into contact'. The site of infection from which the decomposed animal material was absorbed and caused the disease was 'the internal os uteri and upwards from there . . . the inner surface of the uterus'.[24]

There was, as one can see, little difference between the ideas put forward by Simpson, described at the end of the previous chapter, and those of Semmelweis. Simpson saw the process as the transfer of inflammatory exudate on the fingers; Semmelweis saw it as decomposed animal organic matter. Independently, Semmelweis and Simpson had produced a hypothesis that would, when the role of bacteria was discovered, be remarkably close to the truth.

[22] Semmelweis, 'Etiology', trans. Murphy, 429.

[23] Sinclair, *Semmelweis*, 204. Arneth said in Edinburgh that erysipelas could act as the source of infection if it was gangrenous erysipelas; that is, erysipelas that produced decomposing or morbid matter (Arneth, 'Evidence of Puerperal Fever').   [24] Sinclair, *Semmelweis*, 204.

Then Semmelweis started to spoil his work in his determination to make his ideas watertight. The first problem he faced was to explain those cases of puerperal fever that could *not* be explained by the transfer of decomposing animal organic matter from the outside. His answer was auto-infection, or self-infection: that is the production of such decomposing matter within the woman's genital tract. This theory, incidentally, as we shall see, was resuscitated in the late nineteenth and early twentieth centuries, when it was known as the autogenic or endogenous theory.

How commonly did auto-infection occur? To answer that question, Semmelweis used the records of the hospital before 1823 when post-mortems were not carried out (see Table 7.1), arguing that during this period all cases must have been cases of auto-infection. He also used the theory of auto-infection to explain cases of puerperal fever in home deliveries by midwives. Semmelweis calculated that auto-infection accounted for a mortality rate of 'less than 1 per cent of puerpera' or between 90 and 100 per 10,000 births, which he called 'rare' or 'very rare'. He arrived at this figure by looking at the maternal mortality in the Vienna Lying-in Hospital between 1784 and 1822 (see Table 7.1).

If Semmelweis had chosen to look outside the Vienna Lying-in Hospital, he should have seen that the maternal mortality rate in home deliveries throughout Europe from all causes was in the region of 50 per 10,000 births, and deaths from puerperal fever between 20 and 30 per 10,000 births—a much lower figure than the rate in the early days of the Vienna Lying-in Hospital. Semmelweis either failed to realize, or failed to acknowledge, this awkward fact. Instead, he insisted that, apart from the 'rare' cases of auto-infection, *all* cases of puerperal fever could be explained by his second theory of decomposing animal organic matter: 'Puerperal fever is therefore not a species of disease: puerperal fever is a variety of pyaemia . . . I understand by pyaemia a blood-poisoning, produced by a decomposed animal-organic matter.'[25] There remained, however, certain well-established features of the disease that still stood in the way of providing a watertight case for Semmelweis's ideas. Largely because these features were associated with English obstetricians, whom he scorned, Semmelweis decided to deal with these features by the extraordinary step of denying puerperal fever was ever contagious, or that it ever occurred in the form of epidemics.

Puerperal fever is not a contagious disease. By contagious disease we understand the sort of disease which itself produces the contagion by which it is propagated, and this contagion again produces in another individual the same disease. Puerperal fever is not a contagious disease, but puerperal fever is conveyable from a sick to a sound puerpera by means of decomposed animal organic material.[26]

Of course, puerperal fever was never (or only rarely) spread directly from one patient to another, and British and American authors never suggested it was. As Simpson of Edinburgh said:

[25] Sinclair, *Semmelweis*, 206.   [26] Ibid.

Continental accoucheurs generally did not understand exactly the kind or description of evidence upon which British practitioners founded their belief in the contagious communicability of puerperal fever. Some of the Continental writers seem to imagine that British obstetricians believe that puerperal fever was usually propagated directly from one patient to another; and not seeing this . . . they imagine from this fact that they had a disproof of the opinion of the contagious communicability of the disease.[27]

Did Semmelweis really fail to understand the British view of contagion, or did he choose to misrepresent them? It could have been either, but Semmelweis's ability to ignore inconvenient facts was also shown by his insistence that epidemics of puerperal fever were a myth. There never had been any epidemics of puerperal fever, he said, because epidemics were invariably due to 'atmospheric, cosmic, or telluric influences' and he had shown that puerperal fever was never influenced by such factors. Semmelweis scorned all who disagreed (especially the British), labelling them as 'the epidemicists'.[28] Here he may well have been influenced by his intense hatred of Wilhelm Scanzoni, an obstetrician at the Prague Lying-in Hospital who had just published a monograph on the aetiology of puerperal fever and was a firm believer in the importance of epidemic influence.

Semmelweis also faced the difficulty of explaining the seasonality of puerperal fever, a feature that was established beyond doubt, not least from the records of the Vienna Lying-in Hospital. In Vienna, as in all other places, the highest incidence of puerperal fever was always in the winter months. The trouble with seasonality was that it smelt of epidemic theory. So Semmelweis explained seasonality by saying that students were less attentive to their work and less inclined to attend post-mortems in the summer months when they wanted to be out and about in the sunshine; or that fewer students attended courses in the summer.

The misrepresentation of British views on contagion, the denial of epidemics, and the eccentric explanation of the seasonality of puerperal fever show how tenaciously Semmelweis clung to his unitary hypothesis. He believed it was essential to make a clean sweep and destroy the old theories and anything that could remotely be connected with them. By so doing, his original observations were devalued by his dogmatism, his intolerance of criticism, and his failure to consider the views of other obstetricians. He was willing to ignore, or worse to distort, evidence that failed to confirm his theory; and he combined these faults with an extraordinary unwillingness to publish.

The Dissemination of Semmelweis's Doctrines

It would have been as normal in Vienna in the 1840s, as it would be today, to expect any physician who had made such important observations as Semmelweis to publish his work immediately. By 1848 he had formulated his

[27] J. Y. Simpson, *Selected Obstetrical and Gynaecological Works of Sir James Young Simpson Bart.*, ed. J. Watt Black (Edinburgh, 1871), 507. [28] Ibid. 210.

doctrine of 'decomposing animal organic matter' and provided all the evidence he needed. His friend Hebra, who ranked his discoveries alongside those of Jenner, implored him to publish, but Semmelweis failed to do so. Instead, he wrote a number of personal letters to obstetricians in other countries, but that was all.[29]

Apart from these letters, and two occasions on which he addressed medical societies, Semmelweis left the dissemination of his discoveries to a large extent to his friends such as Ferdinand Ritter von Hebra, Josef Skoda, Justus Liebig, Franz Hector Arneth, and Carl Rokitansky, all of whom were distinguished members of the Vienna medical school at a time when the school was at the height of its fame. They were all firm supporters of Semmelweis, and the senior physician of the Vienna General Hospital was enthusiastic about Semmelweis's work.[30] Indeed, the first two published accounts of Semmelweis's work were written by Hebra in 1847 and 1848.[31] Both, incidentally, described Semmelweis's first 'morbid-matter' theory. In 1848 Routh, an English obstetrician who had worked at the first clinic in Vienna as a student, described Semmelweis's doctrines to the Royal Medico-Chirurgical Society of London.[32]

Semmelweis's friends and colleagues continued to spread the news abroad. Franz Arneth, for instance, gave an excellent account that included Semmelweis's second theory in Edinburgh in 1851. The idea, often stated, that Semmelweis stood alone and without friends against the united and implacable opposition of all his colleagues—and that it was this that drove him mad —is plainly untrue. In spite of such missionary work on Semmelweis's behalf, as late as the 1860s many obstetricians believed that Semmelweis still held to the original (largely untenable) cadaveric theory.[33] His second theory of decomposing animal organic matter—a theory that might well have commanded greater respect than the cadaveric theory—was often ignored by those who, having heard of the first theory, were unreceptive to what seemed the rather subtle difference of the second. The consequent misunderstandings were Semmelweis's fault and no one else's.

---

[29] Recently one of the earliest of these letters has come to light. Its significance is discussed by K. Codell Carter and G. S. Tate, 'The Earliest-Known Account of Semmelweis's Initiation of Disinfection at Vienna's Allgemeines Krankenhaus', *Bulletin of the History of Medicine*, 65/2 (1991), 252–7.

[30] Arneth, who later became a successful practitioner in Vienna, was closest to Semmelweis, for he was assistant physician to the second clinic of the Vienna Lying-in Hospital when Semmelweis was assistant to the first. Arneth toured several countries to broadcast the views of Semmelweis.

[31] Ferdinand von Hebra (1816–80) was 'perhaps the most brilliant' member of the New Vienna School and one of the founders of dermatology (F. H. Garrison, *An Introduction to the History of Medicine* (4th edn., Philadelphia, 1929), 434).

[32] Semmelweis, 'Etiology', ed. Murphy, 566. Routh's paper was read by E. W. Murphy, because Routh was not as yet a member of the society. His paper was published in 1849 in the *Medico-Chirurgical Transactions*. It was not, it seems, regarded as an important or momentous communication.

[33] See e.g. the *Medical Times and Gazette* (1862), i. 142–3, 601–2. A German professor had stated that 'M. Semmelweiss [*sic*] even now holds the opinion that the origin of the disease is entirely due to infection with cadaveric poison'. Semmelweis replied in person, refuting this supposition and explaining his second theory of decomposing animal organic matter. It seems that he sent a copy of his treatise to the editor of the *Medical Times and Gazette* so that the editor could see for himself.

Skoda, for example, who gave a number of lectures on Semmelweis's work, remarked that the high puerperal mortality in the Prague Lying-in Hospital appeared to have the same cause as that discovered by Semmelweis, giving the impression that Semmelweis still believed in the theory of 'cadaveric poison'.[34] The news reached Germany, where Professor Schmidt of the Berlin Lying-in Hospital made the reasonable comment that, although 'this mode of infection may be one of the ways in which childbed fever is produced; the only way it certainly is not'. This led Semmelweis to mount a withering attack on Schmidt, saying that 'Schmidt does not possess the ability to make observations'.[35] In numerous instances such as this, Semmelweis displayed a degree of quarrelsomeness that was at best foolish and at worst pathological. As Sinclair, who all but worshipped Semmelweis, remarked: 'in dealing with others he showed a remarkable want of the sense of proportion.'[36]

Why Semmelweis refused to publish is an open question. It is true that Klein, the head of the first clinic and Semmelweis's immediate superior, hated Semmelweis and his doctrines. Josef Skoda (one of Semmelweis's most faithful supporters) suggested a commission to examine Semmelweis's work and the members of the commission were actually nominated, but the plan was vetoed by Klein and the commission never met.[37] Some have suggested that Semmelweis had difficulty with the German language, but he could easily have obtained help from colleagues. We do know, however, that Semmelweis confessed to an 'inborn dislike for everything that can be called writing'.[38] He saw himself as a 'doer' rather than a writer, a medical scientist and clinician, not an author. Perhaps the most likely explanation is that he was so sensitive to criticism that he shied away from committing himself in print.

Semmelweis's first public announcement of his theory consisted of a short series of addresses to the Vienna Medical Society in 1851, which, as far as I can discover, were never published. It was not until the autumn of 1857, more than ten years after his initial observations, that Semmelweis finally decided to publish his work in the form of the 'much quoted but seldom read' treatise on which his reputation is based.

The treatise is an extraordinary work of over 500 pages in which a solid core of clinical observation, deduction, and scientific analysis is interspersed with passages that are muddled, dogmatic, and quarrelsome. For example, about halfway through the treatise Semmelweis inserted the heading 'Correspondence and opinions in the literature for and against my doctrines', which opens with the statement: 'The birthday of my doctrine occurred in the latter half of May 1847. If we put the question to ourselves now after twelve years, did my teachings fulfill their mission, then the answer has a melancholy sound.'[39] This is followed by a series of querulous arguments and attacks on his critics,

[34] Josef Skoda (1805–81) was a physician who taught nearly all his life at the Vienna General Hospital. He was a leading physician of the New Vienna School, and published a treatise on percussion and auscultation (Garrison, *History of Medicine*, 431–2).   [35] Sinclair, *Semmelweis*, 87–8.
[36] Ibid. 102.   [37] Ibid. 83.   [38] Ibid. 196.   [39] Ibid. 558.

including no less than sixty-four pages attacking Scanzoni, the 'epidemicist' at the Lying-in Hospital in Prague.[40] The character of the treatise can be understood when we learn how it was written. Sinclair tells us that Semmelweis worked feverishly through 1858, 1859, and 1860, 'continually writing fresh chapters, all in a great hurry, constantly repeating portions without co-ordination, and hurrying the manuscript off to the printers without revision'.[41] When he heard his views had been disputed, he promptly inserted an account of the dispute in the book at whatever stage the book happened to have reached, which was 'not always in the right place, and seldom with any special heading to intimate to the reader that he was entering upon more or less a digression'.[42] That the style is often clumsy was admitted even by Sinclair, who believed that, 'If Semmelweis could have written like Holmes he would have conquered Europe in twelve months.'[43] As Murphy says in the introduction to his translation of the treatise:

The style is wordy and repetitious; the argument flows back and forth without progressing to any logical point; the author is egotistic and bellicose. We are conscious of signs of Semmelweis' mental abberation and feeling of persecution . . . the book itself discloses the underlying paranoia. If Semmelweis had only spent more time in clearly stating his views and less in argument his book would be twice as good and half as long! But that would not be Semmelweis as he really existed.[44]

Semmelweis's sensitivity to real or imagined criticism and his unwillingness to publish were evident as early as the late 1840s. By the time he was writing his treatise, however (that is from 1857), it seems likely that he was in the early stages of a mental illness, the nature of which has been frequently debated and is still uncertain.

The Illness and Death of Semmelweis

When he first arrived in Vienna, there was nothing to suggest that Semmelweis was anything other than an industrious but cheerful individual in comfortable financial circumstances. As we have seen, in 1847 he had put forward his first 'cadaveric' hypothesis, modified it to his second 'decomposing-animal-organic-matter' hypothesis, and introduced chlorine disinfection. In October 1850 he applied for the position of Privat-Dozent (lecturer) at the hospital. It was eventually granted but with the proviso (probably imposed by Klein) that the appointment should be in theoretical midwifery and all demonstrations should be on the 'phantom' (or model). He was to have no contact with patients. It

[40] Scanzoni asserted that puerperal fever was due to a 'fibrinous crasis of the blood due to cosmic telluric influences'. Having published his views he had no intention of changing them (Murphy, 'Ignaz Philipp Semmelweis: An Annotated Biobibliography', 90).   [41] Sinclair, Semmelweis, 201.
[42] Ibid. 197.   [43] Ibid. 354.
[44] F. P. Murphy, 'Introduction', in Semmelweis, 'Etiology', ed. Murphy, 15.

was an insulting offer and Semmelweis had reason to take offence, but he reacted by promptly leaving Vienna for Budapest. Remembering only his enemies and deciding the world was against him, he rushed off without a word of good-bye to his circle of loyal friends and supporters, to whom he owed so much, and whose work on his behalf he scarcely acknowledged. Skoda, who had done so much to promote Semmelweis, 'was deeply hurt by the ingratitude and folly of Semmelweis. He said nothing, but for him Semmelweis ceased henceforth to exist.'[45]

By leaving Vienna and moving back to Hungary in 1851, Semmelweis lost the support of Rokitansky and Skoda. In Hungary he was appointed as unpaid obstetrician to St Rokus in Budapest and a thirty-seven-bed department of obstetrics was set up. This sounds encouraging until one learns that admissions were confined to gynaecological cases for ten months of the year. Obstetric cases were allowed only in August and September, when the university was closed.[46]

However, Semmelweis was elected Director of Obstetrics at the University of Pest in 1855 and was quite active in promoting obstetric care. But in Hungary, as elsewhere, what was known of his work was his cadaveric theory. So, in 1856, at the urging of his friends, Semmelweis gave a lecture on 'The etiology of puer-peral fever', which was repeated three times and was printed in seven issues of the *Medical Weekly*.[47] This may have had some influence on his reputation in Hungary, but, when his treatise was published, even though it was acknow-ledged in Hungary, reception elsewhere was on the whole hostile.

Semmelweis's abrupt departure from Vienna is not, of course, evidence of anything more than a hot temper and a lack of consideration for his friends. It was this kind of behaviour that led Duka (who published the first bio-graphical account of Semmelweis to appear in Britain in 1886) to remark that Semmelweis was temperamentally unable to cope with adversity and criticism.[48] In 1855 it was said his character and appearance were still very pleasing, and in 1857 he married Maria Weidinhoffer. For a short time all was well. In or about 1858, however, when he had embarked on writing his treatise, it is said that he became odd and eccentric in behaviour. He was irritable and began to look prematurely old, dressing and moving in an eccentric fashion. His behaviour became increasingly unpredictable. He suffered recurrent bouts of depression and became increasingly absent-minded, showing signs of disorien-tation, interspersed with periods of manic energy and great excitement.[49]

[45] Sinclair, *Semmelweis*, 113.   [46] Kápolnai, 'An Overview of University Education', 31.
[47] Ibid. 32.
[48] Theodore Duka, 'Childbed Fever, its Cause and Prevention: A Life's History', *Lancet* (1886), ii. 206–8, 246–8.
[49] Smith, 'Semmelweis—Physician, Martyr, Pioneer'. For this section on the life and death of Semmelweis, the main sources are Sinclair, *Semmelweis*; F. Slaughter, *Immortal Magyar: Semmelweis, Conquerer of Childbed Fever* (New York, 1950); S. B. Nuland, 'The Enigma of Semmelweis—an Interpretation', *Journal of the History of Medicine and Allied Sciences*, 34 (1979), 255–72; Semmelweis, *Etiology*, ed. Carter, and, especially, K. Codell Carter, S. Abbott, and J. L. Siebach, 'Five Documents Relating to the Final Illness and Death of Semmelweis', *Bulletin of the History of Medicine*, 69 (1995),

That the flaws in Semmelweis's treatise may well have been the result of the early stages of mental illness is reinforced by the publication, one year after the *Etiology*, of his embarrassingly scathing *Open Letters to Sundry Professors of Obstetrics*, a work in which he reviled his opponents in the most extreme terms. He accused Scanzoni of slaughtering lying-in women through ignorance and even went so far as to write: 'I denounce you before God as a murderer.' It was a work that did nothing to further Semmelweis's reputation as a scientist. During this period Semmelweis often lectured on gynaecology:

> but even then, his mind was ever preoccupied by his favourite subject to which he loved to allude in the course of his lectures on other subjects . . . Often, when speaking to his class, his excitement rose to such a degree as to cause alarm to those around him. A peculiarity of his conduct, the changeable temper, forgetfulness and carelessness, which characterised him of late, occasioned grave misgivings in the minds of his family and friends. The total breakdown soon followed.[50]

After his death, his widow, Maria, stated that she thought Semmelweis first showed signs of insanity in 1861, although she only realized that in retrospect. She may have regarded earlier signs of eccentric behaviour as not amounting to insanity, or her memory may have been at fault.[51] At all events, it is usually stated that undoubted evidence of a mental breakdown occurred on 21 July 1865, when Semmelweis attended a meeting at which he was to present a report concerning a vacant appointment. It is said that he stood up, took a piece of paper from his pocket, and proceeded to read out the text of the midwives' oath, and was gently removed from the platform by his colleagues.

This famous episode, which may be a myth, was first mentioned by a Dr Fleischer seven years after Semmelweis's death: 'He [Semmelweis] rose, took a piece of paper from his pocket and, to the stupefaction of those present, began to read the text of the midwives oath.' The story was then repeated in the numerous biographical accounts of Semmelweis. But Fleischer was not present at the meeting, so his account is hearsay evidence. It seems unlikely it was invented by Fleischer, and it may have been omitted from the minutes of the meeting for reasons of tact or embarrassment. There is no certainty. It remains, like so many details of Semmelweis's last years, vague and uncertain. The evidence for all this is contained in a series of documents that came to light during the early 1990s and that include an account of that meeting. The incident of reading out the oath is not mentioned. There is no independent corroboration for this story, and for various reasons it is unlikely to be true.[52]

A few days later, however, Semmelweis was examined by a physician who found that Semmelweis was mentally ill, but strongly built with no signs of

---

255–70 (this paper contains the recent evidence of Semmelweis's insanity, final illness, and death; I am grateful to Dr Codell Carter for most generously allowing me to see the manuscript of this paper in May 1993).

[50] Duka, 'Childbed fever', 248.

[51] K. Codell Carter, 'Introduction', in Semmelweis, *Etiology*, ed. Carter.

[52] Carter *et al.*, 'Five Documents', 258–9.

organic disease.[53] This physician believed that Semmelweis's mental affliction was very recent—a matter of weeks or at most months. Previously he had been upright and thoroughly respectable in character. Now, however, he showed indifference to his family, a tendency (not evident before) to heavy drinking, 'a heightened sexual excitement' including 'intercourse with prostitutes after years of faithfulness to his wife, frequent masturbation, and indecency towards both acquaintances and strangers . . .'. He had grandiose ideas such as having a hundred photographs of himself taken and sent out with copies of his treatise. 'He had become wasteful in his expenses, without providing for his family. He estimated his income high and his expenses low.'[54] These features are suggestive of mania.

On 29 July, eight days after the famous meeting where he supposedly read out the midwives' oath, and presumably no more than a day or two after his examination by the physician, Semmelweis left Budapest for Vienna by overnight train. At Vienna, he was met by his old friend Hebra, who, following a plan prearranged by telegraph, persuaded Semmelweis to visit Hebra's own sanitarium. On the pretence of arranging this, Hebra took Semmelweis to a public lunatic asylum, where Semmelweis was forcibly restrained while Hebra walked away.

This is a disturbing story, and there is no reason to doubt it is true. It may be that Hebra felt he was acting in Semmelweis's best interests, but why Semmelweis should have been taken to a common and rough asylum of some 700 inmates instead of a private clinic, why a detaining order was signed by three doctors none of whom was a psychiatrist, and why an expert psychiatric opinion was not obtained for a man who, for all his awkwardness and bellicosity, was still a doctor of high reputation, is impossible to answer. During his incarceration in the asylum Semmelweis was said to be violent, needing forcible restraint. His wife tried to visit him the day after admission but was turned away. A fortnight later Semmelweis was dead. His death was certified as being due to septicaemia from an infected wound sustained in a recent gynaecological operation—a statement that forms the basis of the story that Semmelweis died a martyr to the very disease (septicaemia) to which he had devoted his life.

That Semmelweis was mentally ill seems beyond doubt, but the nature of the illness is obscure. Some favour a diagnosis of Alzheimer's disease, largely on the basis of photographs.[55] Others believe he was suffering either from a manic-depressive psychosis with paranoid features (which is the diagnosis I favour), or an organic brain disease such as neurosyphilis. Syphilis was always an occupational hazard for any obstetrician who did repeated vaginal examinations with an ungloved hand.

[53] The physician, Janos Bokai, was a friend of Semmelweis. But he was not a psychiatrist or neurologist. He was a paediatrician and director of a children's hospital in Budapest: (Carter, Abbott, and Siebach, 'Five Documents').   [54] Ibid.

[55] Nuland, 'The Enigma of Semmelweis'. In my book *Death in Childbirth* I suggested that Alzheimer's disease might be the most likely diagnosis. In view of subsequent evidence, I no longer think so.

As for his death, the newly discovered papers support the suggestion of septicaemia (probably staphylococcal rather than streptococcal, because the notes taken in the asylum describe an illness with multiple septic skin lesions like boils or carbuncles) and the ravings of a man in a fever. The first entry confirms that Semmelweis was tricked into coming to the asylum. On the second day he was confined in a strait-jacket. Six days later it was recorded that 'In a frenzied moment was terribly excited, hit, shoved, breathed with difficulty . . . tongue very dry—the middle finger very gangrenous . . . boils everywhere'. There are frequent references to a rapid pulse, to the gangrenous finger, to difficulty with breathing, a blue colour, and to rambling speech. On the last day, amongst the entries are the words: 'intensive collapsus' [*sic*] and 'pyaemia?'

These records, which sound as if they were written by an attendant with some nursing experience, do not suggest the notes of a doctor.[56] They do, however, suggest that Semmelweis arrived in the asylum with a severe infection of the middle finger of one hand that went gangrenous and that septicaemia may have been the direct cause of death. It has been suggested that the real cause of death was forcible restraint by the asylum attendants: that he was in effect bludgeoned to death and that 'brain disease' was a euphemism for brain injury.[57] Although it is impossible to refute such a suggestion, the records of his admission make this unlikely.[58] In spite of new evidence that raises as many new questions as it answers old ones, the only certainty is that a great deal is still uncertain. We do not know for certain the nature of either Semmelweis's insanity or his death, and, unless new evidence is unearthed, it is unlikely that we ever will.

The Influence of Semmelweis

By the 1850s it would have been difficult for anyone connected with childbirth and maternal care to plead total ignorance of the part that was, or might be, played by contagion. But the concept of contagion (and even more the concept of antisepsis) lay very much at the boundary of orthodox beliefs, although the extent to which this was so varied not only between countries but between individuals. As we have seen, the British were far more ready to accept contagion as part of the accepted canon than their Continental neighbours, especially the French, who seldom saw any necessity to be influenced by what was going on in medicine in other countries.

What Semmelweis was demanding with his 'cadaveric' and 'decomposing-animal-organic-matter' theories was nothing less than throwing out the whole

---

[56] In fact in one place, on 31 July, there is the entry 'recognises the doctor'.

[57] Carter, 'Introduction', in Semmelweis, *Etiology*, ed. Carter, 58. Lancaster is quite definite that this was the cause of Semmelweis's death, but provides no new evidence to support the assertion (H. O. Lancaster, 'Semmelweis: A Re-Reading of *Die Aetiologie . . .*', *Journal of Medical Biography*, 2 (1994), 12–21, at 14).

[58] I have taken the evidence for these statements and the account of Semmelweis's hospital admission directly from Carter *et al.*, 'Five Documents'.

outdated collection of former ideas to replace them with a theory that seemed far too simple to be true. Bruck, the first translator of Semmelweis's treatise, made a very perceptive comment when he pointed out that, if Semmelweis's theories were accepted:

It had to be confessed that all that had been taught for years, about which thick-bellied books full of learning had been written, was error throughout; that a small piece of chloride of lime was sufficient to throw upon the scrap-heap the whole learned apparatus which so many distinguished men of science had been collecting and elaborating for centuries, with the industry of bees; that the application of chloride of lime was sufficient to arrest an outbreak of the disease against which all efforts had hitherto been put forth in vain. All that appeared too simple to be seriously accepted.[59]

Semmelweis failed to convince his contemporaries not only because his theory seemed too simple, but also because of his insistence that every case of puerperal fever was due to the transfer of either 'morbid matter' or 'decomposing animal organic matter'. This made no sense of cases in women who had been delivered at home by midwives, even though Semmelweis would have resorted to his theory of auto-infection to explain such cases. He also damaged his case by refusing to accept that puerperal fever was contagious, or that epidemics of puerperal fever could occur. Most of all he combined a failure to publish in 1847 with what amounted to a genius for making enemies.

Semmelweis, as we have seen, had many supporters in the Viennese medical school until his abrupt departure to Budapest. But he also had formidable opponents. Klein, his immediate superior in Vienna, was one example, and Scanzoni (deeply offended by Semmelweis's attack) was another. He was also opposed by Carl Braun, his successor to the post of assistant to the first clinic. Braun was accused by Semmelweis of ignorance and told he should 'take some semesters in logic' before treating puerperal patients. Professor Créde, Director of Obstetrics and Gynaecology at the Charité in Berlin, and Professor of Obstetrics in Leipzig, opposed Semmelweis and was promptly dismissed by Semmelweis as an 'epidemicist'. In a review of Semmelweis's treatise, Créde complained that 'Semmelweis calls everyone who disagrees with him an ignoramus and a murderer'.[60]

Rudolf Virchow, the founder of cellular pathology whose famous work on that subject was published in 1847, was accused by Semmelweis of being a bad observer and an incompetent pathological anatomist simply because he opposed his (Semmelweis's) doctrines. Not surprisingly, although the two never met, Virchow 'seized almost every opportunity to confront Semmelweis' teaching'.[61] Semmelweis's habit of attacking some of the most famous doctors of his time, and transforming even his mildest critics into enemies by insulting

---

[59] Sinclair, *Semmelweis*, 110–111. Jacob Bruck translated Semmelweis's treatise from the original Hungarian (see Murphy, 'Ignaz Philipp Semmelweis: An Annotated Biobibliography').

[60] Carter, 'Introduction', in Semmelweis, *Etiology*, ed. Carter, 41.

[61] Kápolnai, 'An Overview of University Education', 35.

them, was more than enough to explain why Semmelweis was so often rejected and forgotten And the additional handicap of insanity followed by a grisly death in a common lunatic asylum did nothing to help his reputation as a medical scientist.

What influence, then, did Semmelweis have during his life and in the years following his death? It would be wrong to say none at all. But it does seem that he had little effect on the practice of obstetrics outside Vienna and not much in Vienna once he had left.[62] He probably had most influence in Germany and least in France where 'misunderstanding and prejudice against the teaching of Semmelweis survived for the longest time'. Étienne Tarnier (1828–97), the most progressive French obstetrician, 'attributed the discovery of puerperal fever to an American Obstetrician as late as 1894'.[63] The most telling evidence that his work did not abolish puerperal fever (although it is still believed by many that it did) is that, in every country from which data are available, the mortality due to puerperal fever rose, instead of falling, in the years after his treatise was published, reaching the highest levels ever recorded in the mid-1870s.

In the twenty years after his death, Semmelweis's name was mentioned only on rare occasions, and usually in uncomplimentary terms. In 1875 Robert Lee believed that, while Gordon and Semmelweis were both 'possessed of powers of original thought', Gordon had greater 'intellectual and moral superiority' because 'Semmelweis' work consists chiefly of a series of observations made by himself, without direct reference to the opinions of others . . . it must be acknowledged that he gives proof of possessing very limited knowledge indeed of the literature of his subject, and we cannot feel surprised that he finds but little difficulty in disposing of his opponents to his own satisfaction'.[64]

Semmelweis had a scattering of supporters in the UK and the USA. Murphy of Dublin praised Semmelweis's work, and so did James Young Simpson when he first heard of it in 1851.[65] Both were generous men, ready to acknowledge the work of others. But there was, I suspect, much more hidden support for Semmelweis than we recognize. The reason for saying so—and we will come across this in later chapters—is the frequency with which Semmelweis's views (or statements remarkably close to his views) were repeated by obstetricians without attribution. Some who knew of Semmelweis's work may have found it convincing, but were too embarrassed to admit to association with such a controversial, odd, and difficult man. It is also true, however, that new ideas often

[62] It might be argued that, although Semmelweis's work had little immediate effect, it was seminal in the sense that it led to the introduction of antisepsis in the 1880s. But, as we will see in Chapter 9, the credit for this belongs to Lister, whose method was independent of Semmelweis.

[63] Kápolnai, 'An Overview of University Education', 39. See also A. Hirsch, Handbook of Geographical and Historical Pathology (2nd edn., 1881), trans. Charles Creighton (London, 3 vols.; 1883). The part played by Hirsch is explained in Chapter 9.

[64] R. J. Lee, 'The Gouldstonian Lectures on Puerperal Fever', British Medical Journal (1875), i. 267–70, 304–6, 337–9, 371–3, 408–9, 440–2, at 305, 339.

[65] Murphy, 'Puerperal Fever'; J. Y. Simpson, 'Discussion of Arneth's Paper Read to the Edinburgh Medico-Chirurgical Society, April 16, 1851', Monthly Journal of Medical Science, 13 (1851), 72–80, at 75.

appear separately and independently in science and medicine, especially when climates of opinion change and what previously seemed unreasonable begins to be accepted. Obstetricians who, soon after Semmelweis's death, came up with closely similar notions may have been driven to their conclusion independently because that was the way the tide was flowing.

When Semmelweis was buried in Hungary on 15 August 1865, 'newspapers in Hungary and the medical press hardly took note of Semmelweis' death, and in his native country, his name almost sank into oblivion'. His widow and children even abandoned his name in 1879, changing it to Szemerényi, possibly out of shame over his insanity and the manner of his death.[66] It was a miserable end for a man who, for all his shortcomings, made some brilliantly original observations. But in 1865 no one could possibly have guessed that quite soon Semmelweis would become one of medicine's greatest heroes. Why that extraordinary transformation took place will be discussed at the end of Chapter 9.

Appendix. A Brief Chronology of the Life and Work of Ignaz Semmelweis

1818   Semmelweis was born in Hungary in July 1818, the fourth son of a successful grocer.
1837   Entered Vienna University to study law; changed to medicine.
1844   Qualified as a doctor and obtained the degree of Master of Midwifery.
1844–6 Worked at the pathological department of the Vienna Lying-in Hospital. At the same time he was allowed to work as an aspirant in the first clinic of the maternity department of the Vienna Allgemeines Krankenhaus (General Hospital).
1846   Appointed in February as provisional assistant to Dr Klein at the first clinic.
1847   The death on 13 March of Professor Kolletschka provided Semmelweis with his insight into the cause of the high puerperal mortality in the first clinic, and he formulated his doctrine on the etiology of puerperal fever. In May he introduced chlorine washings in the first clinic.
1848   Semmelweis wrote to several European obstetricians about his work, but refused to publish a paper. In 1847–8 Hebra published two short accounts of Semmelweis's work in the *Transactions of the Medical Society of Vienna* (of which Hebra was the editor). In November 1848 Charles Routh, an English obstetrician who had been to Vienna and studied at the first clinic, wrote a paper about Semmelweis's work, which was presented to the Royal Medico-Chirurgical Society in London by E. W. Murphy.
1850   Semmelweis applied for the post of Privat-Dozent (lecturer). His application was turned down by Klein, the chief of the clinic, who was opposed to Semmelweis's views. Semmelweis reapplied for the post of Privat-Dozent, and this application was granted but hedged round with such restrictions that Semmelweis angrily rejected the offer and returned abruptly to Budapest.

[66] Kápolnai, 'An Overview of University Education', 35.

1850–7   Throughout this period Semmelweis's work became known chiefly through his friends who travelled and described his observations. For example, Arneth, Assistant to the second clinic in Vienna, visited Edinburgh and gave an account of Semmelweis's work and views to the Edinburgh Medico-Chirurgical Society in April 1851.

1851   Semmelweis addressed the Vienna Medical Society on the 'genesis of puerperal fever' in May, June, and July. He was appointed as unpaid director of St Rokus Hospital in Budapest.

1855   Semmelweis was appointed Director of Theoretical and Practical Obstetrics in the University of Pest at the age of 37.

1856   In December Semmelweis addressed the Medical Society of Budapest on the etiology of puerperal fever, and his talk was published in a Budapest medical journal.

1857   Semmelweis married Maria Weidinhoffer (1837–1910), the daughter of a merchant in Pest, and began writing his treatise in the autumn. At this time, or shortly afterwards, he began to show signs of mental illness.

1860   The treatise *Etiology, Concept and Prophylaxis of Childbed Fever* (*Die Aetiologie, der Begriff und die Prophylaxis des Kindbettfiebers*) was published, thirteen years after Semmelweis had made his first observations.

1861   Semmelweis published replies to his critics in a volume entitled *Open Letters to Sundry Professors of Obstetrics*.

1865   In July Semmelweis was taken to Vienna and forcibly detained in a lunatic asylum, where he died on 13 August.

8

Monocausalists, Multicausalists, and Germ Theory

During the twenty years following Semmelweis's death in 1865 books and papers about puerperal fever poured off the presses. Conferences in the UK, France, Germany, and elsewhere, which sometimes lasted for days on end, were devoted solely to this disease. At a meeting in Brussels in 1875, puerperal fever was described as the greatest bone of contention (*pomme de discorde*) in the whole of medicine.[1] British doctors would not have quarrelled with that.

Although these twenty years included the mid-1870s, when mortality from puerperal fever reached the highest level ever recorded, there were many other diseases—phthisis, typhoid, diphtheria, and scarlet fever, for instance—that had much higher rates of mortality. In 1874, for example, there were 3,387 deaths from puerperal fever in England and Wales, but 24,992 deaths from scarlet fever. Why, then, did puerperal fever attract so much attention? Possibly because of the especially tragic nature of maternal deaths, possibly because there was at least a hint that puerperal-fever deaths were preventable, but most of all because puerperal fever seemed to epitomize better than any other disease the rifts of opinions about fevers in general, and the debates surrounding the arrival of germ theory.

Monocausalists and Multicausalists

At the heart of the matter was the division between what I will call for convenience the 'monocausalists' and the 'multicausalists'. The former attributed puerperal fever to a single cause such as putrefaction, contagion, or germs. The latter held tenaciously to a long list of causes, and usually to the notion that puerperal fever was not a single entity but a group of different diseases. The division between the two camps was not absolute. They seldom are in debates of this nature, and there were overlaps and subdivisions. The multicausalists, for instance, were apt to quarrel amongst themselves about the relative importance of different factors, and only a minority of monocausalists insisted on a single cause; most stressed one cause as supremely important, but openly or tacitly admitted there were other factors of minor importance.

---

[1] Anon., 'Discussion, Fièvre Puerpérale', *Compte-Rendu: Congrès Périodique International des Sciences Médicales*, 4th session (1875), 323–4.

To make matters more complex, both groups were changing their views. Before the 1860s, the multicausalists believed that 'epidemic influence' (essentially the seasons and the weather) was one of the key factors in the causation of puerperal fever. After the 1860s we hear less and less about miasmatic theory or epidemic influence and much more about overcrowding, defective drains, and sewer gas. Likewise, predisposition, which was a factor of relatively minor importance in the first half of the nineteenth century, came to occupy a position of supreme importance in the second. Its precise meaning in this context has changed, but in essence it was the belief that pregnant women were highly susceptible or predisposed to puerperal fever purely as a result of a series of physiological changes induced by pregnancy.[2] Furthermore, the contagiousness of puerperal fever, so hotly denied by the multicausalist majority before 1850, was no longer such a contentious issue. It was often included in the multicausalists' agenda. As Evory Kennedy, ex-Master of the Dublin Lying-in Hospital, wrote in 1869: 'The non-contagious furor having pretty well spent itself, reason resumes her sway, and contagion can now be spoken of with calmness and toleration. Whereas twenty years ago the advocate of contagion was worse than an infidel.'[3]

How did medical men deal with the emergence of germ theory? If many were slow to take it on board, it is not surprising. It requires a great effort of imagination to appreciate how medical practitioners must have felt when told that large-scale events such as violent changes in the weather, miasmas, or gases from defective drains, which had been the accepted cause of fevers for generations, were to be abandoned in favour of living microbes so small that they could not even be seen without a powerful microscope. For the monocausalists, who were, of course, adamant that puerperal fever was one and not several diseases, their mainstay—contagion—was expanded to include germ theory, which they saw as a confirmation of their views. The multicausalists, however, believed that, if there were 'germs' in the discharges of patients with puerperal fever, they were either the *consequence* of putrefactive processes and not the cause, or they were secondary causes that came into operation when other processes, such as putrefaction, or exposure to sewer gas, or predisposition due to physiological changes in pregnancy, had initiated the disease.

Although the monocausalists won in the end, during the period with which we are concerned, and judging strictly by the evidence of the time, the debate was evenly balanced. There were times when the multicausalists appeared to have a good case, and the monocausalists a weak one, and vice versa. Hence the heat and complexity of the debates. We will look at several examples, rather than

---

[2] Dr Michael Worboys (personal communication, 1995) has suggested that 'whereas now the word predisposition has connotations of susceptibility, in the 1870s it also carried the meaning of the spontaneous development of disease . . . predisposition in the sense of vulnerability is too passive, it is a notion that smacks of tissues waiting for germs to cause disease rather than the body actively breaking down of its own accord'. Now he has pointed that out, it certainly rings true.

[3] E. Kennedy, 'Zymotic Diseases, as More Especially Illustrated by Puerperal Fever', *Dublin Quarterly Journal of Medical Science*, 47 (1869), 269–307, at 272.

try to summarize everything that was published, which would be tediously repetitive and impossibly lengthy. But we must begin by returning to Vienna and the story of Semmelweis's successor.

Mayrhofer and the Beginnings of Germ Theory in Relation to Puerperal Fever

Although Pasteur is usually credited with being the first to demonstrate the role of bacteria in puerperal fever, his work was preceded by that of several people, of whom one of the most interesting was a little-known Viennese physician Carl Mayrhofer (1837–82).[4] Mayrhofer, who has been called the 'second Semmelweis', occupied the same post as Semmelweis in the Vienna Lying-in Hospital: Semmelweis was assistant to Johannes Klein; Klein was succeeded by Carl Braun as the Professor of the First Clinic, and, in 1862, Braun appointed Mayrhofer as his assistant.

Braun, incidentally, hated Semmelweis, denounced his theories, and stopped the routine of chlorine disinfection. Semmelweis responded with a caustic attack on Braun and his views. By 1862, however, Braun had become so impressed by Pasteur's work that he suggested that airborne germs might be a cause of puerperal fever (the word 'airborne' should be noted, because we meet it again when Lister is discussed in the next chapter). But Braun was no 'monocausalist'. On the contrary, he had constructed an immense list of causes of puerperal fever, to which airborne germs might be added. Braun, therefore, encouraged the young Mayrhofer to search for what were then called 'vibrions' in the uterine discharges of women with puerperal fever, which Braun assumed might be something that would have contaminated patients by airborne infection.

After initial failures, Mayrhofer identified the vibrions and in 1863 sprayed vibrion-infected fluid from uterine discharges into the genital tract of newly delivered rabbits. Most of the rabbits became diseased and died. He then cultured the vibrions in a solution containing sugar and ammonia, filtered the solution to separate the vibrions from other substances in the solution, and repeated the experiment with rabbits. Once again the rabbits became diseased with the rabbit equivalent of puerperal fever.

Braun had long believed that imperfect ventilation was a prime cause of puerperal fever in hospitals, and was encouraged in this view by one of his students, who alleged that the fall in the mortality in the first clinic was due not to disinfection of the hands by Semmelweis's method, but to improved ventilation.[5] Braun believed that Mayrhofer's work offered a rational basis for the supposed effectiveness of ventilation. But Mayrhofer was developing different ideas. In

---

[4] The work of Mayrhofer has become known largely because of the excellent account of his work in K. Codell Carter and B. R. Carter, *Childbed Fever: A Scientific Biography of Ignaz Semmelweis* (Westport, Conn., 1994). I gladly acknowledge my debt to them, and have taken my account of Mayrhofer entirely from this source.   [5] Ibid. 86.

1865 (the year as it happens when Semmelweis died) Mayrhofer had come to the conclusion that puerperal fever was due to tissue decomposition under the influence of vibrions. He also concluded that Semmelweis was correct when he said that infection was conveyed on the hands of doctors and students. Thus he leant towards the 'monocausalist' view that all cases of puerperal fever were due to vibrions, and opposed the view that the disease was due to multiple causes including poor ventilation.[6]

Feelings ran so high in Vienna that Braun regarded Mayrhofer as a traitor and promptly refused to support his research. Mayrhofer went into private practice, where he was dogged by misfortune. In the 1870s he met with difficulties in his practice. Then he developed tuberculosis and also had the misfortune that two of his children died. He became addicted to morphine and went downhill so much that, when he died in 1882, aged 45, his death was described as 'a salvation'. It is odd how many of the major figures in the history of puerperal fever came to an unhappy end.

Amongst others who undertook experimental work, M. D'Espine repeated Mayrhofer's experiments in France in 1872. In 1873 Orth in Bonn found organisms during an epidemic of puerperal fever, and so did Heiberg in Christiana. In Berlin in 1876 Hausmann also injected infected material into the vagina and uterus of rabbits.[7] Thus there was considerable experimental activity on the Continent, and Pasteur was certainly aware of these and other experiments when he attended two meetings of the Academy of Medicine in Paris in 1879 and found himself embroiled in a heated debate that we come to soon. But those who were undertaking scientific and laboratory research were, of course, a small minority, without the immediate influence that medical scientists have today. And almost all of them were on the Continent of Europe. So it might be wise to start with practising obstetricians, as it was they, far more than laboratory scientists, who were the teachers and formers of opinion in their time. I have selected two who were, I believe, representative of many in the UK.

The Views of Dr Barnes and Professor Leishman

Robert Barnes, one of the most prominent members of the London obstetric establishment, published a series of five lectures on puerperal fever in the *Lancet* in 1865.[8] He was an orthodox clinician with an extensive knowledge of

[6] K. Codell Carter and B. R. Carter, *Childbed Fever: A Scientific Biography of Ignaz Semmelweis*, 87–8.

[7] J. A. Doléris, *La Fièvre puerpérale et les organismes infèrieurs: Pathogénie et thérapeutique des accidents infectieux des suites de couches* (Paris, 1880), 45–7.

[8] R. Barnes, 'Lectures on Puerperal Fever', *Lancet* (1865), i. 141–2, 169–70, 279–80, 307–8, 443–4, 527–8; (1865), ii. 531–2, 613–15. In 1865 Robert Barnes FRCP (1817–1907) was Obstetric Physician and Lecturer on Midwifery and the Diseases of Children at St Thomas's Hospital, Physician to the Royal Maternity Charity, and President of the Obstetrical Society of London. During his life he had the unusual distinction of holding the post of Lecturer in Obstetrics at three London teaching hospitals,

European publications and long practical experience of obstetrics, on which he 'held very definite opinions', which he expressed with force and clarity.[9] His classification of puerperal fever was simple. There were two forms of the disease: the *heterogenetic*, in which there was an external cause, and the *autogenetic*, in which there was an internal cause.

He began the first lecture by saying that, 'if we include the continent of Europe, it may be confidently affirmed that puerperal fever destroys more lying-in women than all other causes combined'. Many of these deaths were unnecessary, because puerperal fever stood apart from other fevers as the one most responsive to 'preservative medicine'. He illustrated this by contrasting mortality from puerperal fever in London as a whole with home deliveries undertaken by the Royal Maternity Charity, which undertook home deliveries in the slums of the East End of London, where most patients were poor and lived in appalling housing.

Barnes pointed out (rightly) that the statistics of the Royal Maternity Charity might be challenged on a number of grounds,[10] but the reservations were too minor to account for the wide difference between puerperal fever mortality in hospitals and in lying-in charities. The difference between Queen Charlotte's Hospital, which averaged 221 deliveries a year, and the Royal Maternity Charity, which delivered 3,400 women a year in their own homes, can be seen in Table 8.1. The risk of dying of puerperal fever was *seventeen* times as high for a woman delivered in Queen Charlotte's Hospital (supposedly the leading hospital of its kind in London) as it was for a woman delivered at home by the staff of the Royal Maternity Charity.[11] Similar findings were reported a few years later from Paris and are also shown in Table 8.1. Barnes considered that the 'heterogenetic' species of puerperal fever was synonymous with what he called hospital puerperal fever, and was never seen in home deliveries.

To Barnes, the most important factors in autogenetic puerperal fever (the kind that occurred in home deliveries) were local and constitutional predisposing factors. Essentially they were changes in physiological functions affecting the circulation, the blood, the lungs, the kidneys, the brain, and the nervous system.

---

first at the London Hospital, then at St Thomas's, and finally at St George's. He was a pioneer of operative gynaecology and a man of great mental and physical vigour. He learned Spanish at the age of 85 and he continued his habit of rowing out to sea and bathing from the boat until he was 89 (*Dictionary of National Biography*).

[9] *Dictionary of National Biography*.

[10] Barnes pointed out that the patients of the Royal Maternity Charity were all married women. Since single women had a higher rate of maternal mortality, there was in his words a 'shifting of danger from the Charity'. Charity patients were followed up for only a short time after delivery, and late cases might be attended by poor law medical officers or other doctors, and would not necessarily be known to the Charity. There was also a smaller proportion of first pregnancies amongst the Charity's patients than there was in London as a whole, so again this favoured the Charity. Such factors might account for small differences between hospital and home deliveries by an outpatient charity, but not for the enormous differences that existed.

[11] Barnes, 'Lectures on Puerperal Fever', i. 141. For further details on outpatient charities, see I. Loudon, *Death in Childbirth: An International Study of Maternal Care and Maternal Mortality 1800–1950* (Oxford, 1992), 194–5 and 200, table 12.4 .

TABLE 8.1. *A comparison of the maternal mortality rates in home and hospital deliveries, London and Paris, nineteenth century*

Place and date	Institution	No. of deliveries	Maternal mortality rate
London			
1828–63	Queen Charlotte's Hospital	7,736	263
1853–62	Home deliveries by the Royal Maternity Charity	34,020	27
Paris			
1873–75	Maternity departments in general hospitals	9,298	416
1873–75	Maternity hospitals	6,631	312
1873–75	Home deliveries by midwives employed by charitable outpatient maternity services	28,006	19
1873–75	Home deliveries in Paris by other midwives	5,020	50

Note: Maternal mortality rates are expressed as maternal deaths per 10,000 deliveries.

Sources: London: R. Barnes, 'Lectures on Puerperal Fever', *Lancet* (1865), i. 141; Paris: Léon Le Fort, 'Discussion, Fièvre Puérperale', in *Compte-Rendu: Congrès Périodique International des Sciences Médicales*, 4th session (Brussels, 1875), 334.

'Pregnancy', he said, 'induces a degraded condition of the blood; throws an excessive burden upon the excreting apparatus; impedes the freedom of the circulation; causes hypertrophy of the heart.'[12] This was as clear an exposition as one could wish for of the importance of predisposition.

Barnes was almost alone amongst his contemporaries in referring to Semmelweis, and in his fifth lecture he gave what he called 'a fair summary' of Semmelweis's views.[13] Barnes knew only of Semmelweis's 'cadaveric' theory, and promptly recognized the flaw in Semmelweis's work, for it was now well established that puerperal fever was also rampant in lying-in hospitals in which there were no students and no routine autopsies, showing that cadaveric infection could not be the sole cause of the disease. Barnes agreed that it was wrong for a 'gentleman engaged in midwifery' to carry out autopsies on women who had died of diseases such as puerperal fever, but was it also dangerous to carry out dissections of 'healthy' corpses? Barnes thought it unlikely there was any danger, but it was probably wise for obstetricians to avoid both autopsies and dissections of 'healthy' bodies.[14]

[12] Barnes, 'Lectures on Puerperal Fever', i. 279–80, 307–8.
[13] Ibid. ii. 613–15.   [14] Ibid. 613.

As far as treatment was concerned, Barnes's views were pessimistic. In an era that had lost faith in the virtues of venesection, it was difficult to know what to do. He advised his students to ensure that lying-in women were not exposed to the 'scarlatinal poison', or to poisons that might be carried on the linen or blankets, or the clothes of the medical attendant, the nurse, or visitors. He suggested that 'nurses' (i.e. midwives) should be relieved for two hours every day and allowed to spend that time in the open air, that they should wear cotton gowns (white ones to compel frequent change and washing), and that they should take a warm bath once a week.[15]

It is interesting to note that twenty-two years later, in 1887 when Barnes was aged 70, he published another paper on puerperal fever.[16] In spite of the work of Pasteur, Lister, and the accumulating evidence of the effectiveness of Listerian antisepsis in lying-in hospitals to which we have yet to come, Barnes had scarcely moved an inch from the views he expressed in 1865. He clung to his old ideas, certain that 'fever in a puerperal woman is a complex condition which several factors concur in creating. There is not one cause but a plexus of causes . . . The simplest, the fundamental form of puerperal fever . . . is purely autogenic; I call it endosepsis. The conditions arise entirely within the patient's system.'[17] Once again he said nothing about washing hands, and nothing about antisepsis. In his private practice, his only preventive action was to choose what he judged to be the most 'sanitary' room in the house as the lying-in room, which was sometimes the drawing room because it was furthest from the drains and sewers. He concluded in true Victorian fashion that 'Hard work and exercise', to both of which he was personally addicted, 'are a preventative against the disease'.[18] Here, then, was one of London's leading obstetricians, blissfully untouched by the scientific progress that had occurred in his lifetime and devoted to multiple causation. He never mentioned Pasteur, bacteria, germ theory, or antisepsis in 1887, and this time he even failed to mention Semmelweis. In this he was not alone. Many of his contemporaries held similar views.

Our second obstetrician was William Leishman, Regius Professor of Midwifery in the University of Glasgow. He opened the chapter on puerperal fever in his textbook as follows: 'There is perhaps, in the whole range of obstetrics, no subject which the writer and the teacher approaches with so profound a conviction of difficulties to be encountered, as that group of affections of the puerperal period to which the term Puerperal Fever has, with a somewhat loose signification, been given.'[19] The term 'puerperal fever' implied a specific fever due to a specific poison similar to 'a typhous, an enteric, and a variolous poison'. That, he said, was incorrect. 'Post-partum fevers' was a preferable term for the 'symptoms, far from harmonising, present the most startling contrasts'. Thus:

---

[15] Ibid. 614–15.

[16] R. Barnes, 'On the Causes, Internal and External, of Puerperal Fever', *British Medical Journal* (1887), ii. 1036–42.   [17] Ibid. 1036.

[18] Ibid. 1041.   [19] W. Leishman, *A System of Midwifery* (2nd edn., Glasgow, 1876), 773.

we find one author asserting that, when blood-letting was practised, under the most heroic use of the lancet, almost all his cases recovered; a second has observed that, when blood-letting was practised, almost every case died; while a third describes, under the name of puerperal fever, an affliction so trifling that it was usually checked by a single dose of Dover's powder.[20]

Leishman believed that one form of puerperal fever was due to the introduction of septic matter and the 'absorption of decomposing material', causing what was called either septicaemia, pyaemia, or ichorrhaemeia, which were essentially the same thing. Other forms were caused by a specific poison that was probably identical to the specific poison of erysipelas. But the third and largest group were cases due to 'the peculiar position of the [pregnant] woman, no less in the condition of her blood, than in the newly organised function of lactation and uterine involution'. In this state the woman was susceptible to a wide variety of poisons such as 'the scarlatinal poison' or the poison of 'typhous diseases', and so on. In short the root cause was predisposition. These were examples not of puerperal fever but of 'the puerperal fevers' that he continued to describe in great and confusing detail. He thought that the evidence of Semmelweis (based as it was on a lying-in hospital with students) 'has been considerably exaggerated'.[21] I suggested earlier that historians, intent on interpreting the mentalities of the past, must accept the existence of muddle and uncertainty. Leishman is a case in point. Having said that, we can now turn to the meetings, at home and abroad, that provide us with some insights into the views of some of the leading figures at the forefront of teaching and research in the world of obstetrics.

The Meetings in Paris and London

In 1858 the Academy of Medicine in Paris held no less than eighteen meetings spread over several months to discuss every aspect of puerperal fever. Semmelweis was mentioned very briefly in passing and no firm conclusions were reached. Indeed, so varied and multiple were the views that were expressed that the individual who acted as reporter, taking notes, said with more than a touch of exasperation:

Of the thirteen Academicians who spoke, one could count essentialists, demi-essentialists, involuntary essentialists, unconscious essentialists; absolute localists, half- or one-fourth localists; localists with a tendency to essentialism, essentialists with a passion for localisation; specifists, typhists, traumaticists and non-traumaticists.[22]

[20] W. Leishman, *A System of Midwifery*, 774.   [21] Ibid. 789.
[22] F. P. Murphy, 'Ignaz Philipp Semmelweis: An Annotated Biobibliography', *Bulletin of the History of Medicine*, 20 (1946), 653–707, at 663. Even if the categories such as 'essentialists', 'localists', and so on are unclear, one can at least sense the character of the meeting and the reporter's feelings of exasperation.

Much the same could have been said about the three-day meeting on puerperal fever that was held by the Obstetrical Society of London in 1875.[23] Although there were hints at this meeting that the tide was flowing in the direction of contagion, and that epidemic and miasmatic influence were losing ground, the more closely we look at this meeting the less it seems that old views had been replaced.

It was not as if it was a meeting of a few ill-informed practitioners. Practically all of the British obstetric establishment was there, and the meeting was opened by the well-known surgeon Thomas Spencer Wells, who was, incidentally, a firm believer in Listerian antisepsis in surgery.[24] The discussion was anything but insular. The British may have been mentioned most often, but the work of authorities from other countries such as Bilroth, Weber, Cruveilher, Virchow, Spiegelberg, Schröder, Mayrhofer, and Pasteur was mentioned. So was the work of American authors such as John Bell of Pennsylvania, Thomas Minor of Cincinnati, and Fordyce Barker of Bellevue Hospital, New York. C. H. F. Routh, who, the reader may remember, had been to Vienna and had told the Royal Medico-Chirurgical Society in London about Semmelweis's work in 1848, was the only person to mention Semmelweis, but he might have been referring to Methuselah for all the response he evoked. Indeed, as far as this meeting was concerned, Semmelweis, Gordon, and Holmes might never have existed.[25]

What is most revealing about this meeting is not the conclusions (for, like the Paris meeting seventeen years earlier, nothing remotely like a consensus emerged from the discussions) but the questions that were asked. These were outlined in the opening address by Spencer Wells. And the following is a short summary,[26] with a brief account in italic of the response they evoked:

- Is puerperal fever a specific fever confined to childbearing women in the sense that scarlet fever, or measles, or diphtheria, are specific fevers? *The majority of speakers at this meeting believed it was not.*

---

[23] Obstetrical Society of London, 'Discussion "On the Relation of Puerperal Fever to the Infective Diseases and Pyaemia"', *Transactions of the Obstetrical Society of London*, 17 (1876), 90–165, 178–209, 217–72.

[24] Amongst the speakers were Robert Barnes, Obstetric Physician to St Georges Hospital, W. O. Priestly MD FRCP, Obstetric Physician to King's College Hospital, W. S. Playfair MD FRCP, Professor of Obstetric Medicine at King's College, Grailly Hewitt, Professor of Midwifery at University College London, and Obstetric Physician to University College Hospital, and William Leishman MD, Regius Professor of Midwifery in the University of Glasgow.

[25] By 1875 Routh had become Physician to the Samaritan Hospital for Women and Children. The absence of recognition of Semmelweis is all the more extraordinary when one sees that Grailly Hewitt, Professor of Midwifery, University College London, said: 'It is impossible to escape the conclusion that puerperal fever consists of nothing more nor less than an injection into the general circulating fluid of a poisonous material of animal origin—that is, a form of pyaemia for the production of which the minutest portion of the morbific agent may prove sufficient . . .'. Although that was remarkably close to Semmelweis's views, Hewitt made it clear he was citing James Young Simpson. And he added: 'I entirely disbelieve in the existence of a form of fever which is sufficiently definite and precise to receive a distinct name in the same sense we speak of typhus fever, or typhoid fever, or measles or scarlet fever (Obstetrical Society of London, 'Discussion', 157).   [26] Ibid. 92–6.

- Is it a surgical fever such as erysipelas or pyaemia? *Sometimes, perhaps, but not always.*
- Is it always (or even frequently) due to the poison of a common continuous fever such as typhoid, typhus, scarlet fever, or diphtheria, which is transformed into puerperal fever by the state of pregnancy and lying-in? *The weight of opinion was against this.*
- Is it a form of septicaemia or pyaemia arising from the injection of septic matter or decomposing organic matter, exactly analogous to wound septicaemia, as described by Simpson? *Again, most thought it might be sometimes, but certainly not always.*
- Is there one, or are there several, forms of puerperal fever? *Most believed there were several forms.*
- Is it, therefore, correct to refer to puerperal fever as a fever like other fevers? *Many thought it was wrong to call it a 'fever' and we see here the beginning of the tendency to rename the disease 'puerperal sepsis' rather than 'puerperal fever'.*
- If it was a form of septicaemia, was the septic matter intrinsic in the sense of being already present in the genital tract, or was it introduced from outside? *Most thought that both forms occurred, but the intrinsic/extrinsic or endogenous/exogenous debate was not nearly as heated in 1875 as it became twenty years later.*
- What relation have bacteria and allied organisms to the pyaemic process in the puerperal state? *Almost everyone thought the answer was none at all.*

Four years later, in 1879, a similar but much more interesting meeting was held in Paris. It was the occasion of a clash between two giants of the time: Louis Pasteur and Jacques-François-Édouard Hervieux.

Pasteur and Hervieux

Louis Pasteur (1822–95), who was not a medical practitioner but a chemist and physicist by training, became interested in micro-organisms as a result of research in 1848 on the optical asymmetry of crystals of tartaric acid.[27] By a series of steps with which we need not concern ourselves, this led to his discovery in 1865 that two diseases of silkworms, *pébrine* and *le flacherie*, were due to bacteria. Pasteur then investigated other diseases, both of other animals and of man. By 1877 he had shown that anthrax and chicken cholera were also due to bacteria. Through this work he became one of the two people most responsible for the introduction of germ theory. The other, of course, was the younger of the two, Robert Koch (1843–1910).

By 1879 Pasteur had undertaken a small amount of work on bacteria and puerperal fever, but not enough to feel confident of his findings. For reasons

[27] See W. F. Bynum, *Science and the Practice of Medicine in the Nineteenth Century* (Cambridge, 1994), and F. H. Garrison, *An Introduction to the History of Medicine* (4th edn., Philadelphia, 1929).

that will appear, however, he was forced to announce prematurely that he had found the micro-organism that caused puerperal fever, which he described as resembling a string of beads (it was not yet called the streptococcus). This was announced during a two-day meeting of the Academy of Medicine, held on 11 March and 6 May 1879.[28]

Pasteur's opponent was Jacques-François-Édouard Hervieux (1818–95), 'Médecin Chef' of the Maternité, the largest and most prestigious maternity hospital in Paris, if not the whole of France. Hervieux opened the meeting on 11 March with a long discussion of the causes of puerperal fever, which, he said, were epidemic influence, miasmas, and emanations from newly delivered women, and above all overcrowding of lying-in women in hospitals. He readily acknowledged the prestige of Pasteur but refused to believe in the germ theory.

Pasteur replied at length. In effect, Pasteur presented an all-embracing 'monocausalist' theory of the diseases of animals in general, but at this stage of his career he had produced relatively little evidence of the role of microbes in human diseases apart from his work on anthrax. His famous work on preventive inoculation and rabies, for instance, did not take place until the 1880s. Because Pasteur was not medically qualified, Hervieux may well have felt that he had the crucial advantage of practical experience on the wards of a lying-in hospital. Pasteur, however, was forced to speak about his work on puerperal fever because he was directly challenged by Hervieux, as we can see from his response to the challenge:

M. *Pasteur*. I am really embarrassed to take the floor after the lecture so full of clinical observations by M. Dr Hervieux. But the defence of the theory of germs and of living contagion, in which I firmly believe, forces me to it . . . M. Dr Hervieux said, at the end of his lecture, having learnedly attacked the theory of germs in the etiology of puerperal fever: 'I am afraid I will die before I have seen the microbe [*vibrion*] that produces this fever.' And now, if the Academy will allow me, I will draw before his very eyes the dangerous microbe that I maintain is the cause of this fever. It is likely to be one of the numerous specimens or varieties of these small organisms that I have met so often in my researches since 1860, which have the form of little strings of spherical beads [*chapelets de grains*]. It is to one of these varieties that, in 1861, I reported the fermentation called *viscous* [visqueuse]; it is to one of these varieties that is owed the fermentations of the leaf of the mulberry tree in the intestinal canal of the silkworms, found in the illness called *flacherie*. It is to one of these varieties again that I attributed, in 1862, the ammoniacal fermentation of urine, etc. The German authors, preferring to designate this group of organisms by the Latin names . . . called them the *microsporon* or the *micrococcus*.

A legend has grown up about this incident. It is thought that the drawing on the blackboard was a winning serve by which Pasteur instantly won game, set, and match. Not so. Pasteur had failed to convince Hervieux, and (I suspect) most of the others who attended the meeting.

[28] Anon., 'Discussion, Fièvre puerpérale'.

At this early stage of bacteriology, it was assumed that, if bacteria caused human diseases, each variety or species caused a single specific disease and was found nowhere else but in close association with patients suffering from that disease. Yet here was Pasteur saying that the organism that caused puerperal fever could also be found in numerous other diseases and circumstances. To some of his audience, Pasteur seemed unconvincing, because he had no patience with the business of naming and classifying bacteria; he was more interested in their actions than their form. Pasteur was content to describe what microbes looked like under the microscope. His indifference to classification may have been strengthened by his intense dislike of Germans in general and Koch in particular, who spent much time on a Linnean type of classification of bacteria. Hence his remark that is was the *German* authors who had invented names 'to designate this group of organisms'.[29]

Thus the notion that Pasteur had settled the argument once and for all is wrong. If we put ourselves in the position of those who were present at this meeting in 1879, not knowing what was subsequently known about the streptococcus and bacteria in general, it is easy to see why Hervieux returned to the attack at the second meeting with cogent reasons for rejecting Pasteur's theory.

M. Hervieux: The Academy will remember that my communication of 11 March led to some interesting suggestions from Monsieur Pasteur. Each of us will remember the drawing made by our illustrious colleague of the microbe presumed to be that of puerperal septicaemia. At the end of the following meeting, M. Pasteur left a note on my desk recording the results of new researches he has made in my department at the Maternité. In this note, as in his first thoughts, M. Pasteur puts forward as likely the idea that the microbe in beads [*microbe en chapelet*] was the determining cause of the puerperal infection. With his usual openness and loyalty he recognized that there were certain obscurities and difficulties surrounding this serious question. However, the news of the discovery, not only of the presumed microbe, but of the microbe shown to be of puerperal septicaemia, has gone beyond these walls and the Parisian public has told many of us of the unfortunate rumours. I say unfortunate, because science has nothing to gain from hasty dissemination of a new discovery that certainly requires confirmation . . . I wish today to defend M. Pasteur against his own friends and those overzealous followers who prematurely transform a presumption into certainty, a hypothesis into demonstrated truth . . . from his spoken and written reflection I will show what is still uncertain in the matter of puerperality, the basis on which the germ theory rests.

Hervieux began by saying that Pasteur had conceded that the story of the role of microbes was like 'the eternal story of the chicken and the egg'. In other words, were the micro-organisms the product or the cause of the disease? Pasteur had said the organism was very common. You could find it everywhere. Surely, then, it could not be the cause of puerperal fever because it should only

---

[29] Pasteur had no love for German scientists and in particular Robert Koch, with whom he quarrelled. See Bynum, *Science and the Practice of Medicine in the Nineteenth Century*, 145–6.

be found 'in the places where puerperal septicaemia rages'. Yet 'M. Pasteur has declared, the microbe is very common, it exists everywhere; you can very easily extract it from the common water supply, and in consequence there is not a woman in childbirth who, daily using this water for drinking, douching, and washing, would escape invasion by the infectious organism.' He continued with this theme at length, and ended by saying: 'We can explain the almost exclusive predilection of puerperal fever for certain localities, and in particular for maternity hospitals, by the simple word: overcrowding.' In practical terms, Hervieux saw the danger that acceptance of the germ theory would 'lead to the abandonment of all the hygienic, sanitary, prophylactic measures that had been instituted in the Maternité and everyone would go hunting for microbes instead . . . It is that alone that makes the doctrine of germs so dangerous.'[30] When Hervieux referred to sanitary measures, he had in mind the work of his colleague Étienne Stéphane Tarnier (1828–97), whose work was mentioned briefly in Chapter 5. Before returning to the Paris meeting we must turn briefly to Tarnier, because he showed that effective sanitary measures could be instituted on pragmatic grounds, without the absolute necessity of believing in contagion or germ theory.

Tarnier, who was appointed 'Chef de Clinique' of the Maternité in 1861 and Director in 1867, became France's acknowledged expert on puerperal fever. From 1867 to 1870 Tarnier said he was powerless to alter the stubborn routine and habits of the hospital, so he called this 'the period of inaction'. From 1870, however, he managed to introduce a strict policy of isolation by which the well and the sick were separated. Women who showed the slightest signs of puerperal fever were promptly removed to the general hospital, whose staff were forbidden to enter the Maternité in case they brought infection to the lying-in wards. The principle of isolating the sick was taken further in 1876, when a special pavilion (the 'Pavilion Tarnier') was built as a separate isolation unit. This period, from 1870 to 1881, was called by Tarnier 'the period of isolation'. The mortality rate in the Maternité during the first period, the period of inaction, was 931 per 10,000 deliveries compared with the mortality in the second period, the period of isolation, of only 232 per 10,000 deliveries. At the time it seemed an astonishing success. Tarnier also described a third period, the period of antisepsis from 1881 to 1889, when mortality was reduced to 105 deaths per 10,000 deliveries, as we see in the next chapter.[31] This explains why Hervieux was so emphatic that overcrowding was the cause of puerperal fever, that

---

[30] This remark appears at the end of the second part of the meeting. It was a long meeting, and it was reported at great length. What I have included here is a very small part of the whole. A longer— but still abridged—translation of these two papers can be found in I. Loudon, *Childbed Fever: A Documentary History* (New York, 1995).

[31] The source I have used for this account of Tarnier's work is C. J. Cullingworth, 'Biographical Note on Étienne Stéphane Tarnier', *Transactions of the Obstetrical Society of London*, 40 (1898), 78–89. Incidentally, Tarnier was very careful to see that his figures were accurate. If a patient was moved to a general ward from the lying-in wards and she died, her death was included in Tarnier's statistics, even though she did not die in the maternity hospital.

isolation was a success, and that hunting for bacteria would distract the hospital staff from the strict sanitary measures that had proved so effective.

That ended the long debate. Although they were courteous in their exchanges, Pasteur and Hervieux were miles apart in their views. To an unbiased observer at the time it may well have seemed that, although Pasteur had made a strong case for micro-organisms as the cause of some diseases, his argument that puerperal fever was one of them was not convincing enough to sweep away the long-established theories of the causation of puerperal fever. Just as Semmelweis's theory of decomposing animal organic matter seemed too simple, so Pasteur's theory that a 'microbe en chapelet' was the sole cause of puerperal fever seemed too crude, too simple, to explain such a complex disease as puerperal fever.[32]

Pasteur and Doléris

When Pasteur made his contribution to this meeting, he hinted that he would be undertaking further research on the role of the 'microbe en chapelet' in puerperal fever, but in fact there is no evidence that he did. Pasteur may have lost interest in puerperal fever, but the probable explanation is that he delegated the work to a young colleague, J. Amédée Doléris, who published a treatise on the subject in 1880.[33]

Doléris had been working with Professor Depaul in Paris for six years before he met Pasteur. As he explained:

It was while I was undertaking autopsies of women who had died while under the care of M. Hervieux at the Maternité, around the month of May [1879], that I came into contact for the first time with M. Pasteur, who was at that time searching, by means of culturing of organisms associated with puerperal fever, for the solution to questions raised at the 'tribune académique' . . . After consulting M. Pasteur, and under his guidance, I began to study the lochia [the post-partum vaginal discharges] from the point of view of searching for organisms that were, to a greater or lesser extent, associated with cases of puerperal fever. I will give the results I obtained from more than one hundred observations.[34]

Doléris found various forms of bacteria in the discharges of recently delivered mothers. The most frequent were the diplococcus, consisting of two spherical organisms joined together, and similar spherical organisms in the form of chains, which he called *Micrococcus pyogénique*, thereby anticipating the later name that persists today, *Streptococcus pyogenes*. He showed that the diplococci were found in both normal cases and cases of puerperal fever (although more commonly in

---

[32] Although reports of medical news from abroad were frequently the subject of reports or leading articles in the *British Medical Journal* and the *Lancet*, I have failed to find any mention of this debate in these or any other British medical periodicals.   [33] Doléris, *La Fièvre puerpérale*.

[34] Ibid. 7–8.

the latter) but the chain form—in other words the streptococcus—was found in all cases of puerperal fever but only rarely in normal cases. Further, Doléris isolated these organisms and showed that when they were injected into rabbits and guinea-pigs the animals died and the organisms could be recovered from the dead animals. It was Doléris, not Pasteur, who produced the most convincing evidence that the organism like a chain of beads was the causative organism (or at least the most common organism) of puerperal fever. Although the work of Doléris is rarely cited today, it was painstaking and thorough, and at least moderately well known at the time within, as well as outside, France.[35]

Having reviewed the range of opinions on puerperal fever in the 1870s, we must now return to the state of the lying-in hospitals, picking the subject up where it was left at the end of Chapter 5.

Should Lying-in Hospitals be Abolished?

When an obstetrician as eminent as Barnes had shown that the risk of dying from puerperal fever in a lying-in hospital was seventeen times as great as it was in a home delivery, and had also shown that confounding factors such as social class, marital status, or selection of high-risk cases for hospital delivery could not account for more than a minute fraction of this staggering difference, one is bound to ask two questions. First, why did women agree to be admitted to institutions where they were at such greater risk of dying? Secondly, why on earth were the lying-in hospitals not abolished by obstetricians when it was clear that lying-in hospital mortality was at least as bad, if not worse, than it had been in the late eighteenth and early nineteenth century?

We touched on the answer to the first question in Chapter 5. It is easy to imagine the feelings of a poor woman in a state of advanced pregnancy in the 1870s, living in a slum, exposed to draughts and dirt, cold and hunger. To such a woman, admission to a hospital, where she was provided with a roof over her head, a clean warm bed, obstetric care and advice provided free by midwives and doctors, no housework, and ample meals for a fortnight (about the average length of stay) must have been sheer luxury. It was unreasonable to expect that the poor could have had any appreciation of the statistics of maternal mortality, or the relative risks of a hospital and a home delivery. If lying-in hospitals were closed, women still turned up and begged for admission so that they could enjoy the comforts of which they felt they were being deprived, and which they valued so highly.[36]

Obstetricians, however, were in a different position. They knew the risks. So, how can they be excused for the failure to close the lying-in hospitals? Some

[35] See e.g. A. H. Freeland Barbour, 'Pathology of the Post-Partum Uterus', *Edinburgh Medical Journal*, 31 (1885), 434–44, at 438.
[36] Fleetwood Churchill, 'An Historical Sketch of the Epidemics of Puerperal Fever', in Churchill (ed.), *Essays on the Puerperal Fever, and Other Diseases Peculiar to Women* (London, 1849), 3–42, at 17–20.

argued that hospitals provided an essential form of maternity care for which there was no substitute. But the largest maternity hospitals of Vienna, Paris, and Dublin accounted for only a small proportion—at most 10 per cent—of total deliveries in those cities, and, in England and Wales (and also in France) as a whole, the lying-in hospitals accounted at most for 0.5 per cent of total deliveries in the 1870s. Even in London, where almost all of England's lying-in hospitals were situated, in 1878 there were only four lying-in hospitals with a total of 145 beds (or one bed for every 12,800 of the female population), compared to seventy-five general hospitals with 10,760 beds.[37] The sensible, the humane thing to have done, would have been to abolish the lying-in hospitals and expand the outpatient charities.

A powerful reason for keeping them open, however, was the status they conferred on their medical staff. Throughout the nineteenth century, the London hospitals became the centres of medical teaching, medical research, and medical expertise. An appointment as an honorary physician or surgeon represented the pinnacle of success. So it was with obstetrics. Every ambitious young obstetrician sought a post as an honorary accoucheur at a lying-in hospital. The alternative as a consultant accoucheur at an outpatient charity was second best. The status of obstetricians was low enough as it was. If their hospitals were closed, their status would sink even further. Yet a growing number of authorities recognized that something must be done to reduce the awful mortality.

Robert Lee, a well-known London obstetrician, was one of the first to say openly in the 1830s that lying-in hospitals should be closed.[38] In the 1850s James Young Simpson condemned maternity hospitals without reservation,[39] and coined the term 'Hospitalism', which was defined by Sir John Ericsen, surgeon to University College Hospital, as 'a general morbid condition of the building, or of its atmosphere, productive of disease'.[40] 'Hospitalism' was the cause of high mortality, and Simpson suggested in 1848 that 'medical, surgical and obstetric palaces' should be abolished, and lying-in hospitals replaced by small separate buildings made of iron, which was much easier to wash down and disinfect than brick, stone, or plaster.[41]

In Dublin, Evory Kennedy suggested that the imposing buildings that made up the Rotunda (the Dublin Lying-in Hospital) should be used for administrative purposes and nurses' homes, while the wards should be replaced by a series of small buildings based on the design of Swiss chalets. The plan seemed so comic it was laughed out of court. But the suggestion that the old time-honoured wards should be closed was not a laughing matter. It provoked a

---

[37] A. W. Edis, 'Remarks on the Influence of Obstetric Knowledge on the Mortality of Mothers in Childbed', *British Medical Journal* (1878), ii. 507–11, at 508.

[38] R. Lee, *Researches on the Pathology and Treatment of Some of the Most Important Diseases of Women* (London, 1833).   [39] Edis, 'Remarks'.

[40] Bynum, *Science and the Practice of Medicine in the Nineteenth Century*, 132.

[41] J. Y. Simpson, 'Report of the Edinburgh Maternity Hospital', *Monthly Journal of Medical Science*, 9 (1848–9), 329–38. By 'iron', Simpson meant corrugated iron, which was already available in the 1840s as a building material and was exported to the colonies in large quantities.

storm of outraged protest on both sides of the Atlantic.[42] The superintendent of Glasgow's lying-in hospital spoke for many when he wrote in 1853:

But what are we to do with those poor unfortunates who have not even these insalubrious places of filth and squalor to live in? Are we to shut our hospitals, infirmaries and fever houses against them? . . . Hospitals are necessary evils . . . There may be reasons for shutting hospitals, but not because deaths occur in them.[43]

Florence Nightingale, however, took a different view. In 1862 she used the funds donated by the public for her work in the Crimea to open a lying-in ward at King's College Hospital for the training of midwives. After an epidemic of puerperal fever in 1867 in which nine deaths occurred, she knew she must close the ward and with characteristic decisiveness she did so. Six years' experience had convinced her that 'the mortality is far, far, greater in lying-in hospitals than among women lying-in at home' because of 'foul air, putrid miasms, and predisposition to malignant inflammatory action'.[44] The larger the hospital, the worse the miasmatic influence and the higher the rate of maternal mortality. Like Hervieux, she believed that crowding puerperal patients closely together was the cause of the problem. Home deliveries were safer because, 'however grand, or however humble a home may be in which the birth of the child takes place, there is only one delivery in the home at the time'.[45] Florence Nightingale believed neither in the contagiousness of puerperal fever nor in germ theory, but she believed passionately in sanitary measures and held that, if lying-in hospitals were necessary, they should consist of separate buildings with separate rooms for each patient.

There were similar worries on the Continent. Robert Barnes cited the French physician Trousseau, who complained that the most modern and well-equipped Continental lying-in hospitals were anything but immune to the rages of puerperal fever: 'It is in a model hospital (Beaujon) that there rules a mortality so enormous that if it were the type for the whole country, out of the 900,000 to 950,000 labours taking place yearly, there would be 80,000 deaths, and France would be a desert in less than fifty years.'[46] Likewise, a modern lying-in hospital had just been constructed in Munich at great cost, 'but fever decimates the patients and there is no safety but in the evacuation of the establishment'. After many other examples, Barnes concluded: 'One might have expected that such examples as here collected, which are well known, which have been freely

[42] E. Kennedy, *Hospitalism and Zymotic Diseases as More Especially Illustrated by Puerperal Fever or Metria . . . Also a Reply to the Criticisms of Seventeen Physicians upon this Paper* (2nd edn., London, 1869). See also J. S. Parry, 'Description of a Form of Puerperal Fever which Occurred at the Philadelphia Hospital Characterized by Diphtheritic Deposits of Wounds of the Genital Passages and by Other Peculiar Phenomena', *American Journal of Medical Sciences*, 69 (1875), 46–76, which describes an epidemic of puerperal fever between 1871 and 1874.

[43] J. Wilson, 'Report of the Glasgow Lying-in Hospital for the Year 1851–52 with an Address to the Students Attending the Hospital', *Glasgow Medical Journal*, 1 (1853), 1–10.

[44] Florence Nightingale, *Introductory Notes on Lying-in Hospitals* (London, 1876), 3–4.   [45] Ibid.

[46] Barnes, 'Lectures on Puerperal Fever', i. 169.

and deeply discussed, would have chilled the ardour of the most enthusiastic champion of the hospital system.'[47]

Barnes suggested that, if lying-in hospitals were to continue, they 'ought to be provided on the "cottage" principle of Mr Napper of Cranley when there would never be more than one puerperal woman in one room'.[48] As for the argument that lying-in hospitals must be retained as centres for teaching, and that without hospitals the science of obstetrics would decay, Barnes replied: 'It scarcely seems to enter into the minds of physicians abroad that it is possible to learn the obstetric art elsewhere than in hospitals.' In the UK, many students were taught at home deliveries carried out by the outpatient departments of maternity departments and lying-in charities, and by these means the UK 'turns out every year a body of practitioners who for skill and a tender respect for women are unsurpassed in the world'.[49] He added that many Continental practitioners believed that hospital epidemics of puerperal fever were merely part of general epidemics in the 'population outside as well as inside the hospital'. But he believed that 'In not a few instances it is quite certain that the fever proceeded in the converse direction—that is, from the hospital to the town.'[50]

Some of the most vigorous attacks on the lying-in hospitals came from the USA. Dr Parry, Attending Accoucheur to the Philadelphia Hospital, wrote in 1875:

The records of some hospitals support the opinion that they had better never have been built . . . Year after year the terrible record of their increasing deaths has appealed strongly for investigation, till at last one man, bolder than the rest—a former master and governor of the Dublin Lying-in Hospital [he was of course referring to Evory Kennedy]—rose up and asked whether it would not have been better for these poor women to have been left to the cold charity of the world than to have obtained admission into one of these institutions . . . All remember the storm which raged about him, and what warfare of words followed, a contest more bitter than the most sanguinary encounter . . . Four years have passed since then [but] . . . there is no doubt that many [lying-in hospitals] have year after year been but slaughter-houses in which the lives of a number of unfortunate women have been needlessly sacrificed.[51]

Barton Cooke Hirst, Obstetrician to the Philadelphia Hospital, wrote thirteen years later in 1887: 'It must be conceded that no hospital, whether the community or private charity, has the right to subject its inmates to a danger of death much greater than if they had remained in their own homes, no matter how squalid they might be.' In his view American lying-in hospitals were so appalling (he actually used the word 'murderous') that they ought to come under state or municipal control.[52]

[47] Barnes, 'Lectures on Puerperal Fever', i. 170.
[48] Mr Albert Napper was a country surgeon and the founder of the well-known British system of cottage hospitals. See Meyrick Emrys-Roberts, The Cottage Hospitals, 1859–1990 (Motcombe, Dorset, 1991).   [49] Barnes, 'Lectures on Puerperal Fever', i. 170.
[50] Ibid. i. 142.   [51] Parry, 'Description of a Form of Puerperal Fever'.
[52] B. C. Hirst, 'The Death Rate of Lying-in Hospitals in the United States', Medical News of Philadelphia, 50 (1887), 253–6.

One of the most revealing documents ever published on the problem of lying-in hospitals appeared in 1874. It was written by Dr Steele of Liverpool. Noting the very low mortality of home deliveries undertaken by outpatient lying-in charities in contrast to the appalling mortality in lying-in hospitals, he questioned the justification for hospital delivery, and canvassed the opinion of fifty hospital accoucheurs, asking them whether it was safer in their opinion for 'married women of the class just above pauperism' to be delivered in a lying-in hospital or at home.

Thirty replied, of whom 'twenty-five are in favour of home delivery as safest and best, three are in favour of hospital delivery, under certain conditions, and two prefer hospital unconditionally'. He cited a roll-call of the famous names in late-nineteenth-century obstetrics: Dr Barnes of London 'feels so strongly that he has "refused to associate himself with lying-in hospitals"'; Professor Leishman of Glasgow was convinced home deliveries were safer; Dr Graily Hewitt said: 'At their own homes'; Dr Braxton Hicks expressed the opinion: 'I consider home attendance far superior to hospital attendance, both in a social point of view, as well as regards safety'; and Professor Simpson of Edinburgh replied 'At their own homes.'[53]

A few lying-in hospitals were closed in the provinces. Birmingham closed its lying-in hospital and concluded there was no inconvenience to patients from doing so. Manchester reduced its inpatient deliveries by refusing to admit normal cases and by increasing the outpatient service.[54] In London, however, apart from Florence Nightingale's closure of the lying-in wards in King's College Hospital, they were all kept open in the perpetually frustrated hope that sanitary measures would prove effective, and most of all because of the vested interest of obstetricians in keeping them open.

It is interesting to speculate what might have happened to the lying-in hospitals in the 1880s if the same appalling level of mortality had continued unchecked. Fortunately, it did not. During the meeting of the Obstetrical Society in 1875, the surgeon Spencer Wells suggested that what Lister had done for surgery might be done for obstetrics in the lying-in hospitals; it might be an alternative to closing them:

if traumatic fever and pyaemia can be kept out of a surgical hospital, why should not puerperal fever be kept out of a lying-in hospital, or be prevented from spreading, if it have [sic] been accidentally imported? There has been a great outcry against lying-in hospitals of late; but I trust this Society may be able to guide the feeling rather in the direction of freeing them from puerperal fever than of destroying them.[55]

It was a prophetic remark, for the lying-in hospitals were just about to be saved by the remarkable effects of Listerian antisepsis. How this came about is the subject of the next chapter.

---

[53] A. B. Steele, *Maternity Hospitals, their Mortality, and What Should be Done with them* (London, 1874), 11–13.   [54] Ibid. 25.

[55] Obstetrical Society of London, 'Discussion', 100.

9

Lister and Antisepsis

Joseph (First Baron) Lister (1827–1912), a surgeon who graduated from London in 1852, was appointed Professor of Surgery in Glasgow in 1860, moved to Edinburgh in 1869, and was appointed to King's College in London in 1877. He is famous for the introduction of antisepsis in surgery, which, it is often said, was rapidly adopted by the majority of surgeons throughout Europe and North America. The strength of Lister's method rested on the recognition of the role of bacteria in wound sepsis, and on statistical proof that it reduced surgical mortality so that it became possible to carry out operations (osteotomy, for example) that had previously been avoided because of high septic mortality. This was the essence of the antiseptic revolution.

The Story of Antisepsis

The traditional story, however, has been subjected to close analysis in a series of recent papers, which have shown that the introduction of antisepsis was much more complex than most of us had realized.[1] Here I can provide only a brief summary of recent scholarship, but what is interesting is that none of these recent publications deals with the application of Listerian antisepsis to obstetrics, although the results were as spectacular, if not more so, than they were in general surgery. This may be a reflection of Lister's own apparent lack of interest in antisepsis in childbirth, or the almost universal belief that antisepsis in obstetrics stemmed from Semmelweis and not from Lister. Such a view is mistaken. When antisepsis became routine in lying-in hospitals (which, in the majority

---

[1] Amongst the most recent contributions to the history of Listerism in Britain are L. Granshaw, ' "Upon this principle I have based a practice": The Development and Reception of Antisepsis in Britain, 1867–90', in J. V. Pickstone, *Medical Innovations in Historical Perspective* (Basingstoke, 1992); T. H. Pennington, 'Osteotomy as an Indicator of Antiseptic Surgical Practice', *Medical History*, 38 (1994), 178–88, and 'Listerism, its Decline and its Persistence: The Introduction of Aseptic Surgical Techniques in Three British Teaching Hospitals, 1890–99', *Medical History*, 39 (1995), 35–60. The impact of Listerism in Canada is described in J. T. H. Connor, 'Listerism Unmasked: Antisepsis and Asepsis in Victorian Anglo-Canada', *Journal of the History of Medicine and Allied Sciences*, 49 (1994), 207–39, and its impact in the USA is the subject of a paper by T. P. Gariepy, 'The Introduction and Acceptance of Listerian Antisepsis in the United States', *Journal of the History of Medicine and Allied Sciences*, 49 (1994), 167–206. See also W. F. Bynum, *Science and the Practice of Medicine in the Nineteenth Century* (Cambridge, 1994), 112–13, 144–5.

of hospitals was in the early 1880s), it was done in Lister's name, it was due to Lister's influence, and the method used was closer to that of Lister than of Semmelweis. Any lingering notion that Semmelweis influenced Lister, or that Lister did for surgery what Semmelweis had already done for obstetrics, can be dismissed. In fact Lister had not even heard of Semmelweis, let alone his work, until the mid-1880s, some twenty years after he had introduced his method of antisepsis, and, when he did eventually hear in 1906 that there was a rumour that he owed his ideas to Semmelweis, he firmly replied:

When in 1865 I first applied the antiseptic principle to wounds, I had not heard the name of Semmelweis and knew nothing of his work. When, twenty years later I visited Buda Pesth, where I was received with extraordinary kindness by the medical profession and the students, Semmelweis' name was never mentioned, having been, as it seems, as entirely forgotten in his native city as in the world at large. It was some time after this that my attention was drawn to Semmelweis and his work by Dr Duka, a Hungarian physician practising in London . . . while Semmelweis had no influence on my work, I greatly admire his labours and rejoice that his memory will be at length duly honoured.[2]

In this chapter we will explore three separate but connected themes: the evolution of Listerian antisepsis in surgical practice, the introduction of Listerian antisepsis into obstetrics, and the sudden resurrection of Semmelweis to the position of fame he holds in the history of medicine today.

Listerian Antisepsis in Surgical Practice

Lister's antiseptic method was based on Pasteur's observation that there were living organisms carried on dust particles in the air. Lister (like Braun, mentioned in the previous chapter) believed that airborne particles fell into surgical wounds and caused putrefaction. One minute germ could cause sepsis. 'Upon this principle', he said, 'I have based a practice.'[3] Between 1865 and 1867 he first used German creosote to keep out the germs, and then carbolic acid in dressings applied to wounds. He published two long papers on the antiseptic method in the *Lancet*, one in 1867, the other in 1875.

Initially, Lister believed it was essential to accept germ theory: 'We are guided by the germ theory,' he said.[4] Some of his most ardent followers believed the same, as shown in this statement by a Canadian surgeon:

to carry out the antiseptic treatment thoroughly it is almost necessary that one should be a firm believer in the germ theory, otherwise some necessary precaution is apt to be omitted which may vitiate the whole process. Just as a sentinel to be thoroughly efficient must firmly believe that enemies are hovering round eager to elude his vigilance, and

---

[2] Sir Rickman Godlee, *Lord Lister* (3rd edn., Oxford, 1924), 124. There could hardly be more striking evidence of the extent to which Semmelweis was forgotten.
[3] Granshaw, 'Upon this principle', 21.   [4] Ibid. 22.

a single portal left unguarded or a single moment's neglect may entail the loss of all, however valuable, which may have been committed to his charge.[5]

Others, however, were willing to accept Lister's technique solely on the pragmatic grounds that 'it worked'. They jibbed at having to swallow what seemed to many as the still unproved theory of the role of germs. Lister, seeing this as an obstacle to the acceptance of his method, distanced himself from putrefactive germ theory in the 1870s and invited surgeons to adopt his methods on empirical grounds. Many responded to the invitation.[6]

For some surgeons, seeing just one operation was enough to produce an almost religious conversion to antisepsis.[7] For others, Lister's published results were good enough, even if, by modern standards, the statistics were weak. Lister claimed that the mortality following amputations fell from sixteen out of thirty-five (46 per cent) to six out of forty (15 per cent) after the use of antisepsis. The result may be statistically significant,[8] but the number of cases was small, and more importantly they may have been selected: that is, the pre-antiseptic amputation cases may not have been comparable to the post-antiseptic ones. One recent author has suggested that the fall in surgical mortality associated with antisepsis may have been due to a change in the nutritional status of the patients.[9] Another has suggested more cogently that there may have been a change in the virulence of the organisms causing sepsis, especially the streptococcus.[10] My own feeling is that Lister's method was genuinely effective, and if it had been subjected to a rigorous modern style of clinical trial, its effectiveness would have been confirmed.

But it was not a method to be undertaken lightly. There were practical objections. Carbolic acid was toxic. It burnt healthy skin. Applying antisepsis was not simply a matter of pouring it onto the wound or wiping it on the skin. The frequency and manner of changing dressings, as laid down by Lister, were complicated and tiresome—too complicated for some of his opponents, who were mostly hygienists not yet converted to germ theory and who argued, with some cogency, that it was not the carbolic acid that worked but the insistence on surgical cleanliness.

Nevertheless, Lister's method was rapidly introduced into Boston and New York. Only the time it took to cross the Atlantic separated Lister's announcement of antisepsis from its publication in America, where some accepted Listerism outright, others accepted Listerism but not germ theory, and still others, such as Samuel Gross, dean of American surgeons, had no use for the carbolic acid and Lister's ideas. Some said that surgical mortality was lower in the USA than Britain because Americans were better at sanitary methods such

[5] Connor, 'Listerism unmasked', 211.

[6] Dr Michael Worboys, personal communication, 1995.

[7] As in the case of Alexander Ogston of Aberdeen (Pennington, 'Listerism, its Decline and its Persistence', 43).   [8] By the chi-square test $0.02 > P > 0.01$.

[9] D. Hamilton, 'The Nineteenth-Century Surgical Revolution—Antisepsis or Better Nutrition?' *Bulletin of the History of Medicine*, 56 (1982), 30–40.   [10] Pennington, 'Osteotomy as an Indicator', 180.

as ventilation.[11] Canadian surgeons seem to have been more easily converted to Listerism, possibly because so many of them were graduates of Scottish medical schools.[12]

Faced with such opposition, Lister added to the complexity in 1871 by inventing the famous carbolic-acid spray. Operations were undertaken under a cloud of carbolic acid and dressings consisted of eight layers of gauze impregnated with carbolic acid, with a layer of mackintosh between the two outer layers of gauze. Lister's method had become cumbersome, troublesome, and expensive, yet, paradoxically, its very complexity increased its acceptance, for it convinced many surgeons that Listerism was a surgical method and not just a fancy new dressing.[13]

In the 1870s doubt was thrown on Lister's method by Robert Koch, who showed that anthrax spores could survive immersion in carbolic acid for a week. No wonder, he said, that bacteria are so often found under Lister's dressings.[14] Koch's work led to the substitution of corrosive sublimate (mercuric chloride) for carbolic acid. Although there seemed to be evidence that corrosive sublimate was a more effective antiseptic, it was more toxic than carbolic acid, with the added disadvantage that it reacted with metals and could not be used to sterilize instruments.

Nevertheless, from the time it was introduced, Listerian antisepsis, though frequently criticized, was never in danger; it was increasingly accepted. During the 1880s the gap between the hygienists, who insisted that all that was needed was cleanliness, and the Listerites, who adopted the whole paraphernalia of spray and dressings, began to close. By 1887 Lister had abandoned the spray, and by the end of the 1880s asepsis, with the sterilization of dressings, instruments, and surgical gowns, was increasingly popular, largely as a result of the increasing acceptance of germ theory.[15] The differences of opinion outlined above may seem niggly matters of detail, but they are important in understanding not only the difficulties that surrounded antisepsis in surgery, but the link between its use in surgery and its use in obstetrics. Let me explain.

According to the older versions of the story of Listerism, the introduction of antisepsis into surgery was an overnight revolution, instantly accepted by the medical world because it was based on the widespread acceptance of germ theory. If that were true, why did it take fifteen or more years before most obstetricians followed in the footsteps of the surgeons? The answer, of course, is that there was no overnight revolution. It was a slow process argued back

---

[11] Gariepy, 'The Introduction and Acceptance of Listerian Antisepsis'.

[12] Connor, 'Listerism Unmasked'.   [13] Granshaw, 'Upon this principle', 27–8.

[14] Pennington, 'Listerism, its Decline and its Persistence', 38. In fact anthrax spores were an unfortunate choice, for they are notoriously resistant to destruction by antiseptics and they were not involved in wound sepsis, whereas streptococci and staphylococci, which were involved in wound sepsis, were much more sensitive to antiseptics.

[15] Broadly, germ theory was accepted by most of the American medical establishment by 1885 and the opposition to it had virtually disappeared by the end of the 1880s (Gariepy, 'The Introduction and Acceptance of Listerian Antisepsis', 201).

and forth. Obstetricians would certainly have heard of Listerism, but only as a method of treating surgical wounds. It belonged to surgery. Most obstetricians in Britain were physicians (in the British sense), not surgeons, and there was no immediate or obvious connection between Lister's work and puerperal fever.

Eventually, however, a few obstetricians saw the logic of introducing Lister's method into the lying-in hospitals, and oddly enough most of the early converts to Listerism in obstetrics were Continental rather than British. This may be because most of the early laboratory research in bacteriology took place on the Continent, where Listerism was at least as well known as it was in Britain. Indeed, I would challenge anyone to deny that Lister became by far the most famous British doctor in Europe in the late nineteenth century, if not the whole of the century.

Listerian Antisepsis in Obstetrics

Probably, the first obstetrician to introduce Listerian antisepsis into his lying-in hospital was the Swiss obstetrician Johann Jacob Bischoff (1841–92) of Basle, who visited Lister in Glasgow in 1868. He was so impressed by antisepsis that he went straight home and promptly introduced the same method in his obstetric clinic.[16] Fig. 9.1 shows that the result was a profound and *sustained* reduction in puerperal morbidity (cases of puerperal fever) and puerperal mortality.

Bischoff was followed by Stadfelt, director of the lying-in hospital in Copenhagen, where maternal mortality was horrendous. He was so impressed by the results of Listerian antisepsis in surgical cases in Copenhagen that in 1870 he introduced a method that was both complicated and bizarre. Before attending a midwifery case, every pupil midwife was disinfected by being placed in a small room where a 'hose connected to a window' covered her head and allowed her to breathe while 'her person and wardrobe' was exposed to 'fumes of sulphurous [sic] acid' for a quarter of an hour. Before and after every examination, midwives, and physicians (who were, incidentally, forbidden to undertake post-mortem examinations), washed their hands in a solution of carbolic acid, and instruments and metal catheters were disinfected.

When Lister introduced the carbolic-acid spray, Stadfelt followed suit, and every confinement took place under a carbolic-acid spray. 'Sponges were banished and replaced by oakum' (presumably because oakum was disposable), and the patient lay on a sack filled with chaff. Both the sack and its contents were burnt when the patient was discharged. 'The genitals were covered with carbolised oil which, of late, has been replaced by salicylic acid in ten parts of wheat flour, powdered over the parts two or three times a day.' Every patient was subjected to vaginal injections of carbolic acid twice a day. Patients were

---

[16] H. Stamm, *Ein Rückblick auf die Geschichte des Frauenspitals, Basel* (Basle, 1959), 26.

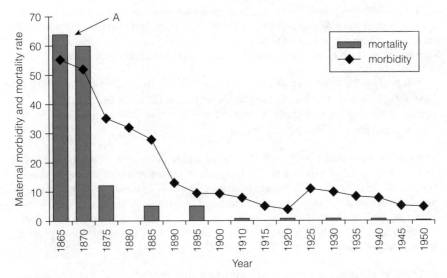

FIG. 9.1 Quinquennial maternal morbidity and mortality rates due to puerperal fever, Basle Obstetric Clinic, 1865–1950

Note: Morbidity rates measured as percentage of deliveries; mortality rates measured as maternal deaths per 10,000 deliveries.

A = introduction of antisepsis.

Source: H. Stamm, *Ein Rückblick auf die Geschichte des Frauenspitals, Basel* (Basle, 1959), 26.

kept in separate rooms and, if possible, when the patient was discharged, the room was left empty for three days and thoroughly disinfected. From 1850 to 1869 the mortality from puerperal fever in the Copenhagen lying-in hospital was 384 per 1,000 deliveries. Following the introduction of these methods, from 1870 to 1874 (inclusive) the mortality was reduced to an average of 114, with a rate of 133 in the worst year and 58 in the best.[17]

It is quite possible that, if Stadfelt had adopted a simpler regime, and in particular omitted the vaginal douching, the mortality would have been even lower. Nevertheless, Stadfelt's and Bischoff's results, when seen against the background of the previous years of awful mortality, were immensely impressive, and were achieved in the early 1870s. In the large majority of British and American lying-in hospitals, Listerian antisepsis was not adopted until the early or mid-1880s, and right up to that time the puerperal fever mortality was as bad as it had ever been. Indeed, what Evory Kennedy said in 1869 was still true in 1880:

[17] Stadfelt, *Les Maternités illustrées par la statistique de 25 ans de la Maternité de Copenhagen*, quoted in H. J. Garrigues, 'On Lying-in Institutions, Especially those of New York', *Transactions of the American Gynaecological Society*, 2 (1878), 593–649, at 606–7. F. P. Murphy, 'Ignaz Philipp Semmelweis: An Annotated Biobibliography', *Bulletin of the History of Medicine*, 20 (1946), 653–707, at 673. Other European examples of antisepsis are mentioned in Garrigues's paper.

Poor women flock to these hospitals under the impression that they are gaining a safe asylum in their hour of trial and distress; little do they imagine that they are, in their ignorance, taking a step that adds to their risks of death, in a ratio, at the very lowest calculation, of three to one, and at the highest at 20 to one, against their lives.[18]

When Listerian antisepsis was established in the majority of lying-in hospitals, however, the murderous levels of puerperal fever mortality that had persisted for 140 years became a thing of the past. By 1888 a genuine revolution had occurred, with the result that:

From being hotbeds of death and disease in which no woman could be confined without serious risk, sometimes hardly less grave than that of a capital surgical operation, in the majority of well-managed lying-in hospitals a woman is now as safe, if not safer, than if she was confined in a large and luxurious private house, with nurse, physician, and all that money can now procure. This is no exaggerated statement. Obstetric literature within the last few years teems with facts and observations proving the accuracy of what I have said.[19]

In 1888 Charles Cullingworth, who had just moved from Manchester to London, gave an address to his students that was published as a pamphlet with the significant title *Puerperal Fever: A Preventible Disease*.[20] Cullingworth, who had a strong historical sense, had just praised the work of Gordon and Semmelweis when he came to the following passage:

The discovery, some years later, of the active part played by micro-organisms in the production of septicaemia furnished the key to the whole situation. Everything was accounted for. The propagation by personal contact, the manner in which the disease dogged the footsteps of individual practitioners, and became the scourge of lying-in hospitals, the fatal results of cadaveric contamination, the deleterious influence of protracted labour, involving, as it did, repeated examinations, the almost entire immunity from the disease of women confined in the streets and elsewhere, in whom no examination was made, the success that attended the purification of the hands by means of chlorine, all these facts were now easily explained . . . How much the knowledge of the dependence of septicaemia on micro-organisms, and the methods of treatment founded upon it, have accomplished for surgery, I need not, in this hospital, remind you. What I desire to impress upon you to-day is, that they are capable of effecting an equally stupendous revolution in midwifery.[21]

This was Cullingworth, a sober, serious, and thoughtful man, at his most triumphant. To him, the sequence of events was clear. Pasteur had laid the theoretical foundations on which Listerian antisepsis was based and the application

---

[18] E. Kennedy, 'Zymotic Diseases, as More Especially Illustrated by Puerperal Fever', *Dublin Quarterly Journal of Medical Science*, 47 (1869), 269–307. Evory Kennedy was one-time Master of the Dublin Lying-in Hospital.

[19] W. S. Playfair, 'Introduction to a Discussion on the Prevention of Puerperal Fever', *British Medical Journal* (1887), ii. 1034–6, at 1034.

[20] C. J. Cullingworth, *Puerperal Fever: A Preventible Disease* (London, 1888).   [21] Ibid. 14–15.

of Lister's work to obstetrics was the basis of the 'stupendous revolution in midwifery'.

It was equally clear to W. L. Richardson, Professor of Obstetrics in Harvard University, in 1887:

Since Lister announced, in 1866, the value of antiseptics in surgical practice, the whole method of operating has been changed [and] . . . the results seem almost incredible . . . What the use of antiseptics has done for surgery it is now doing for obstetrics . . . It was not until Lister, realising the significance of Pasteur's investigations, had announced his views on antiseptic surgery, that Stadfelt, in Copenhagen, endeavoured to introduce the same method of prophylaxis in obstetric practice.[22]

He emphasized that the antiseptic revolution in the lying-in hospitals was based on Lister's method and the acceptance of the role of bacteria in surgical and puerperal sepsis. Old ideas about spontaneous generation were wrong. Bacterial infection was introduced from outside:

Puerperal fever must be considered to be a name given, for convenience, to a group of symptoms which represent an attack upon the system by one *or more* varieties of bacteria . . . The bacteria make their way in from outside. They are not born from nothing in the uterine tissues. There is no spontaneous generation about it. The vagina contains bacteria in health like the mouth, and like the bacteria in the mouth they do no harm . . . [the] pathogenic varieties are *brought* to the uterus. (emphasis in original)[23]

The Effectiveness of Listerian Antisepsis in the Lying-in Hospitals

At the end of the twentieth century we live in an age of evidence-based medicine and randomized controlled trials. We know how easily bias may sway results. Do these claims for Listerian antisepsis stand up to scrutiny? We have seen the results of Bischoff in Basle and Stadfelt in Copenhagen. Table 9.1 shows the effect of introducing antisepsis in the London General Lying-in Hospital in April 1884. It is one of the few reports to measure the effects of antisepsis in several ways, and it shows the striking fall in puerperal morbidity and mortality.

Table 9.2 shows the effect of antisepsis on the mortality in lying-in hospitals in Paris, Vienna, Boston, London, and Sweden. In all there was a dramatic decline in mortality. In the Swedish lying-in hospitals, Högberg estimates that there was a 96 per cent reduction in septic mortality as a result of antisepsis, which prevented 1,632 fatalities from puerperal fever in 69,000 admissions during the period 1881–95.[24]

---

[22] W. L. Richardson, 'The Use of Antiseptics in Obstetric Practice', *Boston Medical and Surgical Journal*, 116 (1887), 73–9, at 73.

[23] Ibid. 74. This section of the paper was written by Harold C. Ernst, Demonstrator at the Harvard Medical School.

[24] U. Högberg, *Maternal Mortality in Sweden* (Umeå University Medical Dissertations, NS 156; Umeå, 1985), 50, table 1.

TABLE 9.1. *Morbidity and Mortality, the General Lying-in Hospital, London, July 1882–April 1884 (before antisepsis) and May 1884–June 1889 (after antisepsis)*

Admissions, morbidity, and mortality	July 1882–April 1884	May 1884–June 1889
Total number of admissions	612	2,150
Maternal mortality rate from all causes (deaths per 10,000 deliveries)	98.0	41.8
Maternal mortality rate from sepsis (deaths per 10,000 deliveries)	98.0	13.9
Percentage of labours followed by fever from all causes	83	40
Percentage of labours followed by septic fever	40	2
Daily percentage of patients in hospital with fever from all causes	39	8
Daily percentage of patients in hospital with septic fever	30	2

Source: R. Boxall, 'Fever in Childbed', *Transactions of the Obstetrical Society of London*, 40 (1890), 283.

Figure 9.2 shows the reduction of mortality in Bellevue Hospital, New York. Figure 9.3 shows the reduction in maternal mortality from all causes in 1865–1902 (and from deaths due to puerperal fever in 1876–1902) in Queen Charlotte's Hospital in London as a result of introducing antisepsis in 1881. Figure 9.4 shows the effect on maternal mortality in the Liège Maternity Hospital of the introduction of antisepsis in the form of phenol (carbolic acid) in 1880 and mercury sublimate in 1884.

Nothing approaching this had occurred in any of the lying-in hospitals before. Listerian antisepsis and asepsis had already produced a remarkable improvement in wound sepsis, but the effect of Lister's method in hospital obstetrics was even more profound, and most importantly it was consistent. In every lying-in hospital that published its rates of maternal mortality and had introduced antisepsis in the early or mid-1880s, there was the same profound reduction in maternal mortality. There were, as far as I can discover, no exceptions. Delivery in lying-in hospitals became, for the first time in their existence, as safe if not safer than home deliveries.

Could the fall in mortality be due to a sudden worldwide decline in the virulence of the streptococcus? This point will be discussed later, but the brief answer is 'no'. In England and Wales, for instance, judging by national mortality rate from puerperal fever (and remembering that in all countries hospital deliveries were then only a tiny proportion of total births), streptococcal

TABLE 9.2. *Maternal mortality rates in various lying-in hospitals before and after the introduction of antisepsis in the 1880s*

Hospital	Maternal mortality rate
Paris, Maternité under Tarnier	
1858–69 (the period of inaction)	931
1870–80 (the period of isolation)	232
1881–95 (the period of antisepsis)	105
Vienna Lying-in Hospital	
1857–62	280
1863–80	160
1881–85	70
Mortality from puerperal fever 1863–80	130
Mortality from puerperal fever 1881–85	40
Boston Lying-in Hospital	
1882	555
1883	458
1884	161
1885	64
1886	0
London, General Lying-in Hospital	
1833–60	308
1861–77	170
1880–87	60
Swedish lying-in hospitals	
1864–80	270
1881–95	9.6

Note: Maternal mortality rates are expressed as maternal deaths per 10,000 deliveries.

Sources: Paris: C. J. Cullingworth, 'Biographical Note on Étienne Stéphane Tarnier', *Transactions of the Obstetrical Society of London*, 40 (1898), 78–89; Vienna, Boston, and London: C. J. Cullingworth, *Puerperal Fever: A Preventible Disease* (London, 1888); Sweden: U. Högberg, *Maternal Mortality in Sweden* (Umeå University Medical Dissertations, NS 156; Umeå, 1985), 50, table 1.

virulence was rising between 1884 and 1894, although this was the first decade that showed a profound decline in lying-in hospital mortality.

Was the decline due to a sudden improvement in the health of mothers, making them more resistant to infection? Again, the answer is 'no', for it would have been very odd if that had occurred simultaneously in all Western countries, and it would have been odder still if the improvement in general health was so great and so sudden that it could account for such a profound fall in mortality, especially when there is no evidence of a sudden worldwide improvement in maternal health during the relevant period. Further, there is firm

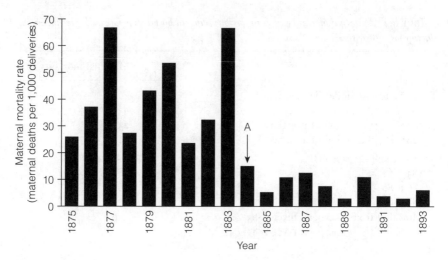

FIG. 9.2 Annual maternal mortality rates, Bellevue Hospital, New York, 1875–1893

Note: A = introduction of antisepsis.

Source: H. J. Garrigues, *The Science and Art of Obstetrics* (Philadelphia, 1902), 721–2.

evidence that changes in the social and economic status of populations had little effect on levels of maternal mortality.[25]

Finally, there is the possibility that the profound fall in mortality was due not to Listerian antisepsis but to improvements in hygiene, including isolation of infected cases. This is an interesting question, because, if one looks closely at mortality levels in some hospitals—notably in Vienna and Paris and the General Lying-in Hospital in London—a substantial fall in the level of maternal mortality had already occurred in the 1860s and 1870s before the introduction of Listerian antisepsis. This can be seen in Table 9.2. As mentioned earlier, some surgeons who initially opposed Listerism said the fall in surgical mortality was due to greater cleanliness and not to the carbolic acid and the complicated routine introduced by Lister. Could the same be said of Listerism in obstetrics?

Certainly, greater cleanliness on the wards, the use of single rooms for midwifery patients, and especially the rigid isolation of infected cases seem to have been partially effective from the evidence of Tarnier in Paris. The most obvious conclusion is that Listerian techniques and general hygienic methods worked in tandem; but it is most unlikely that greater cleanliness alone, without antisepsis, would have produced such universal and profound effects in

[25] I. Loudon, *Death in Childbirth: An International Study of Maternal Care and Maternal Mortality 1800–1950* (Oxford, 1992).

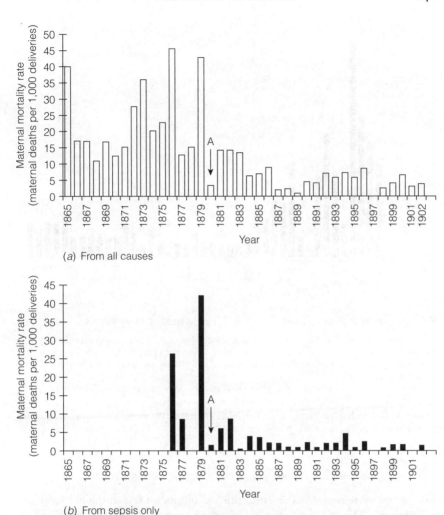

FIG. 9.3 Annual maternal mortality rates, Queen Charlotte's Hospital, London, from all causes, 1865–1902, and from sepsis only, 1876–1902

Note: No data available for maternal mortality rates from sepsis before 1876.
A = introduction of antisepsis.

Source: W. Willams, *Deaths in Childbed* (London, 1904), tables XVIII, XXI.

lying-in hospitals. Both gained credence by the fact that they were underpinned by germ theory based largely on the work of Pasteur and Koch. But it would be mistaken to imagine that, from the 1880s, all the old ideas about the cause of puerperal fever were thrown out of the window.

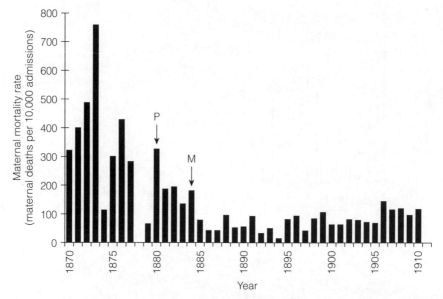

F IG. 9.4 Annual maternal mortality rates, Liège Maternity Hospital, 1870–1910

Note: Data are missing for 1878. The annual number of maternity admissions between 1870 and 1885 was low, in the region of 200–400, which accounts in part for the wide variations in mortality rates. From about 1897, the number of admissions rose from 900 a year to over 1,000 by 1909.

Introduction of antisepsis: P = introduction of phenol; M = introduction of mercury sublimate.

Source: J.-L. Louche, 'La Maternité de Liège ou cent ans de l'évolution d'un hospice', *Annales de la Société Belge d'Histoire des Hôpitaux et de la Santé Publique*, 22 (1984), 5–25.

The Acceptance of Germ Theory and the Adoption of Antisepsis

For senior obstetricians, the antiseptic revolution was a difficult period of adjustment. The views of the multicausalists that they had supported so strongly in 1875 were under attack, but they still persisted. In 1883 a Dr Cory (MD St Andrews) of Essex wrote to the *Lancet* to say that he had known of cases of puerperal fever due to bad drainage, the escape of sewer gas, open gully holes near a house or a bedroom, surface drainage from other houses passing in ditches and watercourses, closets placed over stagnant ponds near the house, especially common at farmhouses, and dirty pigsties near the dwellings of the poor.[26] One might dismiss this as the view of an ignorant provincial doctor, but the eminent obstetrician W. S. Playfair, while allowing that antisepsis was essential, insisted in 1884 that: 'Exposure to sewer gas may, I feel sure, produce the disease . . . the whole question of defective sanitary conditions on the puerperal

---

[26] Correspondence, *Lancet* (1883), i. 230.

state deserves much more serious study than it has ever yet received . . .'[27] In 1887 J. W. Byers laid more stress on defective sanitation and sewer gas than on bacteria,[28] and even Professor C. J. Cullingworth, one of the earliest and strongest converts to germ theory, believed in 1888 that there were two forms of puerperal fever, the bacterial form, and the putrefactive form that could by itself produce a poison independently of bacteria:

The great difference between puerperal fever caused by septic bacteria and that caused by putrefaction is, that whereas in the former there is a living, self-multiplying poison in the system, which, once introduced, must run its course . . . in the latter the poison, though capable, if left to itself, of producing deadly results is, if the source of the poison be removed, and its absorption arrested, quickly eliminated from the system, with entire relief to the dangerous symptoms.[29]

Nevertheless, germ theory was advancing so rapidly that the bacteria that caused puerperal fever were soon identified and classified by their appearance. A. H. Freeland Barbour wrote in 1888 that the 'germs' described in connection with puerperal fever were '1. Monococcus, 2. Diplococcus, 3. Chains of micrococci, 4. Chains of micrococci in S-shaped forms or in larger aggregations, 5. Rod-shaped bacteria. It is category 3 that seems most often associated with puerperal fever.'[30] There were rapid advances in bacteriology, especially the use of aniline dyes to stain bacteria and nuclei, and the recognition of toxins produced by bacteria. The author of an American textbook in 1889 was prepared to go further than most of his colleagues and assert that 'All that class of diseases known as "infectious wound diseases" are today known to be due to the activity of micro-organisms.'[31]

The actual methods of antisepsis and asepsis differed only in detail from one lying-in hospital to another. Most began with phenol but changed to mercurial preparations, especially corrosive sublimate in a strength of 1 in 1,000 or 1 in 2,000 as a result of the work of Koch, who, rather than Pasteur, was usually cited as the authority who had put germ theory on a sound basis.[32]

In the General Lying-in Hospital in London, carbolic acid was replaced by Condy's fluid (potassium permanganate) combined with an emphasis on greater hygiene, 'particularly as regards the midwives and nurses'. But there was no convincing improvement until May 1884, when they changed to sublimate of mercury (the same as corrosive sublimate), when 'septicaemia disappeared entirely, at any rate for a time . . .'.[33] All patients were douched with

---

[27] W. S. Playfair, *A Treatise on the Science and Art of Midwifery* (2 vols.; 5th edn., London, 1884), i. 344.
[28] J. W. Byers, 'The Prevention of Puerperal Fever in Private Practice', *British Medical Journal* (1887), ii. 1042–4. [29] Cullingworth, *Puerperal Fever: A Preventible Disease*, 17.
[30] A. H. Freeland Barbour, 'Pathology of the Post-Partum Uterus', *Edinburgh Medical Journal*, 31 (1885), 434–44, at 441–2.
[31] H. C. Ernst, 'The Etiology of Puerperal Fever', in B. C. Hirst (ed.), *A System of Obstetrics by American Authors* (2 vols.; Edinburgh, 1889), ii. 401–59, at 401.
[32] Barbour, 'Pathology of the Post-Partum Uterus'.
[33] R. Boxall, 'Fever in Childbed', *Transactions of the Obstetrical Society of London*, 40 (1890), 219–43, 264–70, 275–303, at 224.

antiseptic on admission and again after delivery, and there were three basins in each delivery ward—one for washing with soap and water, one for hand-washing in disinfectant, and a third for the disinfection of instruments.[34]

In the USA, the Boston Lying-in Hospital had suffered as much as any other lying-in hospital from recurrent epidemics of puerperal fever, and the hospital was closed for several weeks in 1879, 1880, and again in 1883 so that the wards could be fumigated. Each time the hospital was free from infection for only a few weeks. 'During the ten years preceding 1884, the hospital was rarely free from septic disease of one form or another.'[35] To prevent the intro-duction of septic material from without, and to prevent putrefaction getting a hold within the uterus, obstetricians began in 1883 to use intrauterine injec-tions of phenol, but soon found that this alone was ineffective.[36] In the winter of 1883–4 they changed to corrosive sublimate, both for intrauterine injections and to disinfect the hands of birth attendants. This led to an immediate fall in mortality, but, when they heard of Robert Koch's recent work, they realized that all infection came from without and abandoned the injections, realizing that they did 'as much harm as good'. From 1885 the Boston Lying-in Hos-pital adopted a strict antiseptic and aseptic regime, which included sterilizing instruments, using corrosive sublimate to sterilize the hands of attendants every time before they touched the patient, washing the genitalia of patients with cor-rosive sublimate (but not vaginal douching), and using antiseptic pads during the lying-in period.[37]

Similar methods were described by many authors. There is little doubt that germ theory led to a much greater standard of ordinary cleanliness in the wards and in the delivery rooms, but, unlike the practice of general surgeons, the use of rubber gloves by obstetricians was a rarity and the wearing of sterile gowns unknown. An investigation by Lea in 1910 showed that, in fifteen leading British and European lying-in hospitals, gloves were worn never or rarely in six hospitals, only in cases of infection in two, and always or almost always only in three (in the remainder no information was supplied).[38]

The most disputed part of the antiseptic regime was the dangerous prac-tice (especially when corrosive sublimate was used) of vaginal and intrauterine douching. On this, there were two schools of thought. One, the endogenous (or autogenic-infection) school, held that douching was essential, because in most cases the bacteria that caused puerperal fever were already present in the genital tract of the woman, and had to be eliminated by douching. There was a powerful motive for supporting the endogenous theory of puerperal infection; it exonerated obstetricians and midwives from the accusation that they were responsible for introducing infection.

The other school, the exogenous school, held that puerperal fever was always due to the introduction of bacteria from outside, chiefly on the hands

[34] R. Boxall, 'Fever in Childbed', *Transactions of the Obstetrical Society of London*, 40 (1890), 268–9.
[35] Richardson, 'The Use of Antiseptics'.   [36] Ibid. 75.   [37] Ibid. 76.
[38] A. Lea, *Puerperal Infection* (London, 1910).

or instruments of birth attendants. They agreed with the endogenists that bacteria could be found in the genital tract of healthy parturients, but they said that these were not the bacteria which caused puerperal fever. Thus there was no logical support for douching out the vagina with strong and potentially poisonous antiseptics. The exogenists rightly insisted that hands, instruments, and dressings introduced into the genital tract of women during and after labour must be sterilized and free from bacteria.

The heated debate between the two schools, which began in the 1880s, was still echoing round the hospital corridors in the 1920s. There were endogenists and exogenists in every country, but Germany was at the forefront of the endogenous school, while in Britain and America the majority of obstetricians were exogenists. It is surprising, therefore, that it was a report from Dresden rather than London or New York that first showed that vigorous douching not only failed to reduce, but actually increased, the mortality from puerperal fever. This was followed by other reports that persuaded most British and American obstetricians that vaginal douching was likely to do more harm than good, and, although douching persisted for thirty to forty years in a few lying-in hospitals, in the end it was abandoned.[39]

The success of Listerian antisepsis in the lying-in hospitals leads us to our next subject: the sudden and unexpected 'resurrection' of Semmelweis's reputation, which is a splendid illustration of the process by which accolades are awarded and 'great names' are created in science and medicine.

On Reputations, Statues, and Prizes: The Resurrection of Semmelweis

For the reasons that were discussed at length in Chapter 7, Semmelweis had little influence either in his lifetime or for some twenty or more years after his death in 1865. If mentioned at all, he was seen as a rather obscure minor figure whose dogmatic views were unpleasantly controversial. Spaeth, formerly an opponent of Semmelweis, made an interesting comment in 1864:

What consideration, then, does Semmelweis' theory merit? . . . the minds of men, grown so heated in this controversy, may have again become cooled off to the extent, that one may now speak calmly about it . . . Certainly, the theory would have gained more obstetricians as open friends, if in the beginning Semmelweis had not represented the

---

[39] There are three important papers that span the endogenous debates. The first covers the end of the nineteenth century: C. Jewett, 'The Question of Puerperal Self-Infection', *American Gynaecological and Obstetrical Journal*, 8 (1896), 417–29. The second is a useful review of opinions in the 1920s: G. F. Gibberd, 'Streptococcal Puerperal Sepsis', *Guy's Hospital Reports*, 81 (1931), 29–44. The third produced the decisive evidence showing the exogenous school was right: L. Colebrook, 'The Prevention of Puerperal Sepsis', *Journal of Obstetrics and Gynaecology of the British Empire*, 43 (1936), 691–714.

facts, most obvious to him from one point of view, as the whole, and later defended his theory in a tone which no man of science had been accustomed to up to this time . . . *I also venture to state unreservedly that there is no longer any obstetrician, who is not most deeply convinced of the correctness of Semmelweis' views, even though he may still talk very much against them.* (emphasis added)[40]

An example is provided by the British obstetrician Playfair. In 1884 he wrote that, in puerperal fever, 'just as in surgical pyaemia, any decomposing organic matter, either originating within the generative organs of the patient herself, or coming from without, may set up the morbid action.' That might have been written by Semmelweis himself, but Playfair gave no credit to Semmelweis and only mentioned him briefly in passing.[41]

Nearly all British authors referred warmly to Simpson's 1850 paper on the analogy between surgical fever and puerperal fever, but very few praised Semmelweis before 1885.[42] As late as 1885 a British obstetrician, Dr Priestly, published an account of a tour across the whole of Europe and as far as Russia in which he surveyed puerperal fever in many countries and investigated the success of antisepsis in home and hospital deliveries. But he never once mentioned the name of Semmelweis.[43]

Much the same applies to the French authors.[44] By 1880 almost everyone who wrote about puerperal fever mentioned Louis Pasteur, Robert Koch, and Joseph Lister. A few German authors treated Semmelweis seriously, probably because August Hirsch opened the chapter on puerperal fever in his magnificent work on geographical and historical pathology with a rather charming subtitle: 'The Modern Doctrine started by Semmelweis and continued by Hirsch'. Hirsch allows that Semmelweis's 'view of the causative conditions was one-sided' but he adds that 'he was still a true pioneer . . . and his work was of great service not only to the Vienna Lying-in Hospital but to mankind at large. I take credit to myself for having, in the first edition of this work, stood forward as his exponent and for having directed the attention of the profession in Germany to his writings, which had been little noticed up to that time.'[45] Even

[40] Josef Spaeth, *Med. Jahrbericht*, 20/1 (1864), 145–64, quoted in Murphy, 'Ignaz Philipp Semmelweis: An Annotated Biobibliography', 669–70.

[41] Playfair, *A Treatise on the Science and Art of Midwifery*, ii. 336–7.

[42] J. Y. Simpson, 'Some Notes on the Analogy between Puerperal Fever and Surgical Fever', *London and Edinburgh Monthly Journal of Medical Science* (Nov. 1850), 414–29. Simpson, as we noted before, was one of the few British authors to speak warmly about Semmelweis; but that was before Semmelweis had published his quarrelsome treatise.

[43] W. O. Priestly, 'Notes on a Visit to Some of the Lying-in Hospitals in the North of Europe, and Particularly of the Advantages of the Antiseptic System in Obstetric Practice', *Transactions of the Obstetrical Society of London*, 27 (1885), 197–222.

[44] Léon Le Fort, in his massive work *Des maternités: Études sur les maternités et les institutions charitables d'accouchement à domicile dans les principaux états de l'Europe* (Paris, 1866) fails to give any credit to Semmelweis, and he was not mentioned in the debate between Hervieux and Pasteur or the work by Doléris, both of which were discussed in Chapter 8.

[45] A. Hirsch, *Handbook of Geographical and Historical Pathology* (2nd edn., 1881), trans. C. Creighton (3 vols.; London, 1883), ii. 416.

in Germany, however, the influence of Semmelweis was slight.[46] Beneath the surface, Semmelweis may have had more influence than many cared to admit at the time, but the first sign of impending canonization appeared in a two-part paper published by a fellow Hungarian in the *Lancet* in 1886. The author was a surgeon, Theodore Duka (1825–1908).[47]

Theodore Duka and Semmelweis

Duka, who was born in north-west Hungary, took part as a soldier in the Hungarian war of liberation, and settled *c*.1850 in London, where he learnt English and supported himself by teaching German at the Birkbeck Institution. He became a naturalized British subject, qualified in medicine, holding first the MRCS and then the FRCS by examination, and joined the Indian Medical Service, serving with the Bengal army and reaching the rank of Lieutenant-Colonel.[48]

In writing about Semmelweis he was probably motivated by his Hungarian origin, and may have seen Semmelweis as a fellow liberal. There is no evidence he took part in obstetric practice at any time in his career. Duka, who based his paper on a monograph on Semmelweis written by Jacob Bruck in 1885 and translated into German in 1887,[49] gives a plain account of Semmelweis's work, and presents him as a man who was unjustly neglected and opposed, largely on political grounds. He adds that:

It required far more robustness of intellect and character than Semmelweis possessed to front the opposition which his doctrines evoked . . . Semmelweis became introspective, desponding, irritable and at last unreasonable. He had indomitable industry, a sagacious insight amounting almost to genius, but he had little of the fortitude which enables a man to *labour* and to *wait*.[50]

This paved the way for presenting the story of Semmelweis as it has been presented in countless publications ever since—the story of the neglected genius, great scientist, and pioneer of antisepsis, the man who saved the lives of countless childbearing women, the author of one of the greatest treatises in

---

[46] Schröder wrote a report in 1878 on puerperal fever in Berlin and Prussia in which it is stated the puerperal fever 'is indeed nothing else than the infecting of fresh wounds . . . with organic materials in a state of putrefaction', which may be intrinsic or extrinsic. This is exactly Semmelweis's doctrine, but Semmelweis is not mentioned (C. Schröder *et al.*, 'Report Prepared by the Puerperal Fever Committee of the Berlin Obstetrical Society, and Laid before the Prussian Minister of Public Health, Dr Falk', trans. from the *Zeitschrift für Geburtschülfe und Gynäkologie*, vol. III, part 1, by Dr Charles E. Underhill, *Edinburgh Medical Journal*, 24 (1878), 435–46.

[47] Theodore Duka, 'Childbed Fever, its Cause and Prevention: A Life's History', *Lancet* (1886), ii. 206–8, 246–8. A biographical paper was also published in America in the same year: P. Herdegen, 'Ignaz Philipp Semmelweis (1818–1865)', *American Journal of Obstetrics of New York*, 18 (1886), 248–55.

[48] The biographical details come from the *Medical Directory* for various years and from an obituary notice of Duka published in the *Lancet* (1908), i. 1520.

[49] Duka, 'Childbed Fever', ii. 206. Bruck was described as 'a member of the Board of Health in Buda-Pesth' [*sic*] and provided the first translation into German of Semmelweis's treatise: Jacob Bruck, *Ignaz Philipp Semmelweis: Eine geschichtlich-medicinische Studie* (Vienna, 1887).　　[50] Ibid. 247–8.

the nineteenth century, and the martyr who died of the very disease to which he had devoted his life.

Semmelweis's Rise to Posthumous Fame

In the late 1880s, British obstetricians, excited by the effects of Listerian anti-sepsis on hospital mortality, suddenly discovered (or rediscovered) that anti-sepsis had been practised by Semmelweis forty years previously, and felt guilty at the neglect of the pioneer of antisepsis in midwifery. Cullingworth sang his praises in 1887.[51] Fothergill of Edinburgh presented Semmelweis as a pioneer and misunderstood martyr in his textbook published in 1896.[52] Almost every-one who wrote on puerperal fever after 1887 added their praises, but hero worship reached its greatest heights when Sir William Sinclair published his large and detailed biography of Semmelweis in 1909, which is as blatant an example of hagiography as one could wish to see, and which has formed the basis of numerous accounts of Semmelweis that have appeared ever since.[53]

Obstetricians felt that Semmelweis had suffered so much neglect in his life-time that he deserved a more permanent memorial than a series of articles. Therefore, as noted in the *Lancet* in 1892:

A preliminary meeting was held . . . at the house of Sir Spencer Wells, who occupied the chair, at which it was agreed to call a general meeting in October to consider the best way of promoting a memorial of Semmelweis and his great services to humanity. There were present Sir Joseph Lister, Dr Priestly, Dr Playfair, Dr Grailly Hewitt, Dr Glover, Dr Black, Dr Boxall and Dr Duka.[54]

A series of meetings was held over the next few months. Only the obstetrician Robert Lee, who said (correctly) that Semmelweis had unjustifiably ignored Brit-ish work, added a note of dissent to the chorus of hero worship.[55] Eventually, on 30 September 1906, a statue of Semmelweis was unveiled in Budapest in the presence of his widow. Representatives from all over Europe attended the ceremony. Duka was the British representative.[56]

Why did Semmelweis become a hero at this particular time? Until the mid-1880s the problem of puerperal fever in the lying-in hospitals appeared to be insoluble. When the antiseptic revolution arrived in the 1880s, Semmelweis's dogmatism and other faults were forgotten. Credit was transferred, so to speak, from Lister to Semmelweis, and the fact that Semmelweis had made so little impact on mortality from puerperal fever was conveniently forgotten. Instead, it appeared that at last his theories were justified. Semmelweis was as close to being 'right' as it was possible to have been in the pre-bacterial days of 1847.

[51] Cullingworth, *Puerperal Fever: A Preventible Disease.*
[52] W. E. Fothergill, *Manual of Midwifery* (Edinburgh, 1896).
[53] Sir William Sinclair, *Semmelweis, his Life and his Doctrine* (Manchester, 1909).
[54] *Lancet* (1892), ii. 267. Apart from Spencer Wells, Lister, and Duka (all surgeons), the rest were prominent obstetricians.   [55] Ibid. 897, 1012, 1020, 1116.
[56] *Lancet* (1906), ii. 1020.

But there is another reason of great importance. A revolutionary theory is much more likely to be accepted if it is supported by a demonstrable, or at least a plausible, mechanism or rationale. The old saying: 'It is all very well in practice, but will it work in theory' is more than a neat joke. It encapsulates a way of thinking. Treatments in modern medicine usually demand a rationale before they are accepted, however strong the experimental evidence. And of course the same applies to biological and physical sciences.

In 1912 the German geologist Alfred Wegener (d. 1932), noting that the east coast of South America fitted snugly into the west coast of Africa (and the 'fit' is even more convincing if you map the continents a little below sea level), suggested that they had originally been one continent that had split into two parts and drifted apart. No one took him seriously. The idea of large continents floating about like boats on the ocean seemed ridiculous, until, in the 1960s, the mechanism of continental drift was shown to be due to molten mantle welling up through rifts in the floor of the Atlantic, forcing the sea floor to widen and push the two continents apart. Once this had been accepted, the science of plate tectonics was born.[57]

Lister succeeded where Gordon, Holmes, and Semmelweis had failed, because bacteriology provided a demonstrable mechanism by which puerperal fever was transmitted. Neither Gordon nor Holmes could explain the mechanism of contagion, and, although Semmelweis went some way towards doing so, his theory of 'morbid matter' was inadequate and the defects in his character were no help to the acceptance of his ideas. Nevertheless we are left with the need to explain why Semmelweis, a deeply flawed man almost totally forgotten in 1880, was the subject of such an extraordinary degree of hagiography, for there is almost no one else in the history of medicine who has risen so rapidly and completely from deep neglect and obscurity to extreme fame.

Probably the answer lies in the change in the public image of medicine in the 1880s and 1890s, a period devoted to the creation of the great men and women of medicine and science. It was a period when, in the words of the historian W. F. Bynum, 'medical science goes public', and medical scientists became famous outside as well as inside the profession.[58] It was a period marked by the cult of great men, who were 'showered with national and international awards, decorations, and sometimes high office. On their death they were awarded magnificent state funerals in the national shrine.'[59] It was a time when the streets, avenues, and boulevards were filled with statues of doctors, scientists, and engineers rather than emperors and generals. It was a time when research institutes named after famous doctors were created (Pasteur, Koch, and Lister), when named lectures were created in abundance, when huge International Congresses

[57] I. Asimov, *Asimov's New Guide to Science* (London, 1987), 158.

[58] Bynum, *Science and the Practice of Medicine in the Nineteenth Century*; 'Medical Science Goes Public' is the title of ch. 6, pp. 142–75.

[59] L. Ward, 'The Cult of Relics: Pasteur Material at the Science Museum', *Medical History*, 38 (1994), 54–5.

of Science and Medicine were held in the capitals of the Western world, when rich awards such as the Nobel prizes were given to doctors and scientists. In short, it was a time when the 'great men' of science and medicine were cele-brated with an unselfconscious fervour that is rather less fashionable today.

There were many celebrated physicians and surgeons. But there were no internationally famous obstetricians. The problem was a shortage of suitable candidates. Alexander Gordon of Aberdeen, an obscure general practitioner in a remote Scottish city, was certainly not in the running. Nor was Oliver Wendell Holmes, whose sole contribution to obstetrics was a single essay, unknown in most of Europe. Only Semmelweis had, or seemed to have, the necessary qualities, and he had them in abundance. He was someone with whom the medical élite of the twentieth century could identify, because he was a physician who had worked in a famous teaching hospital and had carried out a clinical trial that—by accident not design—was a randomized trial.[60] He was seen to be modern in the way he used scientific methods, and, although very few had ever read or even seen it, he had published a famous treatise. Above all, he was a man 'before his time' and for that reason had been cruelly rejected and driven to his grave by his less brilliant contemporaries. What more could you ask of a hero? So twentieth-century obstetricians embraced Semmelweis as their very own great historical figure, and presented him as a role model for students. If Semmelweis had failings, it was, in the words of the usually cool and sober Garrison, because 'his sensitive nature was not equal to the strain of violent controversy, and brooding over his wrongs brought on insanity and death. He is one of medicine's martyrs and, in the future, will be one of its far-shining names, for every childbearing woman owes something to him.'[61]

[60] Randomized in the sense that the patients were allocated to the first and second clinics purely on the grounds of the day of the week, and not on clinical grounds.

[61] F. H. Garrison, *An Introduction to the History of Medicine* (4th edn., Philadelphia, 1929), 436–7.

10

Puerperal Fever in the
Early Twentieth Century

During the final years of the nineteenth century, germ theory had established a totally new set of concepts about the nature of infectious or 'zymotic' diseases. There had never been quite such a radical change in medicine. In a remarkably short time preventive treatment was becoming a reality. One aspect was the use of vaccines, which we will explore in the next chapter. The other, of course, was antisepsis.

Although it received little attention outside the world of obstetrics, the undoubted success of antisepsis produced a surge of optimism after years of shameful mortality. Most obstetricians believed that puerperal fever would soon be abolished. Cullingworth told his students that puerperal fever was now a preventible disease, and an American obstetrician wrote in 1902, 'We know that hospital mortality has been reduced almost to *nil* . . . in view of the splendid results which hospitals prove attainable, deaths should be few indeed in the community.'[1]

The Optimism Arising from Antisepsis

In Britain, Dr W. Williams, Medical Officer of Health to the Glamorgan County Council, informed the Royal College of Physicians in the Milroy Lectures in 1904 that mortality in lying-in hospitals had 'decreased to the vanishing point' as a result of antisepsis. Hospital delivery was now at least as safe, if not safer than, home deliveries, and he felt sure that home deliveries would soon follow suit.[2]

Others took up the same theme, showing that the reduction in hospital mortality was occurring everywhere. When an Australian Government Committee issued a report on maternal mortality in 1917, it positively rejoiced at the successes due to antisepsis in lying-in hospitals all over the world:

---

[1] G. J. Englemann, 'Birth and Death Rate as influenced by Obstetric and Gynecic Progress', *Boston Medical and Surgical Journal*, 146 (1902), 505–8, 541–4.

[2] W. Williams, *Deaths in Childbed* (London, 1904), being the Milroy Lectures delivered at the Royal College of Physicians of London, 1904.

In 1907, in Pinard's wards in the Hospital Baudelocque in Paris, there were 3,304 accouchements and only one mother died. Professor O. von Herff in the same year reported that, at his own hospital in Basle, among 6,000 cases confined in the previous fourteen years, not a single woman died of puerperal fever contracted in the hospital . . . At the Rotunda Hospital in Dublin, in 1907–8, 2,060 women were confined, and only three died from puerperal sepsis, and in each of the three the infection occurred outside of the hospital. At the York Lying-in Hospital, Lambeth, during sixteen years, 8,373 deliveries took place, and there was not a single death due to infection occurring inside the hospital . . . The Sydney Women's Hospital in 1904 reported ten years' work with nearly 4,000 cases, and not one death from puerperal sepsis. As Sir Harry Allen pointed out . . . in 1908, 'it is not a question of fine homes or comfortable surroundings. In out-patient practice, amidst the squalor of East London, the British Lying-in Hospital recorded 30,000 cases with only three deaths from septic causes.'[3]

This upbeat report was joined to a stern warning. Those who strayed from the antiseptic pathway were not likely to be forgiven:

Puerperal septicaemia is probably the gravest reproach which any civilized nation can by its own negligence offer to itself. It can be prevented by a degree of care which is not excessive or meticulous, requiring only ordinary intelligence and some careful training. It has been abolished in the hospitals, and it should cease to exist throughout the general community. It should be as rare as sepsis after a surgical operation.[4]

That was the general, the logical, view. Antisepsis in midwifery was relatively simple. It needed no special skills or expensive apparatus. What had been achieved in the hospitals could be, should be, and everyone expected would be, soon achieved in home deliveries. All that was needed was a little training and the will to put that training into practice.

Because the number of women delivered in hospital was such a very small percentage of total births, the reduction in hospital mortality had not produced a visible downturn in the national records of any country, but there was, by 1900, every reason to expect a massive downturn in maternal mortality in the near future. And to everyone's delight, it seemed at first that this was occurring.

The Decline in Puerperal Fever between 1890 and 1912

Between 1890 and the First World War, there was a decline in maternal mortality in England and Wales, as well as in Scotland, as can be seen in Fig. 10.1. It was not nearly as dramatic as the decline in hospital mortality, but it seemed like a reasonable start. At the beginning of the 1890s there were about 25 deaths from puerperal fever for every 10,000 births, with a peak of 33 in 1893. By 1910 the rate had fallen to about 13 or 14 in England and Wales and 16 or 17 in Scotland.

---

[3] Department of Trades and Customs, Commonwealth of Australia, *Committee Concerning Causes of Death and Invalidity in the Commonwealth* (Government Printer for the State of Victoria, 1916). 'Report on Maternal Mortality in Childbirth' (1917), C7867, p. 2.   [4] Ibid. 9.

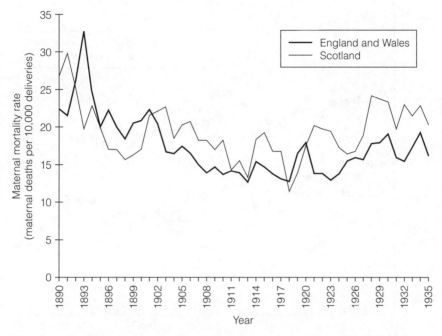

FIG. 10.1. Annual maternal mortality rates due to puerperal fever, England and Wales, and Scotland, 1890–1935

Sources: Annual Reports of the Registrar General for England and Wales; Annual Reports of the Registrar General for Scotland.

The obvious explanation for this decline was antisepsis, but could there be some other explanation? Levels of mortality as low as those around 1910–12 had been recorded long before antisepsis in certain years in the 1860s and again in the years following the all-time peak of 1874. But there had never before been a downward trend that stretched over some twenty years. How, then, can one tell whether this decline was due to medical intervention in the form of antisepsis, or some other factor?

It is a historical commonplace that deaths from a wide range of infectious diseases—tuberculosis, measles, diphtheria, and scarlet fever are examples—began to decline in the late nineteenth or early twentieth century and continued to fall thereafter. Improvements in social and economic conditions are held to be the factors behind this transition. Changes in clinical or bedside medicine played little or no part before the 1930s.

Thus, the post-1890 decline in puerperal fever and erysipelas may simply have followed the general trend for infectious diseases—a trend associated with social and economic improvements. If that was true, then we would expect to see a much steeper fall in deaths from puerperal fever than other infectious diseases, including erysipelas, because puerperal fever was the one infectious

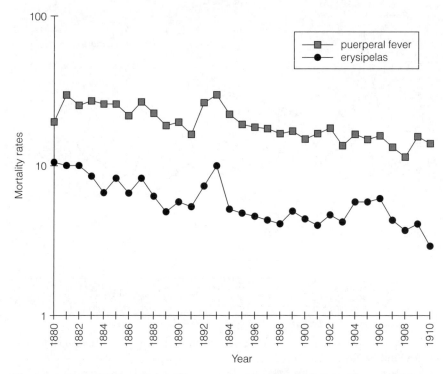

F IG. 10.2 Annual maternal mortality rates due to puerperal fever, and mortality rates due to erysipelas, London, 1880–1910

Note: Maternal mortality rates measured as deaths per 10,000 deliveries; mortality rates measured as annual deaths per 100,000 living; logarithmic scale.

Source: *Annual Reports of the Registrar General for England and Wales.*

disease for which a genuinely effective method of prevention (Listerian anti-sepsis) was available. In fact, there are good reasons for believing that the post-1890 decline in puerperal-fever mortality had little if anything to do either with antisepsis or with improved social and economic conditions. What is the evidence for this?

We have already noted, and will stress again in Chapter 12, the extremely close link between deaths from puerperal fever and deaths from erysipelas, suggesting that these two diseases (but not scarlet fever) were probably caused by the same strains or serotypes of the Group A streptococcus. Fig. 10.2 shows the trend in mortality for puerperal fever and erysipelas in London between 1880 and 1910. The general pattern, and above all the *rate* of fall, in the mortality from these two closely linked diseases were virtually identical.[5] Deaths

---

[5] The same closely linked pattern was seen for England and Wales as a whole.

from erysipelas, however, could not have been affected by the introduction of antisepsis. If antisepsis was a factor in puerperal fever, the decline in deaths from this disease should have been much steeper than it was in erysipelas. Even more telling is the way that the fall in deaths from puerperal fever and erysipelas lasted only until about 1912, when mortality rates of both diseases began to rise again and, as before, to keep in step with each other. Mortality from other infectious diseases, such as those cited above, continued to fall through the 1920s and into the 1930s. Why were puerperal fever and erysipelas different?

The probable reason is that the major determinant of mortality from puerperal fever in any given year was the virulence of the prevailing strains of the Group A streptococcus. It is difficult to find any other explanation for the rapid succession of peaks and troughs in mortality that was so characteristic of the trend in mortality in the nineteenth century in England and Wales (see Fig. 12.1) and also in other countries. The most likely explanation for the decline in mortality from puerperal fever and erysipelas between about 1890 and 1912 is a decline in the virulence of the streptococcal strains that prevailed throughout these years. After 1912 it is likely that new and more virulent strains appeared that led to the reversal of the decline. It is worth noting that what happened in England and Wales also happened in Scotland. There, too, an initial fall in puerperal fever mortality was succeeded by a steep rise from about 1912 (Fig. 10.1).

While the lying-in hospitals were maintaining a low level of puerperal-fever mortality, the situation in home deliveries was quite different. The anticipated fall in puerperal deaths in home deliveries did not occur. At least, not in Britain. Indeed, the suspicion that the fall in deaths from puerperal fever in Britain between 1890 and the First World War had very little to do with antisepsis turns into a near certainty when we see what happened in other countries with different systems of maternal care.

Puerperal Fever and Midwives in North-West Europe

There was a marked difference between Britain and the countries of north-west Europe.[6] In Sweden, Norway, Denmark, and the Netherlands, where a large majority of home deliveries were undertaken by trained and supervised midwives, antisepsis was used conscientiously in home deliveries soon after it was introduced in the period 1880–90. In England and Wales the formal training of midwives did not begin until 1902, and home deliveries were in the hands of untrained midwives and general practitioners, who often used antiseptic techniques imperfectly or not at all.

---

[6] This is explored in detail in I. Loudon, *Death in Childbirth: An International Study of Maternal Care and Maternal Mortality 1800–1950* (Oxford, 1992).

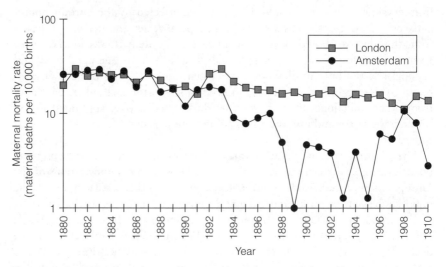

FIG. 10.3 Annual maternal mortality rates due to puerperal fever, London and Amsterdam, 1880–1910

Note: Logarithmic scale.

Sources: *Annual Reports of the Registrar General for England and Wales*, *Amsterdam Statistical Bulletin* (Amsterdam Bureau of Statistics).

Fig. 10.3 compares mortality from puerperal fever in London and Amsterdam. The two towns started at almost exactly the same level in the 1880s, but, from about 1892, the mortality in Amsterdam fell much more steeply than it did in London.[7] In the fifteen years 1896–1910 the average puerperal fever mortality in London was 15.1 per 10,000 births. In Amsterdam it was only 5.2.

Further evidence comes from Denmark, where the regulation of midwives was tightened up by the Royal Board of Health in 1861, and again in 1877, when midwives were required to notify all cases of puerperal fever. In contrast to Britain, medical practitioners in Denmark rarely attended normal deliveries, except in the case of some affluent families, because the highly respected Danish midwife was a state midwife, not an independent, untrained, and unsupervised midwife, as found in Britain before 1902.

Printed leaflets were sent to all Danish midwives in 1871 with instructions on how to avoid infection by boiling instruments, and by the use of antiseptics combined with a high standard of personal cleanliness. From the 1890s there was a steady improvement in the status and image of the midwife, reinforced by new legislation in 1914, which stressed the importance of antisepsis. By the 1920s, although it was common for affluent families to employ the family

---

[7] The wide annual variation in mortality in Amsterdam compared with London is probably due to random variation associated with the small numbers in that city. In 1901 the population of London was 6.6 million, while the population of Amsterdam was only half a million.

TABLE 10.1. *Maternal mortality rates from puerperal fever, Copenhagen and Danish provincial towns, 1860–1899*

Years	Copenhagen including the Lying-in Hospital	Copenhagen excluding the Lying-in Hospital	Provincial towns in Denmark
1860–4	235.5	124.5	45.8
1865–9	107.5	69.4	57.2
1870–4	79.4	69.8	62.2
1875–9	46.9	43.8	41.4
1880–4	36.6	35.1	30.6
1885–9	31.6	31.8	24.4
1890–4	23.5	24.4	28.1
1895–9	18.5	17.2	18.3

Note: Maternal mortality rates are expressed as deaths per 10,000 deliveries.

Source: E. Inglerslev, 'Den Puerperale Mortalitet I Provinsbyerne of Kobenhaven for Tidsrummet 1860–1899', *Tidsskrift for Jordemodre*, 6 (1903), 76, table II.

doctor, a midwife, and a nurse for childbirth, the large majority of births were still attended by a midwife alone.[8]

We can now look at Table 10.1 and Fig. 10.4, which show the mortality rate from puerperal fever (per 10,000 births) in Copenhagen, and in the provincial towns of Denmark from 1860 to 1899. In the first five-year period, 1860–4, what is striking is the very high death rate from puerperal fever. It was 235 deaths per 10,000 births if deaths in the city's lying-in hospital and deaths in home deliveries are added together as total Copenhagen deaths. This is shown in Fig. 10.4 as 'Copenhagen 1'. But it was only 124 in Copenhagen if deaths in the lying-in hospital were excluded; this is shown in Fig. 10.4 as 'Copenhagen 2'.[9]

In contrast the mortality rate in provincial towns, where there were no lying-in hospitals, was much lower. The rate was 46 in 1860–4 rising to a peak of 62 in 1870–4 before starting to decline. But even this was high compared with London and the whole of England and Wales, where the highest annual rate

[8] A. Løkke, 'The Antiseptic Transformation of Danish Midwives 1860–1920', in H. Marland and A.-M. Rafferty (eds.), *Midwives, Society and Childbirth: Debates and Controversies in the Modern Period* (London, 1997), 102–33. I am grateful to the editors and to Anne Løkke for allowing me to read this chapter in manuscript; and I am very grateful to Anne Løkke for sending me the data from which Table 10.1 and Fig. 10.4 were constructed and other data on maternity in Denmark.

[9] That the puerperal fever mortality in the Copenhagen Lying-in Hospital was able to have such an influence on the mortality in the city as a whole is probably due to the fact that the lying-in hospital was large and the city small. By 1900 the population of Copenhagen was under half a million, smaller than Amsterdam and much smaller than London. Moreover, it was common practice for assistant obstetricians at the Copenhagen Lying-in Hospital to be called out to attend complications in home births attended by midwives in private practice in the city. This may have been a source whereby infection spread from the hospital to the community (Anne Løkke, Department of History, University of Copenhagen, personal communication).

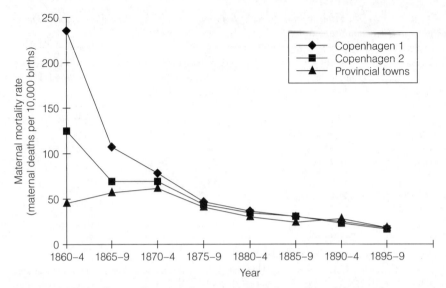

FIG. 10.4 Maternal mortality rates due to puerperal fever, Copenhagen and provincial towns in Denmark, 1860–1899

Note: Copenhagen 1 = Copenhagen including the Lying-in Hospital;
Copenhagen 2 = Copenhagen excluding the Lying-in Hospital.
Sources: See Table 10.1.

of deaths from puerperal fever ever recorded was 36.3 in 1874 compared with 62 in provincial Denmark.

That mortality from puerperal fever was so high in Denmark is unexpected. There is compelling evidence that the standard of maternal care in Denmark during the 1860s, based on well-trained and supervised midwives, was superior to the standard in England and Wales, and yet the rate of puerperal fever mortality was higher in Denmark. Almost certainly, the high Danish rates reflected important differences between the two countries in the accuracy of registering deaths from this disease. The essence of the difference lies in the process of certification and registration of puerperal fever deaths.

In England and Wales there was a well-known tendency to attribute (and certify) deaths from puerperal fever as due to some other cause. This problem, which I have called the problem of 'hidden maternal deaths', is discussed at length in another publication.[10] The extent to which such concealment occurred is difficult to estimate, but in the 1860s and 1870s in England and Wales it may have been as high as 20 per cent of deaths from puerperal fever. Whatever the percentage, it is certain that puerperal fever mortality in England and Wales was under-recorded.

---

[10] Loudon, *Death in Childbirth*, app. 1, 'Hidden Maternal Deaths', pp. 518–24.

In Denmark it was totally different. From the beginning of the nineteenth century, medical officers were appointed to ensure that deaths in epidemics and also maternal and infant mortality were accurately recorded. Every death from fever following childbirth, regardless of the cause of the fever, was registered as a death from puerperal fever. For instance, a death from pneumonia, influenza, or tuberculosis which happened to occur in the puerperium would be registered as a death from puerperal fever. This rule was imposed to prevent midwives from reporting deaths from puerperal fever as deaths from some other cause (as they did in England and Wales); and it appears that midwives felt 'very intimidated' by this rule.

Because of these strict rules, Denmark was probably the only country in the world in which deaths from puerperal fever were not only completely recorded but were actually exaggerated. That the mortality from puerperal fever had, by the end of the nineteenth century, nevertheless fallen well below the levels in · England and Wales, is a tribute to the high standard of care provided by the Danish maternity services.

A similar steep fall in puerperal fever in Sweden from a high peak in 1874 to a low level by 1900 provides further evidence.[11] Here again the fall in mortality was associated with antisepsis. From 1881 all Swedish midwives were required by law to use antisepsis and keep a written record of what antiseptics were used in every delivery, a record that was inspected by a provincial physician appointed for the purpose by the state. In Sweden, however, as in the Netherlands and Denmark, old habits died hard and new ones were only accepted gradually. This led to a campaign in Sweden between 1890 and 1910 to improve the standard of midwives and put an end to midwife care by 'handywomen'. By 1910, 99 per cent of deliveries in Sweden were attended by doctors or by trained and supervised midwives, all of whom were fully trained in the use of antisepsis.[12]

Compared with Britain, these Northern European countries had a long tradition of maternity care based on midwives who were trained and supervised by the state and trained to use antisepsis intelligently during the last two or three decades of the nineteenth century. This is probably why, by about 1910, deaths from puerperal fever in these countries had fallen to a low level and often remained at that level until the mid-1930s. The contrast with England and Wales is striking. Here, the number of deliveries in the voluntary maternity hospitals[13] and deliveries of private patients by consultant obstetricians— the deliveries in which antisepsis was most likely to have been used—amounted to at most 5 per cent of all deliveries. General practitioners undertook rather

[11] U. Högberg, *Maternal Mortality in Sweden* (Umeå University Medical Dissertations, NS 156; Umeå, 1985).

[12] I am grateful to Ms Lisa Öberg, of the Department of History, Stockholm University, for this information on Swedish midwives.

[13] These were the maternity hospitals staffed by obstetricians as opposed to the much larger numbers of poor-law maternity wards where medical care was almost always provided by general practitioners.

less than half of the remaining 95 per cent, and midwives, most of whom had no formal training and were totally unsupervised before the introduction of the Midwives Act of 1902, undertook the rest.

The poor standard of maternal care in Britain was revealed when the decline in maternal mortality between the 1890s and 1912 turned around, began to rise, and continued to rise until the mid-1930s. Part of the rise was due to an increase in septic abortion, but deaths from puerperal sepsis also rose.[14] This was more than a bitter disappointment. It was a scandal, for it was widely recognized that many British deaths from puerperal fever could have been prevented.

Puerperal Fever, Midwives, and General Practitioners

It has been said that 'a scientific truth does not triumph by convincing its opponents and making them see the light, but rather because its opponents eventually die, and a new generation grows up which is familiar with it'.[15] That this was true of obstetric antisepsis was suggested by an American obstetrician who, in 1905, published a paper on puerperal sepsis in private practice in which he divided birth attendants into four classes. The first class, who graduated before 1870, were the older practitioners who, if still in practice, rarely if ever used antisepsis. Most of the second and larger class, who graduated between 1870 and 1890, used antisepsis conscientiously, but others 'go through [it as] a disagreeable and tiresome task with as little personal labour as possible'. The third class, those who had graduated since 1890, were all 'avowedly antiseptists', and many were 'enthusiasts'; but there were still some who were 'careless in technic and do poor work'. The fourth class were the midwives. 'Here and there among this group is a graduate of a maternity nursing school . . . who does her duty under the most trying conditions with honor to herself and safety to the patient', but most were women whose knowledge consisted solely of 'ancestral folk lore and servility . . . It is among patients attended by this class that sepsis and death riots, a fact which daily observation and reading warrants.'[16]

What was the position in England and Wales as far as midwives, general practitioners, and home deliveries were concerned? Apart from a small minority of midwives who had been trained in lying-in hospitals or taken the midwives' examination of the Obstetrical Society of London, midwives were neither trained nor supervised until the Midwives Act of 1902. Few would have heard of, let alone understood, germ theory. Many had never even heard of puerperal fever and very few would have known about antisepsis. Here, as in the USA, the

[14] Loudon, *Death in Childbirth*, ch. 14.
[15] Attributed to Max Planck, who encountered great difficulty in persuading his seniors 'to understand, to respond to, even to read' his work, which led to quantum theory (E. J. Hobsbawm, *The Age of Empire, 1875–1914* (London, 1987; paperback edn., 1994), 250).
[16] S. P. Warren, 'The Prevalence of Puerperal Septicaemia in Private Practice at the Present Time Contrasted with that of a Generation ago', *American Journal of Obstetrics*, 51 (1905), 301–31.

untrained midwives were frequently accused of causing unnecessary deaths from puerperal fever. The Medical Officer of Health to the Glamorgan County Council, Dr W. Williams, said in 1904 that:

It is well within my knowledge that most of the confinements amongst the poorer women are attended by untrained women in the country districts of Merionethshire and Cardigan; in fact in all the country districts, villages and small towns of Wales; and, from my experience in Glamorgan . . . I can prove without a doubt that they often spread puerperal fever broadcast and often are not interfered with.[17]

Detailed information on the standards of obstetric practice in the beginning of the twentieth century is scarce, and much of what can be found tends to consist of prejudiced assertions. Manchester, however, is a rich source of data, because it had, in the early years of the century, one of the most advanced systems of maternal care in Britain.[18] In 1901 the population of Manchester was 543,000 (slightly more than Copenhagen or Amsterdam) and it contained a number of obstetricians with international reputations who were supporters of the Midwives Act of 1902 and active in their attempts to improve the standard of midwifery.[19] Because it was well supplied with maternity hospitals, Manchester possessed a larger proportion of trained midwives than anywhere else in Britain. Of the 18,000 births in Manchester in 1902, about 60 per cent were delivered by midwives, and, by 1905, 92 out of 151 registered midwives had received formal training. The remaining fifty-nine consisted of the 'bona fides' midwives.[20]

A vigorous campaign by the obstetricians and the medical officers of health in Manchester was instituted to train the midwives in antiseptic technique and turn them into 'smart, hygienic professionals'. It was uphill work. Many of the older 'bona fides' midwives were unreceptive to new ideas and reluctant to report cases of puerperal fever because of the threat of suspension and disinfection. If complications arose in a midwife delivery, the midwife was required to call in a medical practitioner, but sometimes patients in the poorest areas were unable to pay a doctor's fee, and some refused to attend when called. Many general practitioners were bitterly opposed, for financial reasons, to improving the status and efficiency of midwives. They would rather have seen the midwife abolished and replaced by an obstetric nurse who would assist the general

---

[17] Williams, *Deaths in Childbed*, 33.

[18] The following account of midwifery in Manchester is based on J. Mottram, 'State Control in Local Context: The Early Years of Midwife Regulation in Manchester, 1900–1914' in Marland and Rafferty (eds.), *Midwives, Society and Childbirth*, 134–52. I am grateful to the editors and Joan Mottram for permission to cite this chapter.

[19] Examples were Sir William Sinclair, Professor of Obstetrics and Gynaecology and author of the standard biography of Semmelweis, Arnold Lea, University Lecturer in Obstetrics and Gynaecology, who was the author of a standard English work on puerperal fever, *Puerperal Infection* (London, 1910), and Charles Cullingworth, who had moved from Manchester to St Thomas's Hospital in London in 1888, but whose influence was still felt in the twentieth century.

[20] *Annual Report of the Medical Officer of Health for Manchester for 1907* (Manchester, 1908). 'Bona fides' midwives were women who had acted as untrained midwives for a number of years and were considered to be sufficiently experienced and reliable to be registered under the Midwives Act of 1902.

TABLE 10.2. *Midwives and puerperal fever, Manchester, 1907*

Data	Qualifications of midwives			
	'Bona fides'	Hospital trained[a]	CMB[b]	Totals
Midwives practising in Manchester in 1907				
no.	58	89	6	153
percentage of total	38	58	4	
Home births attended by midwives:				
no.	3,297	7,345	486	11,128
percentage of total	30	66	4	
Cases of puerperal fever reported				
no.	9	41	3	53
rate per 10,000 births	27	55	61	47
Deaths from puerperal fever				
no.	2	8	1	11
rate per 10,000 births	6	11	20	10
Deaths from puerperal fever in Manchester as a whole[c]				
no.				20
rate per 10,000 births				11

[a] The group of hospital-trained nurses included thirty-three who held the qualification in midwifery of the London Obstetrical Society.

[b] CMB—Central Midwives Board—was the official qualification for a midwife trained and examined under the 1902 Act.

[c] These included deaths due to puerperal fever in home deliveries attended by midwives and general practitioners, and deaths in hospitals.

Note: Rates are given to the nearest whole number.

Source: Data extracted from the *Annual Report of the Medical Officer of Health for Manchester for 1907* (Manchester, 1908), 286, 289, tables A and B.

practitioner but would not be allowed to undertake deliveries on her own.[21] These were some of the problems that beset the authorities that tried to introduce a modern and integrated system of maternal care that could bear comparison with the Netherlands and Scandinavia. Table 10.2 shows the distribution of deliveries amongst midwives in Manchester in 1907. Although the number of cases and deaths from puerperal fever is too small for statistical confidence, the accusation that the 'bona fides' were responsible for most of the puerperal fever is not borne out.[22]

[21] Mottram, 'State Control in Local Context'.

[22] *Annual Report of the Medical Officer of Health for Manchester for 1907*, 290.

Manchester was, however, better than most of Britain by the yardstick of maternal mortality. The official rates of maternal mortality from all causes in 1907 were 10.9 deaths per 10,000 births in Manchester, 12.5 in London, 15.9 in England and Wales, 16.0 in Ireland, and 18.2 in Scotland. Arnold Lea of Manchester echoed others before him such as Williams of Cardiff, and Cullingworth of Manchester and London, when he wrote in 1910 that:

In the last quarter of a century our knowledge of prevention of septic disease has become almost complete, and surgical practice . . . has undergone a complete revolution . . . This unfortunately cannot be said of obstetric practice, with the exception of lying-in hospitals, in which the mortality has been reduced to a minimum.[23]

He noted that the Registrar General reported between 1,500 and 2,000 deaths a year from puerperal sepsis in England, but he distrusted the official figures and quoted Sir William Sinclair, who believed 'We do no violence to statistics if we put down the septic mortality in England and Wales at between 3,000 and 5,000 per annum.'[24]

From the late nineteenth century to the 1930s, puerperal fever became a highly contentious issue and the main source of conflict between the three arms of the maternity service, the midwives, general practitioners, and obstetricians. Obstetricians blamed general practitioners for what Williams called 'the ridiculous parody which in many practitioners' hands stands for antisepsis'[25] and were apt to scorn the standard of care provided by general practitioners. General practitioners replied by accusing obstetricians of patronizing 'ivory-tower' attitudes to midwifery in general practice, where conditions were totally different from hospitals. General practitioners also tended to accuse midwives' ignorance, while midwives resented such criticisms and complained of lack of cooperation by general practitioners called to difficult home deliveries.

Much of the blame lay squarely on the teaching hospitals, where, in the late nineteenth century and the early years of the twentieth, medicine, surgery, and pathology were regarded as the supremely important subjects, while obstetrics (and the same could be said of psychiatry) was regarded as an unscientific subject of little importance. 'Get your "midder" out of the way as soon as you can so that you can concentrate on the real subjects' was the kind of advice given to students by the deans of medical schools.[26] The attitudes of medical students are profoundly influenced by the attitudes—explicit and implicit—of their teachers. If consultants in teaching hospitals deplored the standard of midwifery care in the community, they (the teachers) were largely to blame.

---

[23] Lea, *Puerperal Infection*, 16.

[24] Ibid. 20–1. Sir William, however, was prone to sweeping statements and gives no evidence to support the round numbers, which he may have plucked from the air.

[25] Williams, *Deaths in Childbed*. The phrase was actually used by the Edinburgh obstetrician, Professor Milne Murray, in the 1890s.

[26] On the standards of teaching in Britain and the USA during the late nineteenth century and the early decades of the twentieth, see Loudon, *Death in Childbirth*, 229–31, 295–7.

The importance of this is obvious in countries such as Britain where general-practitioner deliveries formed a large proportion of the total. Nothing is more difficult than trying to generalize about such standards in the past, except that they varied very widely, not only between different parts of the country, but even between partners in the same practice. No doubt many general practitioners practised a high standard of midwifery, intervening only when really necessary and being meticulous in antiseptic practice. That criticisms of general practice were sometimes well founded, however, is suggested by the astonishing response to a lecture on antisepsis in midwifery.

General Practice and Midwifery in the Early 1900s

In 1906 Peter Horrocks, the senior obstetrician to Guy's Hospital, delivered this lecture to the Lambeth division of the British Medical Association. The title was 'Midwifery of the Present Day', and the lecture was published in the *British Medical Journal*.[27] It was a model of orthodox views on what constituted good obstetric practice. There was nothing controversial about it. He described the impressive results of the antiseptic revolution and offered advice on how deliveries should be conducted in general practice, stressing the importance of very careful antisepsis in all deliveries because, as 'more and more facts were discovered, it was found that the germs were not so much in the air as on the fingers of the accoucheur', which explained the marvellous results of disinfection.[28] He reminded his audience that childbirth was a physiological process that in the vast majority of cases could be left to proceed on its own. Interference in normal labours was rarely justified and he implored his audience of general practitioners to use minimal interference, and avoid syringing of the uterine cavity after labour, which had been shown to be dangerous. He spoke at length on other details, but his main points were meticulous antisepsis and minimal interference.

The publication of his lecture provoked an extraordinarily hostile correspondence in the columns of the *British Medical Journal*. There was the familiar cry that hospital obstetricians lived in ivory towers and knew nothing of the nature of general practice. Most correspondents utterly rejected the doctrine of minimal interference. 'Twelve years ago', said Dr Rees of Wigan, 'I knew an able practitioner in a large practice who gave chloroform and used forceps in the large majority of his midwifery cases. He argued that his mission was to save his patients as much pain as possible, so long as he could do it with safety to mother and child.' Horrocks's objections to interference in normal labours

[27] P. Horrocks, 'An Address on the Midwifery of the Present Day', *British Medical Journal* (1906), i. 541–5. Subsequent correspondence in *British Medical Journal* (1906), i: F. Rees, 712–13; W. W. Williams, 713; F. E. Wynne, 773; F. C. Mears, 773; J. R. Leeson, 831; J. Cameron, 831–2; A. L. Scott, 892; A. M. Thomas, 892; J. M. M. 949; 'Colliery surgeon', 949; B. T. Lownes, 950; F. J. Geoghegan, 1012; B. Jordan, 1012–13; C. E. Douglas, 1255.   [28] Horrocks, 'Address', i. 542.

were condemned as 'barbaric'. Modern civilized women in towns, said Dr Rees, could not be expected to give birth without medical assistance. 'The civilised woman is not in a normal environment', wrote Dr Wynne of Leigh in Lancashire; she was totally different from 'an Indian squaw or an Esquimaux mother'. 'Nature intended women to deliver themselves easily,' wrote Dr Mears of North Shields, 'but civilization, injudicious breeding, and modes of dress and occupation have interfered, and the art of midwifery must come to the rescue.'

Other and less respectable reasons floated to the surface. Interference saved time and justified a high fee. 'The crux of the matter', said Dr Leeson of Twickenham, 'is to wait, and inside this problem is another—the fee. This waiting midwifery, this scientific midwifery, cannot be done at the price, and the public must be taught this—the remuneration he [a general practitioner] receives is probably a fraction of what a cabman would obtain for waiting at the gate.' 'I use chloroform and forceps in every possible case', said Dr Mears, 'and have done so for many years. The whole procedure occupies from 15 to 40 minutes according to the difficulty of the case.'

This description of midwifery in general practice is even more alarming when one hears what these general practitioners had to say about germ theory and antisepsis. 'Antiseptics are worse than useless,' said Dr Mears. 'Wash the hands at the patient's house before examining. Having observed these rules, do not bother about micro-organisms.' Several correspondents said that soap and water were all that was necessary and upbraided Horrocks for being out of touch with the realities of general practice by advocating antisepsis. It took too much time, it was unnecessary, and it was just not possible in home deliveries. Dr Bert Jordan (of King's Norton) used forceps very frequently, and he too advocated simple washing in soap and water.

What is surprising is not only the way these general practitioners practised midwifery but the fact that they were willing to parade their views in the correspondence columns of the *British Medical Journal*. It is true that there were other correspondents who agreed with most of what Horrocks had said in his lecture, but the majority showed that they were happy to continue using forceps and chloroform in a large majority of normal labours and were far from convinced that antisepsis was necessary in general practice. It is, of course, impossible to say which of the correspondents were 'typical' general practitioners, or even if the word 'typical' has any meaning in this context. But there is no reason to doubt that a substantial number of general practitioners practised midwifery in a way that was known to be dangerous at a time when virulent streptococci were prevalent in the community.

Puerperal Fever, 1910–1935

It is now, perhaps, easier to understand why so little was achieved in the UK in the war against puerperal fever between 1900 and 1935. Many of the maternity hospitals and departments in the UK continued to achieve the low levels of mortality they had reached by 1910. Midwives improved (especially from 1930) as the number who were trained and examined increased while the untrained retired or died. Nevertheless, the undeniable feature is that, far from falling, deaths from puerperal sepsis rose steadily during this period. In the USA excessive intervention and high maternal mortality were a feature of many maternity hospitals and maternity departments up to the mid-1930s. A series of reports on maternal mortality in the UK and the USA confirmed the scandal of high maternal mortality and showed that many deaths, especially deaths from puerperal sepsis, were due to bad obstetric practice.[29] It was a deplorable state of affairs.

By the 1920s all but a tiny minority of medical practitioners and trained midwives knew that puerperal fever was due to infection with 'germs'. The endogenist/exogenist debate rumbled on in the background (it will be recalled that the endogenists believed that the germs came from within the patient's genital tract, the exogenists that infection was introduced from outside); but the evidence against the endogenists, who clung desperately to a theory that removed the blame for infection from the birth attendant, became overwhelming.

It was known by the 1930s that the source of the infection was sometimes the nose or throat of the patient herself, sometimes a member of her family such as one of her children, but in the majority of cases the midwife or doctor who attended her at her delivery or during her lying-in. What was only slowly realized was the ubiquity of the streptococcus and the need for quite elaborate precautions if infection was to be prevented. Most general practitioners who attended a delivery, and frequently applied forceps, contented themselves with a bowl of antiseptic in which they dipped their fingers and their forceps for a few seconds. Few, if any, carried sterile drapes; few carried sterile rubber gloves; very few wore masks, and if they did so the masks were usually inadequate.[30] Most took off their coat, rolled up their sleeves, and perhaps put on an apron.

---

[29] There were many government reports on maternal mortality, which are listed in Loudon, *Death in Childbirth*. The most influential were: Ministry of Health, *Interim Report of Departmental Committee on Maternal Mortality and Morbidity* (London: HMSO, 1930); J. Smith, *Causation and Source of Infection in Puerperal Fever, Department of Health for Scotland* (Edinburgh: HMSO, 1931); Ministry of Health, *Final Report of Departmental Committee on Maternal Mortality and Morbidity* (London: HMSO, 1932). In the USA the most notable were three publications by the Children's Bureau, US Dept. of Labor, Washington, DC, Govt. Printing Office: (1) No. 19 Grace Meigs, *Maternal Mortality from all Conditions Connected with Childbirth in the United States and Certain Other Countries* (1917); (2) No. 152 Robert Morse Woodbury, *Maternal Mortality: The Risk of Death in Childbirth and from all the Diseases Caused by Pregnancy and Confinement* (1926), and (3) No. 223 *Maternal Mortality in Fifteen States* (1934). The report of the New York City Public Health Committee and New York Academy of Medicine, *Maternal Mortality in New York, 1930, 1931, 1932* (New York, 1933), was probably the most influential of all the American reports.
[30] See the paper by G. F. Gibberd, Assistant Obstetric Surgeon to Guy's Hospital London, 'Streptococcal Puerperal Sepsis', *Guy's Hospital Reports*, 81 (1931), 29–44. Gibberd pointed out that, while it had become standard practice to wear masks in general surgery, masks were seldom worn in obstetrics. He said that they should be worn and should be properly constructed out of sixteen thicknesses of gauze.

The Maternity Committee of the College of Obstetricians and Gynaecologists minuted in 1929–30: 'We assume that all in attendance on a case in labour wear a sterilised gown with sleeves and a mask and rubber gloves. We would recommend that rubber gloves used in maternity work should reach the elbows. A sterilised outfit should always be provided when poor class women are attended at home.'[31] Most general practitioners would have said this was a totally impractical and unnecessarily fussy way of carrying out midwifery in general practice.

The only way to achieve a reduction in deaths from puerperal fever was prevention. Before 1937 puerperal fever was resistant to all treatments, although medical periodicals were littered with claims that this or that treatment was effective. Medical remedies such as antimony or mercury, and others such as venesection, had been abandoned by most practitioners by 1870. Instead, a large number of surgical procedures were tried. Some washed out the uterine cavity with antiseptics. Some packed the post-partum uterus with gauze and pessaries containing carbolic acid, or iodine, or mercurchrome. Intravenous injections of formalin or an aqueous solution of silver or carbolic acid (all terribly dangerous) were tried. In the 1920s there was a vogue for instilling glycerine into the uterine cavity, which was at least safer than strong antiseptics, but it was ineffective.[32] Some obstetricians advised curetage. A few were so desperate that they suggested hysterectomy as a treatment for puerperal fever. The multiplicity of treatments and the fact that none was shown to work were profoundly depressing.

In April 1925 the Fifth British Congress of Obstetrics and Gynaecology was held in London. One of those who attended and spoke was John Whitridge Williams of Johns Hopkins Hospital in Baltimore (1866–1931), one of the greatest and most experienced of all American obstetricians, and a man of considered and moderate opinions. There was a prolonged discussion on the treatment of puerperal fever, and this is what Williams had to say on the subject:

When a person has general streptococcal peritonitis she will die whatever you do for her. Two thirds of those with very acute general sepsis [and] pyaemia (the thromboembolic form) will die. Of women subjected to intrauterine manipulation when infected 80 per cent will die. Others if left alone will generally recover if we do not help to kill them. I say that an average infection, if left alone, takes care of itself. If you have a virulent organism and a non-resistant woman, death is the almost universal outcome, no matter what you do, and there is no use deceiving ourselves and using sixty remedies for such cases as are mentioned in the London paper.[33]

---

[31] Royal College of Obstetricians and Gynaecologists, London, Archives, Minute book B7, Minutes of the Maternity Committee. [32] Gibberd, 'Streptococcal Puerperal Sepsis'.
[33] The papers of the Fifth British Congress of Obstetrics and Gynaecology exist in manuscript form in the archives of the Royal College of Obstetricians and Gynaecologists in London. A slightly abbreviated account of the proceedings was published in the *Journal of Obstetrics and Gynaecology of the British Empire*, 23 (1925), 239–58.

Few obstetricians had the seniority, experience, or the courage to state openly such a therapeutically nihilistic conclusion. Although there were no therapeutic advances of any note on the prevention or treatment of puerperal fever during the fifty years between the 1880s and the mid-1930s, a great deal of basic scientific research had been carried out, especially on the Group A streptococcus.

Rebecca Lancefield in the USA played the leading role in the 1920s in classifying the genus Streptococcus, and discovering the M-antigens of the Group A streptococcus (see Chapter 12). In Britain two of the leading figures were Leonard Colebrook and his sister, Dora Colebrook. In 1936 a paper by Leonard Colebrook on the prevention of puerperal fever was published.[34] It is probably the most clear and comprehensive account of all aspects of puerperal fever in the 1930s just before the introduction of the sulphonamides. Colebrook stressed many of the points that have been covered in this and previous chapters, especially the ubiquity of the Group A streptococcus. He described the work that had been carried out on the nature and infectivity of this organism, and laid to rest the endogenous theory of the causation of puerperal fever; it is interesting that, as late as 1936, Colebrook still felt it necessary to do so. Like Whitridge Williams ten years earlier, Colebrook stressed that puerperal fever was a disease for which there was no treatment and that could only be prevented by meticulous antiseptic and aseptic care.

At the time that Colebrook gave the lecture on which this paper was based, he was probably unaware that within a few months he would have embarked on the trial of the sulphonamides that turned out to be so effective that they virtually brought an end to puerperal fever within a few decades. That is the subject of the next chapter.

---

[34] L. Colebrook, 'The Prevention of Puerperal Sepsis', *Journal of Obstetrics and Gynaecology of the British Empire*, 43 (1936), 691–714. This paper was based on a lecture, but when the lecture was given is not recorded. It was probably in late 1935 or early 1936.

11

Puerperal Fever: A Curable Disease

To understand the pathway that led to the discovery of a cure for puerperal fever we must go back briefly to the late nineteenth and early twentieth centuries and the work that followed from the discoveries of Pasteur, Koch, and their colleagues. The first step was the realization that the effects of infection by micro-organisms were sometimes due to the production of poisonous substances called toxins. This explained why, in diseases such as diphtheria, where the organisms are confined to a localized area such as the throat, damage can occur to distant organs such as the heart, or liver, or kidneys. The next step was the discovery that the body responded to the toxins by producing substances that opposed their action—the antitoxins or, as they were later called, the antibodies.

Immunotherapy and Chemotherapy

These observations were the key to immunotherapy. If antitoxins could be produced artificially, they could be used to prevent or cure infectious diseases. One way of doing this was to inject bacteria that were either killed, or attenuated to such an extent that they did not cause illness but still retained the faculty of provoking the body into producing antitoxins. This process became known as active immunization, which it was thought could work by either or both of two mechanisms. Most thought that active immunization simply led to the presence of specific antitoxins in the circulation waiting to attack the specific toxins should the immunized individual contract the disease in question. Another possible mechanism was based on the observation of the Russian zoologist Elie Metchnikoff (1845–1916) that mammalian blood cells could ingest micro-organisms, a process that he called phagocytosis, and the white cells in the blood that possessed this property came to be known as phagocytes. Some, notably Almroth Wright, to whom we come shortly, believed that the main function of antitoxins was to stimulate the phagocytes.

Obviously, active immunization was primarily a means of prevention. For most diseases it was not an effective means of treatment. If vaccines were given to a patient already ill, the patient might be dead (or recovered) before the body had time to produce antitoxins. Pasteur's successful use of active vaccination as a treatment for rabies was really an example of prevention because the disease has such a long incubation period. If he gave the vaccine immediately after someone was bitten by a rabid dog, there was enough time to develop antibodies before the disease began.[1]

The other method was passive immunization. This involves the injection of disease-specific antitoxins and could be used to treat ill patients. The problem was how to get hold of such antitoxins in sufficient volume for clinical use. To do so, animals (usually horses) were injected with enough toxins to provoke anti-toxin production, but not so much as to make the animal ill. Blood was taken from the horse, and the horse serum with its rich content of specific antitoxins was administered to the patient. It was a crude method with dangerous side effects, particularly anaphylactic (allergic) reactions against substances other than the antitoxins in the serum. Such adverse reactions were called 'serum sickness'.

This method of passive immunization was already well established in the 1890s. It is said that diphtheria antitoxin was first used (successfully) to treat a girl dying from diphtheria in Berlin in 1891.[2] During the 1890s reports on the use of diphtheria antitoxin or 'serum' therapy were contradictory. By 1896, however, sufficient antitoxin was available to carry out a clinical trial in Denmark. Here, only eight out of 239 patients with diphtheria died in the treated group, while thirty died out of the control group of 245 cases. The difference was highly significant, but 60 per cent of the treated group showed signs of serum sickness. This trial was carried out by Johannes A. G. Fibiger (1867–1928), and is of great interest as a very early example of a controlled trial, used expressly to eliminate bias. Treatment or control depended on the day of admission, so that on one day all admissions were allocated to the treatment group, and on the next day to the control group, and so on.[3]

Paul Ehrlich and German Research

In the first thirty years of the twentieth century, it was believed in most countries that immunotherapy, combined with constitutional remedies, held out most hope for the prevention and treatment of infective diseases.[4] A great deal of the early work on the production of antitoxins was carried out in Germany, where

---

[1] For a more detailed discussion of the history of immunotherapy, see M. Weatherall, *In Search of a Cure* (Oxford, 1990), esp. chs. 3 and 8; also P. Weindling 'The Immunological Tradition', and M. Weatherall, 'Drug Therapies', chs. 10 and 39 in W. F. Bynum and R. Porter (eds.), *Companion Encyclopaedia to the History of Medicine* (London, 1993). For an excellent account of the history and modern knowledge concerning immunology, see W. R. Clark, *At War Within* (Oxford, 1995; paperback edn., 1997). [2] Weatherall, *In Search of a Cure*, 52.

[3] A. Hróbjartsson, P. C. Gøtzsche, and C. Gluud, 'The Controlled Trial Turns 100 Years: Fibiger's Trial of Serum Treatment of Diphtheria', *British Medical Journal*, 317 (1998), 1243–5.

[4] For a discussion of the multiple approach to treatment of bacterial disease before chemotherapy, see M. Worboys, 'Treatments for Pneumonia in Britain, 1910–1940', in *Medicine and Change: Historical and Sociological Studies of Medical Innovation* (Proceedings of the Symposium INERM held in Paris, 21–23 April, 1992), 317–35, at 320–6.

there was a strong chemical industry with academic connections to institutions such as the Koch Institute for Infectious Diseases, which was opened in Berlin in 1891. In the 1890s, Paul Ehrlich (1854–1915) joined the Koch Institute and was later provided with a research institute of his own. At first he worked on methods of purification and the assay of antitoxins. Then he began to wonder if simpler substances could be used to inactivate or destroy bacteria.[5]

One of the techniques that had been developed in bacteriology was the use of dyes to stain microbes so that they were easier to see and identify under the microscope. Koch had noted that certain dyes would stain microbes but not the tissues of the infected host, and Ehrlich asked himself the question—why do certain dyes combine selectively with micro-organisms? He decided that 'parasites possess a whole series of chemo-receptors', which, if they have 'no analogue in the organs of the body', could be targeted by chemotherapy like aiming a 'poisoned arrow' or a 'magic bullet' at one or more of the receptors on the parasite.[6] Thus, if a dye or some other chemical could be synthesized that not only adhered to receptors on microbes, but in the process interfered with their normal activity, they might destroy the microbe. This was an extremely prescient observation, because, to jump ahead for a moment, shortly after the sulphonamides were discovered in the 1930s it was shown that bacteria that were sensitive to the sulphonamides did indeed have receptors for a substance, p-aminobenzoic acid (PABA), which they needed as a building block. Because the sulphonamides were closely related chemically to PABA (the first sulphonamide was p-aminobenzenesulphonamide), they were able to occupy and block the site in the bacterium at which PABA operated. Thus, as Ehrlich had forecast, they were able to interfere with the ability of bacteria to reproduce and cause disease.

Following up this idea of dyes that were lethal to microbes, Ehrlich found that the dye methylene blue, which stained malarial parasites, had a therapeutic effect on two patients with malaria. The effect was modest compared with the effect of quinine, but this and subsequent research led Ehrlich to name this process 'chemotherapy' as opposed to antitoxin therapy. Early attempts to find chemicals that would be lethal to micro-organisms but harmless to human beings ('magic bullets') were modestly successful. A dye called trypan red was found to be active against trypanosomal infections in mice but not unfortunately in cattle or human beings. By a long and tortuous process that included 605 failed experiments, the details of which need not concern us here, Ehrlich discovered that a certain arsenical, known as compound '606' (its other names were Salvarsan and arsphenamine), was effective against the spirochaete *Treponema pallidum*, the causative agent of syphilis. Salvarsan and its successor Neosalvarsan were used extensively, but they were difficult and dangerous drugs. Salvarsan

    [5] Weatherall, *In Search of a Cure*, 55–62.
    [6] P. Ehrlich, 'Chemotherapeutics: Scientific Principles, Methods and Results', *Lancet* (1913), ii. 445–51, 447. In this paper, 'magic bullet' was rendered as 'bewitched balls'. See also Weatherall, 'Drug Therapies'.

was unstable and so toxic that it could be given only once a week at most, and, if some of the solution leaked out under the skin during injection, it could cause necrosis and even the loss of an arm. But it was moderately successful and certainly better than any previous form of treatment for syphilis.

The discovery of compound 606 was announced in 1910. A short time later two effective anti-malarials were discovered, Plasmoquine and Atebrine.[7] And, when the two forms of dysentery—bacterial dysentery and amoebic dysentery—were separated, it was shown that a substance called 'emetine', isolated from the South American plant ipecachuana, was effective against amoebic dysentery but not against bacterial. Thus there were two chemotherapeutic compounds, quinine and emetine, that were derived from plants, and others, such as trypan red, the new anti-malarials, and Salvarsan, that were manufactured in the laboratory.

Note that during this period, the late nineteenth and early twentieth centuries, Germany was the leader in advances in immunotherapy and chemotherapy. This was largely, as mentioned above, because of strong links between academic research and the German chemical industry (especially the dye industry, as we will see), and the brilliant work of Ehrlich. It is also important to note that the early successes in chemotherapy were against microbes such as the trypansomes, the malarial parasites, the spirochaete of syphilis, and the amoebae of amoebic dysentery. Although the spirochaete is a bacterium, albeit a rather curious one, in general during the first three decades of the twentieth century no chemotherapeutic agents had been discovered that were effective against bacteria, and many believed that chemotherapy against bacteria such as the streptococcus or staphylococcus would never work because (it was believed) bacteria were too small, and too uncomplicated in their structure.

Almroth Wright and British Research

In contrast to Germany, British research was centred on immunotherapy and there was very little interest in chemotherapy. Some of this was due to the relative absence of traditional links between medical research and the pharmaceutical industry, which, in any case, was in its infancy at the time.[8] But the main reason was the domination of bacteriology and immunology by the formidable and arrogant bacteriologist Sir Almroth Wright (1861–1947) at St Mary's Hospital. Wright was convinced the future lay in immunotherapy, and he concentrated on therapy that aimed to stimulate the phagocytes. Those who have read or seen *The Doctor's Dilemma* by George Bernard Shaw will remember

---

[7] L. Colebrook, 'Gerhard Domagk', *Biographical Memoirs of Fellows of the Royal Society*, 10 (1964), 38–44, at 39.

[8] Even in the 1990s, doctors who qualify in medicine in the normal way and then choose a career in the pharmaceutical industry are apt to be accused by their colleagues of selling their professional independence by joining the drug industry.

that this appears as a catchphrase uttered by the character based on Wright, Sir Colenso Ridgeon.[9] Wright came to believe that medical science should be carried out by sitting in the privacy of one's study and working out a problem by the powers of reason untrammelled by experiments. When the answer was obtained, all that was needed was one single experiment to prove the theory was right. No other experiments were necessary, and he was utterly scornful of work such as Ehrlich's, which consisted of experimenting with large numbers of chemicals in the hope of finding one that worked.

Wright's work on immunization was criticized on statistical grounds by the mathematician Karl Pearson, leading to what was, at the time, quite a famous debate. Characteristically, Wright asserted that the claims of a clinician and laboratory researcher were superior to those of a mathematician. Using the analogy of shipbuilding, Wright asserted that: 'It is exactly as if a calculator, whose office it was to compute the strength of certain shipbuilding materials, were to contend that he, and not the practical seaman, was the proper judge of the performances of a shipbuilder'.[10] Wright's scorn for the mathematical approach was combined with the belief that chemotherapy and the search for magic bullets were not only useless but a form of sacrilege.[11] To him, vaccines were far superior, partly at least because of the gradual development of his idea that, if vaccines stimulated the phagocytes, the vaccine need not necessarily be specific for the disease in question. If that were true, vaccine therapy would have two advantages over chemotherapy. Active immunization would be long lasting or even permanent for the immunized patient. Chemotherapy would last only as long as the chemotherapeutic agent was given. Further, vaccines could not only prevent disease when given to a healthy individual; they could be used as a form of therapy in the sense that a vaccine would aid the body to overcome a disease. Vaccines could have a general as well as a specific effect.

Wright believed this so strongly that he put it into practice on a considerable scale. He was able to do so when he was provided by St Mary's Hospital with a research institute at which his vaccines could be produced and marketed by Parke Davis and Co., providing a rich source of income for his department. Wright claimed that his vaccines could cure conditions as diverse as acne, pyorrhoea, boils, pneumonia, bronchial colds, influenza, gonorrhoea, sore throats, intestinal troubles, and even cancer.[12] Since the sales of vaccines were so profitable, it might be said that the outrageous claims for Wright's vaccines

---

[9] Wright and Shaw knew each other well, and often argued with each other, taking opposite points of view on almost everything. Shaw was a formidable debater, but it is said that Wright was sometimes more than his equal (G. Macfarlane, *Alexander Fleming* (paperback edn., Oxford, 1985), 76–7).

[10] Cited in J. Rosser Matthews, *Quantification and the Quest for Medical Certainty* (Princeton, NJ, 1995), 97–103. Matthews has written an excellent account of the debate and of Wright's essential scorn for what he saw as interference in medical research by mathematicians and statisticians.

[11] Macfarlane, *Alexander Fleming*, 148. Michael Worboys remarks that 'One reason why chemotherapy was in such bad odour in Britain was the constant stream of dubious agents emanating from Germany in the 1920s and early 1930s' (personal communication, 1995).

[12] Macfarlane, *Alexander Fleming*, 67.

bordered on downright dishonesty. However, Wright was completely convinced of the truth of his theories, and the money went not into Wright's pocket but into the funds of his institute.

Amongst the members of Wright's group were two who were, sooner or later, to become interested in chemotherapy in spite of Wright's disapproval. One was Alexander Fleming of penicillin fame; the other was Leonard Colebrook.[13] The importance of Colebrook's work will soon be evident.

Domagk and Prontosil

Before the nineteenth century, dyes used in the clothing industry were derived from vegetable or animal products. In 1856 the English chemist William Perkin (1838–1907), who was just 18 at the time, set up a makeshift laboratory in his home and in Easter 1856 tried to synthesize quinine from coal-tar products, a messy by-product from the growing gas industry. He failed as far as quinine was concerned, but accidentally synthesized an aniline dye that he named 'mauve' from the French for mallow, a plant that has purple flowers. The dye, which became very popular, was patented by Perkin. It was the first aniline dye to be produced. From the failed attempt to synthesize quinine, there was, as we will see, a thread connecting quinine to aniline dyes to chemotherapy and ultimately in a rather roundabout way to penicillin.[14]

One of the many to exploit the dye-making potential of the coal-tar industry was Friedrich Bayer (1825–80), whose father was a milliner and great-grandfather a dyer and draper in Bavaria.[15] He founded the firm of Bayer in 1863, whose rapid growth was initially due to the large-scale production of a wide range of brilliant dyes. With the synthesis of phenacetin in 1888, and acetyl-salicylic acid (for which 'Aspirin' was Bayer's patented trade name in Germany and which was first marketed in 1899), Bayer developed a large and successful pharmaceutical division that played a very large part in this story.[16]

In 1916 a number of different firms involved in the dye industry, failing to agree to a merger, formed the Interessengemeinschaft der deutschen Teer-farbenindustrie (literally the Community of Interests of the German Coal-Tar Dyestuffs Industry), which became known as the I. G. Farbenindustrie, or simply I. G. Farben, *färben* being the German for a dye. In this loose confederation, Bayer was the leading player, and this explains why one often sees the work that follows as being attributed either to Bayer or to the I. G. Farbenindustrie. Both attributions are correct.[17] The important point is that the work to be described was undertaken within a firm deeply involved with dyes, and within a country, Germany, in which there was a totally different attitude

[13] R. Hare, *The Birth of Penicillin* (London, 1970), 52.
[14] D. Greenwood, 'The Quinine Connection', *Journal of Antimicrobial Chemotherapy*, 30 (1992), 417–27, at 424.   [15] E. Verg, *Milestones: The Bayer Story, 1863–1988* (Wilmington, Mass., 1988), 24.
[16] Ibid. 90–3, 136.   [17] Ibid. 222, 230–2.

to chemotherapy from that in Britain. This brings us to Gerhard Domagk (1895–1964), who was strongly influenced by the ideas of Ehrlich.

Domagk fought in the First World War, was wounded in 1915, and transferred from a grenadier regiment to the medical corps. After the war he studied medicine in Kiel, graduating in 1921, and, following work in several pathology departments, he was appointed in 1927 as the director of Bayer's newly established Institute of Experimental Pathology and Bacteriology.[18] Domagk shared Ehrlich's belief that, if a chemotherapeutic agent was active against bacteria, it would have to be an agent capable of sticking to cells. Dyestuffs were by their very nature the substances most likely to stick to things. Bayer produced numerous dyes for commercial purposes, and Domagk tapped this extensive group of azo-dyes in his slow but systematic search for an antibacterial agent. In 1932 two of Domagk's chemist colleagues (Fritz Mietzsch and Josef Klarer) synthesized a red dye first known as D 4145, which included a sulphonamide group 'for the chemically logical reason that this improved the colourfastness in fabrics'.[19] This dye, which was later named Prontosil rubrum, was tested by Domagk for antibacterial activity.[20]

Domagk's usual method was to test numerous substances by seeing if they were active *in vitro* (which means 'in glass')—that is, to see if they killed bacteria grown in culture in a test tube or Petri dish in the laboratory. If they seemed to be active, they were tested *in vivo* on animals. If they were effective in animals, testing them on patients would be the final step. Prontosil was first tried on streptococci growing in a Petri dish. There was no effect, and this might have seemed to rule it out. But Domagk broke his usual rule and proceeded to test it on mice. Initial tests suggested that it was effective, and its toxicity for mice was low, so he proceeded to a proper experiment.

In late December 1932 a virulent strain of the streptococcus was injected into the peritoneum of twenty-six mice. Fourteen were kept as controls. The other twelve were treated one and a half hours after the injection of streptococci with a single dose of Prontosil red administered by stomach tube. The fourteen untreated mice died within four days, most dying on the second day. The twelve treated mice survived.[21] It was an amazingly clear-cut result. Domagk then tested numerous other dyes and carried out many animal experiments, only to find that none was as effective as Prontosil. For this reason, and also, it is said, because of the need to secure patents, it was not until February 1935 that he published his work.[22]

However, news of the successful experiment soon leaked out. Domagk treated his own daughter (successfully) with Prontosil for a severe streptococcal infection, and workers in other countries asked for samples of Prontosil

---

[18] For various accounts of the work of Domagk, see Colebrook, 'Gerhard Domagk', Hare, *The Birth of Penicillin*, Weatherall, *In Search of a Cure*, Verg, *Milestones*, and Anon., 'A Medical Revolution', *Bayer Review*, special anniversary edition (Mar. 1988), 58–9.

[19] Greenwood, 'The Quinine Connection', 425.   [20] Anon., 'A Medical Revolution'.

[21] Weatherall, *In Search of a Cure*, 50.   [22] Anon., 'A Medical Revolution', 59.

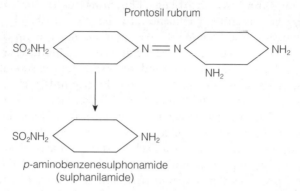

FIG. 11.1 The chemical structure of Prontosil rubrum and Sulphanilamide

but were refused, presumably because of the potential for huge profits from the discovery.[23] Domagk was awarded the Nobel Prize for Medicine in 1939, but the Nazi government forced him to decline the award, which was eventually presented to him in 1947, although by this time the prize money had reverted to the Foundation's funds and he was able to receive the medal but not the money.[24]

Although scientists at the Pasteur Institute in Paris failed, after repeated requests, to obtain any Prontosil, the patent specifications were used at the Pasteur Institute to synthesize a red crystalline substance in 1935 that was closely similar to Prontosil and that also cured streptococcal infections in mice.[25] Most importantly, Tréfouëls and his colleagues showed how Prontosil worked. Prontosil is a molecule consisting of two parts joined in the middle by a double bond (see Fig. 11.1). When administered to an animal, this bond is broken, yielding two separate smaller molecules. One was tri-amino-benzene, which gave the colour to Prontosil rubrum: the other was p-aminobenzenesulphonamide, which became known as sulphanilamide. It was one of the first examples of what is sometimes known as a 'pro-drug'—that is, a drug that has to be broken down in the body before it can act as a chemotherapeutic agent. Thus it was the sulphanilamide component that was the therapeutically active agent, and it was active against bacteria *in vitro* and *in vivo*. This, of course, explained why Prontosil had no effect *in vitro*.

From one point of view this was good news. Sulphanilamide was easy and inexpensive to manufacture—much more so than Prontosil. But the bad news for Bayer was that sulphanilamide could not be patented, because it had been synthesized in 1908 by a chemist, Paul Gelmo, and its chemical structure was published as part of his work for a doctoral thesis. It had been thought to be

---

[23] Hare, *Birth of Penicillin*.　　[24] Colebrook, 'Gerhard Domagk', 41.
[25] H. Hörlein, 'The Chemotherapy of Infectious Diseases Caused by Protozoa and Bacteria', *Proceedings of the Royal Society of Medicine*, 29 (1936), 313–24, at 320–4.

of no importance and by 1935 this chemist, who so narrowly missed fame and a fortune, was working in a small and obscure firm that produced printing inks.[26] Because sulphanilamide could not be patented, any pharmaceutical firm was free to market the drug under its own trade name, and soon many would be doing just that.

Although it appears that few convincing clinical trials of Prontosil were carried out on the Continent, a number of case reports appeared. By October 1935 it is possible that as many as 1,500 patients had been treated with Prontosil in Germany.[27] There were not, however, any convincing trials of any sulphonamide before those carried out in England by Leonard Colebrook.

Colebrook and the Introduction of the Sulphonamides

Leonard Colebrook (1883–1967) graduated in medicine from St Mary's Hospital in 1906. A year later he joined Alexander Fleming as an assistant in Almroth Wright's department, and in 1911 Fleming and Colebrook published a paper on the use of arsenicals in syphilis.[28] Later the Wright Institute was renamed as the Wright–Fleming Institute.

Wright and Colebrook could hardly have been more different in character and temperament. Colebrook (known invariably to his friends as 'Coli') was modest and idealistic. His original intention was to become a medical missionary. He was the very opposite of the egotistical, quarrelsome, and dogmatic Almroth Wright. Colebrook always said that any success he achieved was due to his team as a whole and not just to himself. Moreover, unlike Almroth Wright, he was a scientist who believed in experimental medicine and careful clinical trials. When Colebrook came to a conclusion, he did so with great caution, considering all the possibilities of what are now called 'confounding factors'. And yet, as sometimes happens with complete opposites, Wright and Colebrook were firm friends, and Colebrook's loyalty and admiration for Wright lasted throughout his life.[29]

In 1919 Colebrook was appointed a member of the scientific staff of the Medical Research Council and continued to work at St Mary's Hospital. He turned to the problem of puerperal fever in the 1920s when the wife of a close

---

[26] Ibid. 157. Although sulphanilamide had not been used therapeutically, Hare mentions that in 1919 it was shown that sulphanilamide combined with quinine could kill bacteria in the test tube. The source of this information was a Dr Michael Heidelberger of New York, who came to Hare's house in order to play the Brahms horn trio, which Heidelberger had transposed for his clarinet. The other two members of the trio were Hare's wife and a friend who was a violinist.   [27] Ibid. 156.

[28] A. Fleming and L. Colebrook, 'On the Use of Salvarsan in the Treatment of Syphilis', *Lancet* (1911), i. 1631–4.

[29] Leonard Colebrook wrote the entry on Almroth Wright for the *Dictionary of National Biography (Supplement, 1901–1960)*. As an account of Wright it is, to say the least, excessively kind to the memory of his chief, who is put on a par with Pasteur and Ehrlich. No hint is given of Wright's faults or failures as a scientist.

friend died of the disease, and Colebrook saw the intense distress of a death in childbirth of a potentially preventible disease. True to the philosophy of his chief, Colebrook tried to find a vaccine that could be used for the active immunization of pregnant women against puerperal fever. The attempt was a failure, because of the large number of serotypes of the Group A streptococcus (see Chapter 12) and the fact that vaccines were strain specific. Producing a single vaccine against all strains was in fact impossible.

Colebrook then tried the effect of arsenical drugs, similar to those used for syphilis, for the treatment of puerperal fever. The drugs were so poisonous that it was necessary to wait for several days before a second dose could be given, until a chemist at May and Baker, the pharmaceutical manufacturers, produced another arsenical called Metarsenobillon, which could be given daily. This was tested extensively by Colebrook and Ronald Hare, but it proved to be a complete failure.[30] In 1930 Colebrook left St Mary's to take up the post of director of the research laboratories at Queen Charlotte's (maternity) Hospital, a unit that had been established specifically for research into puerperal fever.[31]

It is astonishing to learn that, when Colebrook arrived at Queen Charlotte's Hospital, generally regarded as the Mecca of obstetrics in Britain, he found that it was not customary to wear gloves or masks or even to sterilize instruments. Colebrook knew better than anyone the danger of such negligence and at once enforced proper aseptic precautions at the hospital. There was a prompt fall in the incidence of puerperal fever in the hospital, but, of course, preventive measures had no effect on patients who had already contracted the disease.[32] Colebrook continued with various lines of research but with absolutely no success until 1935, when news of Domagk's work had reached England. At first, neither Wright nor Colebrook was impressed by the news: Wright because he hated chemotherapy, Colebrook partly because his own unhappy experience with the trial of arsenicals for puerperal fever had made him very cautious indeed, and partly because he felt the new drug had not been properly tested.[33] Admittedly there were some hopeful reports from the Continent, but, as Colebrook was to say later: 'their evidential value must be regarded as small since, in most cases, the recovery of patients is unhesitatingly ascribed to treatment, and too little allowance is made for the tendency to spontaneous cure of these infections.'[34] Nevertheless, Colebrook was determined to get hold of some Prontosil, and he managed to do so with great difficulty.[35]

In England in 1935 there appears to have been little appreciation of the significance of Domagk's work. Quite an extensive account of Domagk's experiment

[30] Hare, The Birth of Penicillin, 53.   [31] Dictionary of National Biography for 1961–1970.

[32] V. Colebrook, 'Leonard Colebrook: Reminiscences on the Occasion of the 25th Anniversary of the Birmingham Burns Unit', Injury: The British Journal of Accident Surgery, 2/3 (Jan. 1971), 182–4.

[33] Macfarlane, Alexander Fleming, 148–9.

[34] L. Colebrook and M. Kenny, 'Treatment of Human Puerperal Infections, and of Experimental Infections in Mice, with Prontosil', Lancet (1936), i. 1279–86, at 1279.

[35] V. Colebrook, 'Leonard Colebrook', 182.

with mice was given to a British audience in October 1935, and published in the *Proceedings of the Royal Society of Medicine* in 1936.[36] A short note on Prontosil, published in the *Lancet* of 1 February 1936, reported that an agent called Prontosil had been discovered in Germany that was said to be effective against streptococci but not against any other organisms, adding that British workers had been able to confirm only part of the reported findings. The report was given no prominence and the way it was written was unexciting. There was nothing to suggest that this was the beginning of a revolution in the treatment of infectious disease.[37]

The clinical trials by Colebrook

All this was to change, however, in the next few months. In the *Lancet* of 6 June 1936 two important papers were published. One was by Buttle, Gray, and Stephenson of the Wellcome Physiological Research Laboratories in Beckenham, reporting experiments on mice. The other was by Colebrook and Meave Kenny—who was the resident medical officer at Queen Charlotte's Hospital—using mice first, and then trying the new drug on patients.[38] Both papers reported the successful treatment of mice injected with streptococci. Colebrook and Kenny did not use exactly the same form of Prontosil as that used by Domagk. They used Prontosil soluble by injection (obtained from Bayer in Germany) and the French equivalent of Prontosil by mouth. They also used sulphanilamide in their mice experiments, but not yet in the treatment of patients. Buttle and his colleagues used sulphanilamide in their mice experiments, which they reported under its pharmaceutical name, *p*-aminobenzene-sulphonamide. They also compared sulphanilamide with Prontosil, finding that both were active against streptococci but sulphanilamide seemed to be the less toxic of the two.

In the first of three trials in close succession, Colebrook treated his patients with two forms of Prontosil simultaneously: Prontosil red was given by mouth and another form, Prontosil soluble, by injection. Vera Colebrook (Leonard Colebrook's wife) recalled in 1971 that Colebrook had been nervous about using Prontosil red for patients on the grounds of its safety. It had 'turned mice pink and patients blue', and there was a suspicion it could cause kidney damage. However, these were minor objections to their use in desperate cases. The first case in which Prontosil was used by Colebrook was a woman admitted to Queen Charlotte's Hospital. She was desperately ill and virtually certain to die of puerperal fever. Prontosil was administered in the evening and she was watched at intervals through the night by staff 'in the oddest assortment of nightwear'.

[36] Hörlein, 'The Chemotherapy of Infectious Diseases'.
[37] Anon., 'An Anti-Streptococcal Agent', *Lancet* (1936), i. 269–70.
[38] G. A. H. Buttle, W. H. Gray, and D. Stephenson, 'Protection of Mice against Streptococcal and Other Infections by *p*-aminobenzenesulphonamide and Related Substances', *Lancet* (1936), i. 1286–90; Colebrook and Kenny, 'Treatment of human puerperal infections'.

The next morning her temperature had fallen from 104°F to normal. The same occurred with the next patient, who had a temperature of 106°F and a 'raging septicaemia'. She too recovered promptly.[39]

These were the first two cases in the first trial of Prontosil on patients with puerperal fever. The total number of cases in the trial was thirty-eight, and there were three deaths, giving a mortality rate of 8 per cent. This compared favourably with a mortality of 26.3 per cent in the thirty-eight cases admitted to the hospital immediately before the trial began. However, Colebrook, as always, was cautious. Nearly half of the cases in the trial would, in his opinion, have recovered anyway. Amongst the other half, however, there were several who had been seriously ill with signs of peritonitis and septicaemia. It is most unlikely that they would have recovered without Prontosil, for, as Colebrook remarked, in ten years' experience of the disease he had never seen a case with severe septicaemia proven by a positive blood culture that recovered spontaneously.[40]

But the trial was by no means as clear and definite as Domagk's original trial of the drug on mice in 1932. In fact, there were three severe cases who died in spite of Prontosil. Nevertheless, there were some remarkable recoveries. Many researchers at the time would have been happy to throw their hats in the air with delight at a reduction of mortality from 26 per cent to 8 per cent combined with the striking evidence that severe streptococcal septicaemia—virtually a death sentence up to that time—could be cured. Not Colebrook. He went no further than to suggest that the results were sufficiently encouraging to justify a careful clinical trial. A fortnight later the *Lancet* published a letter from Colebrook asking for cases of puerperal fever to be sent to his unit in Queen Charlotte's Hospital. 'In view of the promising results reported in THE LANCET of June 6th', he said, it was 'very desirable to complete our clinical trial of Prontosil treatment . . .'.[41]

From our present standpoint it may be difficult to realize just how revolutionary these papers were. There had been many previous but unsuccessful attempts to treat bacterial infections by chemotherapy, which, for reasons of space, have not been mentioned here. They were, indeed, a catalogue of failures and an apparent justification for Almroth Wright's scorn for chemotherapy. Hence the tone of the leading article that accompanied the publication of these two papers in the issue of the *Lancet* on 6 June 1936:

The history of attempted chemotherapy in bacterial infections is so discouraging that any indisputable success in this direction is almost totally unexpected. It has seemed hitherto that some radical difference between protozoal and bacterial infections offers an insuperable bar to the treatment of the latter by chemical means. Nothing in therapeutics is more certain than the disappearance of malarial parasites or trypanosomes

---

[39] V. Colebrook, 'Leonard Colebrook', 182.

[40] L. Colebrook, 'The Story of Puerperal Fever, 1800–1950', *British Medical Journal* (1956), i. 247–52, at 250.   [41] L. Colebrook, correspondence, *Lancet* (1936), i. 1441.

under the influence of appropriate drugs; nothing has been more uncertain or perhaps more frankly disappointing than the effect on such a condition as streptococcal septi-caemia of administering all kinds of supposedly bactericidal compounds.[42]

The article continued by emphasizing the importance of the two papers, and mentioned that Colebrook had already embarked on his promised clinical trial. In fact Colebrook began the second trial in May 1936, using Prontosil supplied by Bayer, and the results were published in the *Lancet* in December 1936.[43] The paper, entitled 'Treatment with Prontosil of Puerperal Infections due to Haemolytic Streptococci', began as follows:

In a previous paper we reported the treatment of streptococcal peritonitis in mice by the injection of Prontosil soluble, and gave an account of 38 cases of human puerperal fever treated by injections of the dye together with oral administration of the less soluble compound, Prontosil [red]. The present paper deals with our experience in treating a further series of 26 consecutive cases, and summarises the impressions gained to date. During the next few months it is proposed to treat a new series of patients with the nearly related compound, *p*-aminobenzene-sulphonamide, which has given results even better than Prontosil in experimental infections of animals, and confers a much greater bactericidal power upon the blood. A comparison of the clinical results obtained with the two substances will be published later.

The results with these twenty-six cases were:

None of the patients has died. In one patient, admitted on the 25th day with an abdomino-pelvic mass, the treatment appeared to have no beneficial effect, but the inflammatory mass slowly resolved. Eleven others (42 per cent.) were mild cases which would almost certainly have recovered without any special treatment. The rapid and complete recovery of the remaining 14, more severe, cases makes it seem probable that the treat-ment assisted recovery. In at least three cases it was more than probable. Six of these 14 cases (23 per cent of the whole series) gave a positive blood culture (haemolytic streptococci) on admission; in one case the signs and symptoms pointed definitely to a generalised peritonitis, while in one other there was reason to suspect the beginning of that condition.

The overall mortality rate of the two trials combined—a total of sixty-four cases—was 4.7 per cent. In the five years before the first trial the mortality rate had varied between 16.6 per cent and 31.6 per cent, with an average of about 25 per cent.[44] Colebrook was cautious to a fault in his conclusions. He carefully considered the possibility that the results were due to a decrease in streptococcal virulence and showed why this was unlikely. He concluded that, on the evidence so far obtained, Prontosil was a highly effective treatment of streptococcal puerperal fever. Colebrook knew that sulphanilamide was the active agent of Prontosil, but—cautious as ever—he decided the next step must be to test sulphanilamide.

[42] Anon., leading article, 'The Chemotherapy of Streptococcal Infections', *Lancet* (1936), i. 1303–4.
[43] L. Colebrook and M. Kenny, 'Treatment with Prontosil of Puerperal Infections due to Haemolytic Streptococci', *Lancet* (1936), ii. 1319–22.   [44] Colebrook, 'The Story of Puerperal Fever', 250.

The third trial was reported in two papers in the *Lancet* in November and December 1937 [45] Altogether, 106 cases of streptococcal puerperal fever were treated with sulphanilamide. In nearly all cases the drug was administered by mouth. There were eight deaths, but only three were due solely to puerperal fever.[46] In the other five, conditions such as generalized peritonitis, pulmonary embolus, cerebral infarct, and a perforated gastric ulcer were partly or wholly the cause of death. In the three fatal cases in which death was due solely to puerperal fever, the disease was already at an advanced stage when they were admitted.

The main purpose of this, the third trial, was to compare the effects of sulphanilamide with Prontosil red and Prontosil soluble. Essentially, there was no significant difference. There were side effects from all three, especially cyanosis and methaemoglobinaemia, and in a few cases a recurrence of the fever seemed to be due to the drug itself and was called 'drug fever'. But none of the side effects was life threatening. Once again Colebrook dealt with the possibility that the fall in mortality was due to a change in the virulence of the streptococcus, noting that the obstetrician G. F. Gibberd was suggesting in 1937 that the virulence of the streptococcus might have declined over the past few years. Thus it might be that Colebrook's trials of Prontosil and sulphanilamide owed their success to a larger fall in the incidence of streptococcal septicaemia than formerly.

This was a suggestion that worried Colebrook greatly. He responded by comparing the mortality of all cases of puerperal septicaemia in Queen Charlotte's Hospital between 1932 and 1935 (that is, *before* the sulphonamides were available) in which there was a positive blood culture (evidence of invasion), with those cases in which there was a positive blood culture treated with sulphonamides in all three of the trials. There were eighty-two cases in the pre-sulphonamide group and the mortality rate was 71 per cent. In the group treated with sulphonamides there were twenty-two cases and the mortality rate was 27.3 per cent.[47] This was decisive. Taken together, these three careful and methodical trials carried out by Colebrook are one of the landmarks in the history of therapeutics. They showed for the first time that it was possible to cure bacterial diseases (other than syphilis) by chemotherapy. And what was so startling was this: after years of testing a vast number of chemical agents, many of them of great complexity, the successful one turned out to be a relatively simple chemical, easy to manufacture, which had been described in 1908 and promptly forgotten because there had been no hint of its therapeutic possibilities.

---

[45] L. Colebrook and A. W. Purdie, 'Treatment of 106 cases of Puerperal Fever by Sulphanilamide', *Lancet* (1937), ii. 1237–42, 1291–3.

[46] By the time the paper was published, a further fifteen cases had been treated with no deaths: 'The death-rate for all cases of infection by haemolytic streptococci, therefore, since August, 1936, has been 7 per cent' (ibid. 1293 n.).   [47] Ibid. 1291, table III.

The Impact of the Sulphonamides

The introduction of the sulphonamides summons up such hackneyed phrases as 'a miracle drug', 'a breakthrough', or 'the dawn of a new era in medicine'. Hackneyed they may be, but they are not an exaggeration. A general practitioner who became a partner in a market town in the Cotswolds in the 1960s recalls how one of his predecessors in the practice ('Jimmie') told him the following story:

Jimmie, as he was always known . . . was very much of the old school, brought up in an age when there were few active pharmaceuticals . . . In his cottage hospital, he had a maternity unit, of course, and the patients were confined to the hospital for several days *post-partum* in case they developed puerperal fever. He told me that those of us working in the 1960s with modern antibiotics aplenty could not begin to understand the feeling of horror of watching the swingeing fever take grip of a fit young woman, who had just given birth to her child, and realise you could do precious little but pray. One such tragedy was beginning to unfold in the mid-1930s when Jimmie happened to read the letters section of the *BMJ* over breakfast [circumstantial evidence suggests this was probably in the summer of 1936]. He saw a report from a London teaching hospital of a dye which appeared to have antibacterial properties. He picked up the telephone and managed to contact the author of the letter, demanded a sample of his dye to use on his patient, and suggested that if it was put on the noon train from Paddington he would meet the train personally. Not expecting any response he met the train, and the guard handed him a neatly wrapped brown paper parcel in which there was a vial of crystals without any instructions. He had read that he would need two to three days worth of treatment, so he divided the crystals into three, and dissolved a portion in sterile water. By this time the patient was almost comatose with a high fever, but Jimmie gave her the injections, and could hardly believe his own eyes when the fever receded. 'And she's still around the town to this day,' he would tell me, with a twinkle in his eye.[48]

Jimmie would soon have been able to obtain sulphonamides by orthodox prescribing, for, with a rapidity that would be unlikely in the late twentieth century, sulphonamides were on the market and widely used in hospital and general practice even before the third of Colebrook's papers was published.

In 1936 and 1937 there were reports from several British hospitals confirming Colebrook's results. At the Simpson Memorial (maternity) Hospital every patient delivered was given a prophylactic course of a sulphonamide.[49] Other reports came from hospitals in London,[50] Glasgow,[51] and Liverpool.[52] The

---

[48] A. Crowther, 'An Influential Doctor', *British Medical Journal* (1996), ii. 1530. I am grateful to Dr Crowther and the *British Medical Journal* for permission to publish this account.

[49] Edinburgh Medical Archives Centre, Records of the Edinburgh Royal Maternity and Simpson Memorial Hospital, *Annual Report for 1938*.

[50] G. F. Gibberd, 'Prontosil in Puerperal Infection', *British Medical Journal* (1937), ii. 229–30.

[51] M. A. Foulis and J. B. Barr, 'Prontosil Album in Puerperal Sepsis', *British Medical Journal* (1937), i. 445–6.   [52] B. Williams, 'Obstetrics and Gynaecology', *British Medical Journal* (1939), i. 39.

general practitioners' journal *Practitioner* published articles on the sulphonamides, and by the spring of 1937 it also carried advertisements of a variety
of sulphonamides produced by various drug companies. A survey of general
practitioners carried out in December 1937 showed that the sulphonamides
were widely used in general practice.[53] In a careful Medical Research Council
trial in 1936–7 involving 312 cases, it was shown that Prontosil was highly
effective against erysipelas.[54]

Prontosil rubrum was widely used on the Continent during and after 1935.
Roussel in France marketed a variant under the name of Rubiazol (*chlorhydrate
de sulfamido-chrysoidine*) in May 1935. In England sulphanilamide was marketed in 1936 or 1937 by Burroughs Wellcome as Sulphonamide, by Evans as
Streptoside, by British Drug Houses as Sulphonamide P, and by Allen and
Hanbury as Sulphonamide A&H. Variants were synthesized by drug companies in the hope of finding patentable versions that were as effective as
sulphanilamide and Prontosil, if not more so, and that had fewer side-effects.
There was one notable success.

May and Baker produced Sulphapyridine in 1938 giving it the name M&B
693 (693 was simply the number of the compound in the company's production schedules). Highly successful advertising made this such a household
name that all sulphonamides became known to most of the public as 'M&B',
just as the trade name Hoover became synonymous with vacuum cleaners.
Sulphapyridine was said to be much more effective against pneumococcal infections than sulphanilamide at a time when pneumococcal pneumonia was common amongst young people and carried a high mortality rate of about 24 per
cent. By 1943 it had been shown that the sulphonamides were effective against
erysipelas and puerperal sepsis, the pneumonias, meningococcal and gonococcal
infections, and bacillary dysentery.[55] All of these were common diseases in the
1930s and 1940s, and some were frequently fatal. The sulphonamides saved a
very large number of lives, and were used extensively by the services in the
Second World War, but in the early days the sulphonamides were not accepted
so readily in the USA as in Britain because of a disaster that occurred in 1937.
An American firm produced a formulation of sulphanilamide (called 'Elixir
Sulfanilamide') in which diethylene glycol was used as a diluent, and out of 353
patients treated with this medicine 105 died from the poisonous effects of the
diethylene glycol.[56]

As far as puerperal fever was concerned, however, unfortunately a small
proportion of severe cases were due to *Staphylococcus aureus* and these did

---

[53] Anon., 'Report of the Results of a Questionnaire Sent out to Practitioners on the Use of
Sulphonamides in General Practice', *Practitioner*, 140 (1938), 484–92.
[54] W. R. Snodgrass and T. Anderson, 'Prontosil in the Treatment of Erysipelas: A Controlled Trial
of 312 Cases', *British Medical Journal* (1937), ii. 101–4.
[55] Anon., editorial, 'The Medical Use of the Sulphonamides', *Public Health*, 57 (1943), 1–2.
[56] P. Wax, 'Elixirs, Diluents, and the Passage of the 1938 Federal Food, Drug and Cosmetic Act',
Annals of Internal Medicine, 122 (1995), 456–61.

not respond to the sulphonamides. Thus, when penicillin became available in 1944–5, it replaced the sulphonamides as the treatment of choice for puerperal fever, because penicillin was active against *Staphylococcus aureus* as well as *Streptococcus pyogenes*. Penicillin (but not the sulphonamides) was also effective against certain other organisms such as the gas-gangrene bacterium *Clostridium perfingens*, which was not uncommon (but virtually always fatal when accompanied by septicaemia) in cases of septic abortion, although it was rare in puerperal fever.[57] Penicillin had the additional advantage of being more active and less toxic than the sulphonamides.

The introduction of penicillin was accompanied by enormous publicity. Alexander Fleming was showered with honours from all over the world—a process, for all that he was genuinely a modest and unassuming man, that he greatly enjoyed—while the greater contribution of Florey and his colleagues in Oxford was largely ignored.[58] Penicillin is still used today. Everyone has heard of it. Fleming, and to a lesser extent Florey, are 'household names'. But who has heard of Domagk and Colebrook? For that matter, very few people today have even heard of the sulphonamides, apart, perhaps, from those old enough to associate the magic letters 'M&B' with their childhood.

Because the introduction of the sulphonamides did not provoke the intense publicity that surrounded the introduction of penicillin, the latter completely 'upstaged' the sulphonamides. It is true that penicillin was the better drug in many ways, even though the sulphonamides were active against certain bacteria such as the coliform organisms, and the organisms of bacterial dysentery, that did not respond to penicillin. Today, however, few are aware that the sulphonamides saved thousands of lives before penicillin became available. Doctors who were in clinical practice when the sulphonamides were introduced remember it as a more striking advance than the introduction of penicillin. Those who had for so many years scorned the possibility of ever discovering a 'magic bullet' that was effective against a range of bacteria were finally proved wrong, and the effect of this on medical research cannot be exaggerated.

Looking back, we can trace a thread of ideas from Perkin's attempt to synthesize quinine and his accidental discovery of mauve, to the growing connections between the dye industry and the pharmaceutical industry, especially in Germany. This, in turn, led to Ehrlich's work and his brilliant insights into receptors on bacteria that could be attacked or blocked by 'magic bullets', and thus to the notion of chemotherapy. Domagk's work arose directly from Ehrlich's, and the discovery of the sulphonamides led, at least in part, to penicillin. For, as Ronald Hare, who worked with Alexander Fleming and was involved in the introduction of penicillin, wrote in 1970: 'Let there be no doubt

---

[57] The first successful treatment with penicillin of gas-gangrene septicaemia in a case of septic abortion was carried out in the Radcliffe Infirmary, Oxford, in 1944 (the late Professor Sir John Stallworthy, personal communication, 1989).

[58] An excellent account of all this can be found in Macfarlane, *Alexander Fleming*.

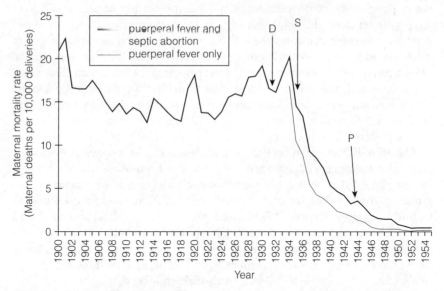

FIG. 11.2 Annual maternal mortality rates due to puerperal fever and septic abortion, England and Wales, 1900–1955, with the introduction of the sulphonamides and penicillin

Note: D = Domagk's experiment; S = the time when sulphonamides became available in hospital and general practice; P = the introduction of penicillin.

Source: A. Macfarlane and M. Mugford, *Birth Counts: Statistics of Pregnancy and Childbirth* (2 vols.; London 1984), ii, tables A.10.1, A.10.2.

about it, without the sulphonamides to show the way, it is improbable that penicillin would have emerged from its obscurity.'[59]

As far as puerperal fever is concerned, the sulphonamides were responsible for the initial part of the steep and sustained fall in deaths from puerperal fever that has continued ever since. In 1935 there were about 200 deaths from puerperal fever in England and Wales for every 100,000 births; in Scotland the rate was 230 per 100,000. By 1940 the mortality from puerperal fever (in England and Wales) had fallen to 30 per 100,000 births. By 1944, when penicillin was becoming generally available, puerperal-fever deaths had fallen to about ten, by 1950 to four, and by 1960 to only one per 100,000 births. In the years 1967–78 inclusive there were six years in which the rate of death from puerperal fever in England and Wales was one, and six in which it was zero. This decline, up to 1955, can be seen in Fig. 11.2.

This, then, seems to be the end of the story of puerperal fever. But not quite.

[59] Hare, *The Birth of Penicillin*, 161.

Post-antibiotic Epidemics of Puerperal Fever

By the 1960s a majority (often a large majority) of women in developed countries were delivered in hospital; the main exception was the Netherlands. Cases of puerperal fever outside hospitals would have been rare if only because so few women were delivered at home; and in the hospitals few doubted that hospital epidemics of puerperal fever had gone for ever. In May 1965, however, there was a rude awakening at the prestigious Lying-in Division of the Boston Hospital for Women when they suffered a sudden and totally unexpected epidemic of puerperal fever.[60] Twenty mothers and five babies were involved. There were no deaths, but many of the mothers were very ill indeed, in spite of prompt treatment with large intravenous doses of penicillin without which some would almost certainly have died.

As soon as the outbreak started, an intensive search began. Eight hundred personnel in the hospital, and many others (including visitors), were investigated as potential carriers. Using what was then a new technique for serotyping Group A streptococci, the offending serotype was found to be T-type 28. This type was not found in the initial (and very comprehensive) searches, and prophylactic penicillin (or other antibiotics) were given to all the maternity staff and to all maternity patients on admission in the hope of halting the epidemic. But it continued.

Eventually only one individual was found to be the carrier of the T-type 28 Group A streptococcus. He was a 'physician-anaesthetist'. Only two of the puerperal patients who were infected with the T-type 28 organism had *not* been exposed to him during their hospital stay. The oddest feature of all is that this anaesthetist was not a nose or throat carrier of the organism. The organism was isolated from beneath a small scab on the back of his hand and another on his shin. He had acquired these trivial scratches while pruning some rose bushes and they were so slight, so unimpressive, that they had escaped his attention until the survey was made. In his attendance on the affected patients he had never carried out a rectal or vaginal examination. All he had done was to hold the patients' hands for reassurance and help them when they were moved from the delivery table to a trolley or bed. Apart from providing an anaesthetic, this was his sole physical contact with the women who had developed puerperal fever.

There may have been similar post-1960 epidemics elsewhere, but I have not been able to find any. This appears to have been an isolated outbreak. The more one thinks about this epidemic (which has acquired the title the 'Rosebush-scratch' epidemic) the more it seems to be the oddest outbreak of an epidemic of puerperal fever ever recorded. Testing medical and nursing personnel revealed that 5 per cent were carriers of the Group A streptococcus, but none

[60] J. F. Jewett, D. E. Reid, L. E. Safon, and C. L. Easterday, 'Childbed Fever—a Continuing Entity', *Journal of the American Medical Association*, 206/2 (1968), 344–50. Another chattier account of this epidemic is J. A. Fitzgerald, 'Rosebud Scratch', *New York State Journal of Medicine*, 1 May 1972, 1077–80.

carried T-type 28 except the anaesthetist. Only this serotype, the T-type 28, proved capable of provoking the outbreak, and it had such an extraordinary degree of infectivity that it managed to leap, as it were, from two trivial scratches on the hand and leg of the anaesthetist to the genital tract of some twenty women, most of whom developed puerperal fever of a severity not seen for many decades.

Other people in the hospital must have been exposed to what seems to have been an extraordinarily virulent streptococcus, but there is no record of any becoming ill, except for the children of one of the patients who had puerperal fever in hospital; two of her children had acute pharyngitis due to T-type 28, which, it was thought, was brought home to them by the patient's husband after a hospital visit. Apart from this, only lying-in women were affected. It was almost as if this particular organism was disease-specific: that it could cause puerperal fever but no other form of streptococcal disease, although such a suggestion is not consistent with modern knowledge of the Group A streptococcus. We will refer to this epidemic briefly in the next and final chapter on the epidemiology of puerperal fever and streptococcal disease.

12

The Epidemiology of Puerperal Fever

Let us begin this chapter by reviewing some of the main features of the history of childbed or puerperal fever. Although it is probable that this disease had always existed, it was not until the end of the first half of the eighteenth century, when midwifery started to become part of regular medical practice and lying-in hospitals were established, that puerperal fever became recognized as a specific disease.

Endemic and Epidemic Puerperal Fever

It soon became apparent that it was a contagious disease, but one that stood apart from all other infectious or contagious diseases. It was not transmitted by direct contact, case to case. It was nearly always transmitted by those in attendance on the patient—doctors and midwives. By the end of the nineteenth century, obstetricians gradually became aware that midwives were, on the whole, less likely to transmit puerperal fever than doctors, because midwives interfered with labour to a lesser extent than doctors, and were less likely to come into contact with cases of sepsis such as erysipelas and septic wounds.

Because the poor were most often delivered by midwives, and the middle and upper classes by doctors, puerperal fever was unique in its social-class distribution. Whereas death rates from infectious disease were almost invariably higher amongst the poor and lowest amongst the upper and professional classes, the opposite was true of puerperal fever. This can be seen in Table 12.1, where the social-class gradients of death rates for maternal mortality (all causes) and of deaths from puerperal fever are contrasted with the social-class gradient of infant mortality in the 1930s.

We have seen that puerperal fever occurred in sporadic (or endemic) form and also in epidemics. A list of epidemics from 1770 to 1849 can be found in Table 4.1, but Hirsch, on whose work this table is largely based, identified a few much earlier epidemics of puerperal fever.[1] It seems safe to assume there were other epidemics, unrecognized and therefore unrecorded, in earlier periods.

[1] See Ch. 4 n. 2.

TABLE 12.1. *Maternal mortality rates from all causes and from puerperal sepsis, and infant mortality rates, England and Wales, 1930–1932*

Social class	Maternal mortality rate[a]		Infant mortality rate[b]
	All causes	Puerperal sepsis	
I	44.4[c] ⎫	14.5[c] ⎫	33
II	⎬	⎬	45
III	41.1	13.3	58
IV	41.6	12.1	67
V	38.9	11.6	77

  [a] Maternal mortality rates are expressed as maternal deaths per 10,000 deliveries.
  [b] Infant mortality rates are expressed as infant deaths per 1,000 deliveries.
  [c] Social classes I and II combined.

Sources: Maternal mortality: *Annual Statistical Review of the Registrar General for England and Wales* (1934), 131; infant mortality: R. Titmuss, *Birth Poverty and Wealth: A Study of Infant Mortality* (London, 1943), 26, 37.

In epidemics, the case fatality rate tended to be highest at the beginning of the epidemic, sometimes reaching levels of 70 to 80 per cent, but the rates tailed off over a period of a year or two. Data on case fatality rates in sporadic cases are relatively sparse, but it seems likely that they were on average in the region of 25 to 30 per cent up to the introduction of the sulphonamides in the mid-1930s. Incidentally, the shorter the time between delivery and the onset of the disease, the higher the mortality, and also the shorter the interval between onset and death. Rapid onset and death were a feature of epidemics.

The 'ferocity' of epidemics (by which I mean the case fatality rate and the severity of illness) was at least as great in the second half of the eighteenth century when there are several descriptions of whole wards being 'swept away', as it was in the early and mid-nineteenth century. By the late nineteenth and early twentieth centuries, it seems that epidemics had become less common, but that, as we will see, may be a partial illusion.

In numerous accounts of town epidemics, there were striking stories of medical practitioners (or occasionally midwives) who suddenly had a large number of successive cases of puerperal fever while their colleagues had few or none. We cited several examples of this from the UK, the USA, and France in Chapter 4. Oliver Wendell Holmes stressed this aspect of puerperal fever, roundly condemning medical practitioners who, having had two or more cases of puerperal fever in their private practice, continued to attend deliveries. Hence the title of his publication, *Puerperal Fever as a Private Pestilence*, meaning that puerperal fever was a disease spread by practitioners in their private practice.

Holmes's work (published in 1843, and republished in 1855) reflected a growing tendency from the mid-nineteenth century for practitioners to be blamed and accused of negligence if they had a case, or, worse, a series of cases, of puerperal fever in their practice. With the introduction of Listerian antisepsis in the 1880s, this tendency increased, for it became abundantly clear that to a large extent puerperal fever should be regarded as a preventable disease. It is, therefore, not surprising that some doctors were tempted to deflect blame by resorting to means of concealing deaths due to puerperal fever by entering a different cause of death on death certificates. Some would certify the cause of death as obstetric haemorrhage, or enter the terms 'peritonitis' or 'septicaemia' on the death certificate while deliberately failing to mention childbirth.[2] In England and Wales the Registrar General's office knew this was occurring and, by some detective work, managed to estimate the extent to which it occurred, concluding that the consequent under-certification of deaths from puerperal fever was slight.

We can be sure that the number of deaths from puerperal fever was never exaggerated, and the same motive—concealment through fear of blame—may have prevented some doctors from publishing accounts of epidemics of puerperal fever. This may have contributed to the apparent cessation of epidemics in the twentieth century. Cullingworth knew of at least one extensive but unpublished epidemic in the practice of a doctor in Sussex in 1906.[3] Likewise, when Watson reported an outbreak of puerperal fever in a New York hospital in 1928 and remarked that 'an occurrence of this nature is now happily rare',[4] the famous American obstetrician Joseph B. DeLee remarked that he had collected evidence on '29 outbreaks of puerperal fever in the country at large but only one institution [the New York hospital] had had the scientific candor to report the epidemic'.[5] Nevertheless, it is likely that there was a real decline in epidemics of puerperal fever from the late nineteenth century and through the first thirty years of the twentieth.

Mortality due to Puerperal Fever

The trend in deaths from puerperal fever in England and Wales from 1850 to 1940 is shown in Fig. 12.1, where it can be seen that mortality remained on a high plateau until the mid-1930s and then began to fall steeply. The striking difference between mortality from puerperal fever and from most other

---

[2] This difficult problem is discussed in I. Loudon, *Death in Childbirth: An International Study of Maternal Care and Maternal Mortality 1800–1950* (Oxford, 1992) in app. I, 'Hidden Maternal Deaths', pp. 518–24, where reasons are given for believing that, although the true mortality rate from puerperal fever was underestimated, the extent to which this occurred was relatively slight.

[3] C. J. Cullingworth, *Oliver Wendell Holmes and the Contagiousness of Puerperal Fever* (London, 1906), 27 n.

[4] B. P. Watson, 'An Outbreak of Puerperal Sepsis in New York City', *American Journal of Obstetrics and Gynaecology*, 16 (1928), 157–79, at 157.

[5] J. F. Jewett, D. E. Reid, L. E. Safon, and C. L. Easterday, 'Childbed Fever—a Continuing Entity', *Journal of the American Medical Association*, 206/2 (1968), 344–50, at 350.

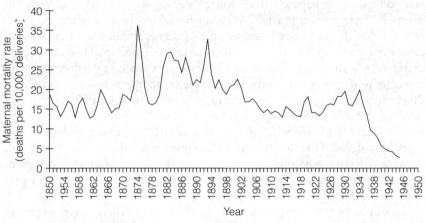

(a) Arithmetic scale

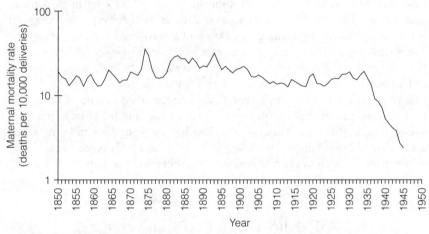

(b) Logarithmic scale

FIG. 12.1 Annual maternal mortality rates due to puerperal fever, England and Wales, 1850–1946

Sources: Annual Reports of the Registrar General for England and Wales; Statistical Reviews of the Registrar General for England and Wales.

infectious diseases such as diphtheria, typhoid, measles, scarlet fever, and tuberculosis is the *absence* of a sustained decline of puerperal-fever deaths from the end of the nineteenth century to the mid-1930s. The chance of a child dying of scarlet fever or diphtheria was very much lower in the 1930s than it had been in the mid-nineteenth century, but the risk of a woman dying of puerperal fever in Britain in the first half of the 1930s was as high as it had been in the 1860s, and actually higher than in 1910. The other striking features of Figs. 12.1 and 12.2

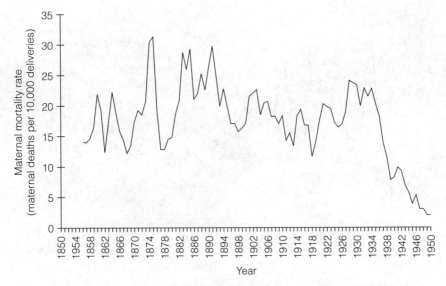

FIG. 12.2 Annual maternal mortality rates due to puerperal fever, Scotland, 1855–1950; arithmetic scale

Source: I. Loudon, *Death in Childbirth: An International Study of Maternal Care and Maternal Mortality* (Oxford, 1992), 546–9, app. 6, table 3.

are the 'spikiness' (that is, surges of mortality above and below the average) of the graphs in the nineteenth century and the partial reduction of that 'spikiness' in the twentieth.

What happened in other countries? Puerperal fever was on the whole as prevalent in all developed countries as it was in the UK. Exact comparisons of international secular trends would be easy if most Western countries (and cities) had routinely collected and published data from the mid-nineteenth century on annual deaths from puerperal fever in a consistent manner. Very few did. However, many countries published data on maternal mortality rates as a whole, and mortality trends of puerperal fever can often be inferred from trends of total maternal mortality. The reason for saying so is that, in contrast with the 'spikiness' of mortality rates of puerperal fever, maternal deaths from causes other than puerperal fever were relatively constant, rumbling along at much the same level year after year. Wide variations in maternal mortality over short periods were always due to puerperal fever.[6]

In countries of north-west Europe such as Scandinavia and the Netherlands, rates of maternal mortality (and probably of puerperal fever) were of the same order as those found in Britain during the second half of the nineteenth

---

[6] Trends in maternal mortality in various countries can be found in Loudon, *Death in Childbirth*, app. 6, pp. 542–84.

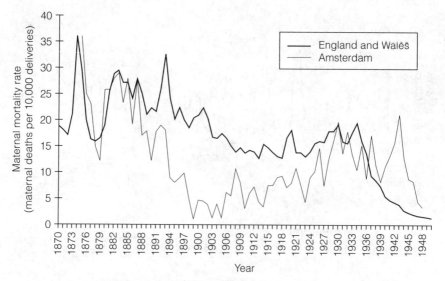

FIG. 12.3 Annual maternal mortality rates due to puerperal fever, England and Wales, 1870–1946, and Amsterdam, 1875–1950

Sources: England and Wales: see Fig. 12.1; Amsterdam: Loudon, *Death in Childbirth*, 564–5, app. 6, table 15.

century. From about 1880–1900, however, maternal mortality in north-west Europe fell steeply until about 1910, owing to the widespread use of antisepsis (see Chapter 9) and then levelled out to form a plateau as in Britain, but a plateau at a lower level. The steep fall from 1880–1910 was due to a reduction of deaths from puerperal fever rather than a reduction of deaths from other causes. Amsterdam, unlike most cities, kept records of deaths from puerperal fever over a long period, and the pattern of mortality in that city is shown in Fig. 12.3 together with the pattern seen in England and Wales.

The trend in puerperal-fever deaths in Amsterdam has two interesting features. After the steep fall between 1880 and 1910, the rise in puerperal-fever mortality between 1910 and the mid-1930s was unusually steep. It is probable that this rise was due to an increasing rate of deaths from septic abortion.[7] The second feature is the effect of wartime occupation in the Netherlands, which, because it disrupted maternal care and morale and led to a scarcity of sulphonamides, prevented the steep fall in puerperal-fever mortality seen in unoccupied countries.[8] After the war, however, puerperal-fever mortality in Amsterdam rapidly fell to the same levels as in England and Wales and other Western countries.

[7] Trends in maternal mortality in various countries can be found in Loudon, *Death in Childbirth*, app. 6, pp. 542–84.   [8] Ibid. 443–4, 456–8.

In other European countries, as well as in the Commonwealth countries such as Australia and New Zealand, the same general pattern of deaths from puerperal fever occurred: a high rate throughout the nineteenth century, usually a continuing high plateau from 1900 to the mid-1930s, and then, more or less at the same time, a steep downturn in mortality with the introduction of the sulphonamides.

As Fig. 12.3 shows, there was a close correspondence between the peaks and troughs of mortality in England and Wales and in Amsterdam during the nineteenth century. It is a matter of some interest that, from the time national records began, the highest peak of puerperal-fever mortality ever recorded in England and Wales occurred in 1874–5 and was accompanied by simultaneous record highs in Scotland, in Norway and Sweden, the Netherlands, and Belgium, and also in Massachusetts and probably in Montreal, New York, and Philadelphia.[9] Whether other countries or cities were similarly affected is unknown, because data on national rates of maternal mortality in the 1870s were not recorded.

That the two years 1874 and 1875 (and occasionally 1873 as well) seem to have been notable for what was probably the most deadly pandemic of puerperal fever ever recorded suggests the possibility that some seasonal global influence may have been responsible, or that an exceptionally virulent serotype of the Group A streptococcus travelled widely and rapidly round a large part of the world. To make matters more difficult, however, it should be noted that not all peaks followed such a pattern. Thus the second highest peak of deaths from puerperal fever in England and Wales and in Scotland occurred in 1893 (Figs. 12.1 and 12.2), but an 1893 peak does not appear to have occurred in other countries.

These are some of the main features of the epidemiology of puerperal fever. Why did the trend in puerperal-fever deaths follow the pattern described above? Why was the secular trend so 'spiky' in the nineteenth century? Why did some practitioners have dozens of patients with puerperal fever while others had none? Why were there close links between puerperal fever and erysipelas, but not between puerperal fever and scarlet fever? I believe the key to understanding such questions is the versatile and complex micro-organism, the Group A streptococcus. This was not, as we have seen, the only micro-organism capable of producing puerperal fever, but it was the cause of all epidemics, and of a large majority of deaths in sporadic cases. Table 12.2 is based on a bacteriological report that is typical of many produced before the Second World War. It suggests that, for all practical purposes—and it was an opinion shared by

---

[9] Ibid., app. 6; J. S. Parry, 'Description of a Form of Puerperal Fever which Occurred at the Philadelphia Hospital Characterized by Diphtheritic Deposits of Wounds of the Genital Passages and by other Peculiar Phenomena', *American Journal of Medical Sciences*, 69 (1875), 46–76; Massachusetts, Reports to the State Board of Health; D. C. McCallum, 'Report of the University Lying-in Hospital, Montreal, from Oct.1 1867 to Oct. 1 1875', *Transactions of the Obstetrical Society of London*, 20 (1878), 35–51.

TABLE 12.2. *Bacteriological findings in eighty-eight cases of puerperal fever, Aberdeen, 1918–1927*

Bacteriological findings	Died	Recovered
Results obtained from blood culture, uterine culture, or culture from secondary suppurative processes		
Streptococcus haemolyticus, alone or in combination with other organisms	28	26
Staphylococcus		1
Staphylococcus and B. Coli		4
Streptococcus viridans and B. Coli		1
B. faecalis		1
B. coli		2
Gonococcus		1
All cultures sterile		23
No bacteriological evidence obtained	1	
TOTALS	29	59
Results of blood culture		
Streptococcus haemolyticus	22	6
Other organisms	0	3
Blood culture sterile	6	50
Blood culture not carried out	1	0
TOTALS	29	59

Sources: Scottish Board of Health; J. P. Kinloch, J. Smith, and J. A. Stephen, *Maternal Mortality: Report on Maternal Mortality in Aberdeen, 1918–1927, with Special Reference to Puerperal Sepsis* (Edinburgh, 1928), 52–4.

the leading bacteriologists of the 1930s—puerperal fever should be regarded as essentially a streptococcal disease.[10]

The Group A Streptococcus

The streptococci are spherical or ovoid bacteria joined together like a chain. Pasteur referred to them as the 'microbe en chapelet' (the microbe like a rosary).[11] The streptococci comprise a very large family, but we are concerned with only one member, properly called *Streptococcus pyogenes* but commonly

---

[10] W. W. C. Topley and G. S. Wilson, *Principles of Bacteriology and Immunity* (2nd edn., London, 1936), 1170.

[11] Streptococcus comes from the Greek *streptos*, which came to mean a chain formed of links or a necklace of beads. *Coccus* meant a round berry. The cocci are 0.5–0.75 microns in diameter, a micron being 1/1000th of a millimetre, and the number in a chain varies but is often about ten (A. B. Christie, *Infectious Diseases, Epidemiology and Clinical Practice* (2nd edn., London, 1974, 1009).

TABLE 12.3. *Some of the diseases associated with infection by the Group A streptococcus*

Diseases always due to the Group A streptococcus	Diseases usually or sometimes due to the Group A streptococcus, but which can also be due to other bacteria or to viruses
Scarlet fever	Puerperal fever/sepsis
Erysipelas	Cellulitis and impetigo
Streptococcal toxic shock-like syndrome	Necrotizing fasciitis
Acute glomerular nephritis[a]	Pharyngitis and tonsillitis
Rheumatic fever[a]	Otitis media and mastoiditis
	Pneumonia
	Meningitis
	Endocarditis
	Septic arthritis
	Osteomyelitis
	Septicaemia

[a] Strictly speaking, these are sequelae to streptococcal infection.

known as the Group A streptococcus or, to give it its full name, the ß-haemolytic streptococcus Lancefield Group A.[12] In the past it was often called *Streptococcus haemolyticus*. The main diseases associated with the Group A streptococcus are listed in Table 12.3.

Although Rokitansky in 1864 and Mayrhofer in 1865 found unidentified microbes in the vaginal discharges of women with puerperal fever,[13] streptococci were probably first recognized by Pasteur in 1879 when he described them at a meeting in Paris, and his findings were confirmed soon afterwards by Doléris, as described in Chapter 8. The term *Streptococcus pyogenes* was first used by Rosenbach in 1884 in recognition of the presence of these organisms in suppurative lesions; Schottmüller distinguished haemolytic from non-haemolytic streptococci in 1903, and in 1907 Schick recognized the connection between scarlet fever and subsequent rheumatic fever and acute glomerulonephritis. It was not until 1924 that Dick proved what had long been suspected —that scarlet fever was indeed due to the Group A streptococcus.[14]

In the 1920s Griffiths in England and Lancefield in America classified streptococci by their surface antigens. Lancefield divided streptococci into Group A, Group B, Group C, and so on, by means of their polysaccharide antigens, and showed that the protein antigens, used for classification by Griffiths,

[12] The full name was given by Rebecca Lancefield, an American bacteriologist who, in the 1920s, was largely responsible for the classification of the streptococci.

[13] J. H. Burtenshaw, 'The Fever of the Puerperium (Puerperal Infection)', *New York Journal and Philadelphia Medical Journal*, 79 (1904), 1073–9, 1134–8, 1189–94, 1234–8; 80 (1904), 20–5.

[14] G. F. Dick and G. H. Dick, 'The Etiology of Scarlet Fever', *Journal of the American Medical Association*, 82 (1924), 301–2.

could be divided into T and M antigens. T antigens are useful for differentiating serotypes of the Group A streptococcus, but it is the M antigens by which the serotypes are usually known, and which play a large part in determining virulence. Immunity tends to be serotype specific, so that anyone attempting to produce a vaccine against the Group A streptococcus would find that the vaccine was effective against only one specific serotype. Likewise, people who suffered a streptococcal disease due to one serotype would not, when they recovered, be immune to other serotypes, and by the late 1990s over ninety different T or M serotypes have been identified.[15]

Although the work of Lancefield and Griffiths enabled bacteriologists to trace the origin of cases or epidemics of streptococcal diseases, it proved impossible to identify any given M serotype (or group of M serotypes) as the invariable cause of one type of streptococcal disease rather than another, although some M serotypes tended to appear more frequently than others in certain outbreaks of streptococcal disease. Likewise it was impossible to identify certain M or T serotypes as being invariably virulent, or others that were weakly virulent.

By the 1970s, however, it often seemed in clinical practice that detailed serotyping was unnecessary, because severe streptococcal disease was thought to have disappeared. Rheumatic fever and acute nephritis had virtually ceased to exist. Scarlet fever had changed from a deadly disease into a minor one. Serious epidemics due to group A streptococci were very rare, and puerperal fever had almost totally disappeared as a life-threatening disease.[16] Moreover, unlike organisms such as *Staphlyococcus aureus*, whose ability rapidly to produce resistance to a wide range of antibiotics is well known, the Group A streptococcus remains sensitive to penicillin. Clinicians who encountered streptococcal disease were usually content to identify the offending organism as the Group A streptococcus on clinical and/or bacteriological grounds, regardless of serotype, in the knowledge that penicillin would nearly always cure the patient rapidly.[17]

From the early 1980s, however, there has been a surge of interest in the Group A streptococcus following the startling reappearance of rheumatic fever in the

---

[15] G. H. Stollerman, 'Changing Streptococci and Prospects for the Global Eradication of Rheumatic Fever', *Perspectives in Biology and Medicine*, 40/2 (1997), 165–87, and 'Streptococcus Pyogenes', in S. L. Gorbach, J. H. Bartlett, and N. R. Blacklow (eds.), *Infectious Diseases* (2nd edn., Philadelphia, 1998) ch. 192, 1703–19.

[16] This, however, only applies to the developed world in the second half of the twentieth century. Serious streptococcal disease in the developing world, and rheumatic fever in particular, is still common. In the 1970s the prevalence of rheumatic heart disease per 1,000 schoolchildren was 0.1 in the USA, 1.5 in China, 10 in Egypt, 6–11 in India, 1.8–11 in Pakistan, and 1.2–21 in Thailand (G. H. Stollerman, 'Rheumatogenic Group A Streptococci and the Return of Rheumatic Fever', *Advances in Internal Medicine*, 35/1 (1990), 1–25).

[17] In 1997 I asked a senior London obstetrician with an appointment in a teaching hospital when he had last seen a case of puerperal fever? He said that he had not used the term for years. If one of his patients ran a fever, he simply gave her antibiotics and if he named the cause of the fever he said it was 'metritis', which was a nice resuscitation of a term often used in the early nineteenth century.

USA in 1984, and a marked rise in the incidence of invasive streptococcal infection since 1987. The sudden appearance of streptococcal toxic shock syndrome —a syndrome previously associated solely with *Staphlyococcus aureus*—was also a total surprise.[18] Deaths and severe illness due to Group A streptococcus diseases have reappeared not only in the USA but in other developed countries.[19] Some microbiologists have even suggested that we may be on the edge of seeing a resurgence of streptococcal disease similar in severity to the nineteenth century.

In a review of this unexpected reappearance of Group A streptococcus disease, Musser and Krause in 1998 listed some of the features of the microorganism that had become known:

Wild-type strains isolated world-wide possess substantial chromosomal and allelic diversity and cause an unusually diverse range of infection types. In part due to this diversity we lack a comprehensive understanding of the molecular pathogenesis of Group A streptococcus virulence . . . Evidence suggests that the following streptococcal molecules contribute to one or more phases of Group A streptococcus pathogenesis: M protein, M-like protein, hyaluronic acid capsule, C5a peptidase, streptokinase, streptolysin O, and hyaluronidase . . . The tissue destruction in many patients [with invasive streptococcal disease] is extensive, rapidly progressive, and characterized by a virtual total destruction of the extracellular matrix. This histopathology occurs at many distant sites where bacteria are not present.[20]

The effect of research since 1980 has been to reveal the complexity of this formidable and versatile organism. The array of armaments available to the Group A streptococcus includes virulent M antigens, spreading factors such as hyaluronidase, which liquefy pus and facilitate the rapid spread of infection and destruction, and exotoxins, which extend the damage beyond the actual presence of bacteria. Three distinct toxins, known as erythrogenic toxins SPE A, SPE B, and SPE C, have been identified. These are 'superantigens' that can cause 'fever, shock and tissue damage'.[21] It is now known that the same M-type may exist in several forms depending on the presence or absence of such factors as the A, B, and C erythrogenic toxins, streptolysins, and streptokinase. In an outbreak of invasive streptococcal disease in Sweden in 1989, predominantly due to the M1T1 serotype, patients with uncomplicated infections were

[18] M. M. Musser and R. M. Krause, 'The Revival of Group A Streptococcal Diseases with a Commentary on Staphylococcal Toxic Shock Syndrome', in R. M. Krause (ed.), *Emerging Infections* (New York, 1998), 185–218, at 185.

[19] R. M. Krause, 'Dynamics of Emergence', *Journal of Infectious Diseases*, 170 (1994) 265–71. Krause believes the re-emergence of severe streptococcal infections causing the toxic shock-like syndrome (TSLS) suggests it may be due to 'the cascade of toxic events released by "superantigens", the erythrogenic toxins or exotoxins'. See also Musser and Krause, 'The Revival of Group A Streptococcal Diseases'.

[20] Musser and Krause, 'The Revival of Group A Streptococcal Diseases', 189, 190, 191.

[21] P. W. Ross, 'Streptococcus and Enterococcus', in D. Greenwood, R. C. B. Slack, and J. F. Peutherer (eds.), *Medical Microbiology* (15th edn., London, 1997), 175–87, at 175–7.

found to have high serum antibody levels to pyrogenic exotoxins B and C, while patients with bacteriaemia or fatal infections had low levels. Here, the virulence appeared to be related not only to the M proteins but also to the SPE exotoxins.[22]

There is also some new evidence linking specific streptococcal diseases to specific strains. Stollerman has shown there are serotypes that are invariably associated with rheumatic fever—the rheumatogenic serotypes—making it feasible at last to produce a vaccine against rheumatic fever. It is also known that rheumatic fever and acute nephritis (the two major sequelae of some forms of Group A streptococcal disease) never occur together, have a different natural history, and are due to different serotypes. Serotypes associated with acute nephritis are related to those that cause pyoderma—that is, skin infection—while those that cause rheumatic fever are kin to serotypes causing pharyngitis.[23] In general, however, 'Although a few M-type strains have appeared more frequently than expected in series of isolates associated with severe streptococcal disease, among recent severe cases no single M- or T-type strain has predominated.'[24]

This glance at the pathological features of the Group A streptococcus is, of course, not intended to be in any way comprehensive. It may, however, be sufficient to help us to understand some of the mechanisms that shaped the epidemiology of puerperal fever in the eighteenth and nineteenth centuries. New work on the molecular structure, and thus the specificity and virulence of certain serotypes of the Group A streptococcus, may help in understanding the rapidity with which the disease could kill, the high proportion of peritonitis in fatal cases of puerperal fever,[25] and the connections between streptococcal diseases.

In the study of diseases such as typhoid and cholera, historians look for epidemiological clues in such factors as the water supply and sewage disposal. In diseases such as typhus, conditions that encouraged the spread of lice, such as close contact and overcrowding, are seen as a prime epidemiological factor. Streptococcal diseases are different because of two factors that, although not unique, play a larger part in determining the distribution, incidence, and fatality of streptococcal disease than they do in any other disease or group of diseases. The two factors are wide-ranging differences in virulence between serotypes, and the vital importance of the carrier state.

---

[22] Musser and Krause, 'The Revival of Group A Streptococcal Diseases', 209.

[23] Stollerman, 'Changing Streptococci'.

[24] A. R. Katz and D. M. Morens, 'Severe Streptococcal Infections in Historical Perspective', *Clinical Infectious Diseases*, 14 (1992), 298–307, at 298.

[25] In some instances, as many as 90% of cases examined at post-mortem showed signs of invasive infection and peritonitis. In 1830 Tonnellé in Paris found post-mortem evidence of peritonitis in 193 out of 222 dissections of fatal cases of puerperal fever (M. Tonnellé, 'Des fièvres puerpérales observés à la Maternité pendant l'année 1829', originally published as four papers in *Archives Générales de Médecin* (Mar., Apr., May, and June 1830); repr. in 'Critical Analysis', *Edinburgh Medical and Surgical Journal*, 34 (1830), 325–49).

The Carrier State

The natural habitat of the Group A streptococcus is the nose and throat of human beings, where it adheres by the hair-like projections or 'fimbriae' on the surface of the organism, which contain lipoteichoic acid allowing the fimbriae to bind avidly with the epithelial cells.[26] Group A streptococci may survive for a few days outside the body under damp conditions such as damp clothing or surgical dressings, but they die rapidly under dry conditions. In general, however, the organism is content to live in a state of peaceful symbiosis in the nose and throat of human beings.

The carrier state of the Group A streptococcus has been recognized since the late 1920s, and various studies during the inter-war period came up with different estimates of the proportion of carriers in the population. One of the pioneers of streptococcal pathology, Ronald Hare, wrote in 1935: 'It would appear that from 5 to 40 per cent of apparently normal individuals living in the temperate zone have haemolytic streptococci in the upper respiratory tract.' He found, however, that only about a third of the streptococci belonged to group A, and it has been known for some time that not all the group A serotypes isolated from human beings are pathogenic. Hare also mentioned that, amongst doctors, nurses, and attendants on parturient women, potentially pathogenic haemolytic streptococci could be found in the throat of 20.3 per cent, and in the nose of 5.4 per cent.[27] Hare thought that nasal carriers were more dangerous than throat carriers as a source of infection.[28] Topley and Wilson reported in 1946 that investigations in Melbourne in Australia showed that 4.5 per cent of healthy children and adults were streptococcal carriers in 1939 and 13.3 per cent of children in 1940.[29] Many other reports in this period came up with similar findings.

One might well imagine that, since the Second World War, widespread use of antibiotics, better standards of living and general health, better hygiene, and the decline in severe streptococcal disease (for which there is no certain explanation) would have been accompanied by a profound fall in the proportion of carriers in the population. This appears not to be the case. In England, Barnham wrote in 1997 that 'recent studies in Yorkshire' showed a general carrier rate of 6.4 per cent of all streptococci and 1.5 per cent of Group A streptococci, but in closed communities—residential schools and detention centres—carrier rates of 50 per cent may be found.[30] In the USA, Gray and

---

[26] Stollerman, 'Streptococcus Pyogenes'.

[27] This was cited by Hare as unpublished work by Elizabeth White (R. Hare, 'The Classification of Haemolytic Streptococci from the Nose and Throat of Normal Human Beings by Means of Precipitin and Biochemical Tests', *Journal of Pathology and Bacteriology*, 41 (1935), 499–512).   [28] Ibid. 511.

[29] W. W. C. Topley and G. S. Wilson, *Principles of Bacteriology and Immunity*, rev. G. S. Wilson and A. A. Miles (3rd edn., London, 1946), 1469.

[30] M. Barnham, 'ß-Haemolytic Streptococci', in A. M. Emmerson, P. M. Hawkey, and S. H. Gillespie (eds.), *Principles and Practice of Clinical Bacteriology* (Chichester, 1997), 37–71.

colleagues, writing in 1991, reported that, in an investigation carried out in Rochester, New York, between 1967 and 1988, out of 23,000 throat cultures 18–25 per cent were positive for Group A streptococci. They were surprised to find that the annual rates of carriers had remained more or less constant, even though cases of rheumatic fever and glomerulonephritis had fallen profoundly during this period. They also found that in most carriers who were infectious there was evidence of recent overt streptococcal infection, although the infection may have been of a minor nature.[31]

Thus, even under the healthier conditions of the developed world at the end of the twentieth century, a large number of people are, at any given time, carriers of Group A streptococci. A carrier rate as low as 5 per cent may sound trivial, but it would mean that the streptococcus is carried by about two and a half million people in Britain. In the eighteenth and nineteenth centuries, when streptococcal disease was much more common and severe, it is probable that carrier rates of virulent strains were much higher.

Carrier rates usually vary with season, with the presence or absence of streptococcal outbreaks, with crowded living conditions, and, most importantly for puerperal fever and erysipelas, with occupation. Thus the rate will usually rise in the winter months when streptococcal outbreaks are most frequent, and high carrier rates are often found in institutions such as boarding schools and military barracks. Surprisingly few reports of the carrier state amongst medical personnel exist, but those there are consistently report a higher rate than prevails in the general population. In 1946, Topley and Wilson reported that amongst patients and nurses in the Birmingham Accident Hospital in 1944 the carrier rate was 19.2 per cent, whereas the rate in the general population was between 4 per cent and 8 per cent.[32]

Many of the features of puerperal fever that were so puzzling to our predecessors can be explained by the carrier state. Birth attendants, such as the unfortunate Dr Rutter of Philadelphia in the 1840s (see Chapter 4), who had case after case in their practice and carried infection with them wherever they went, were almost certainly people who probably had a recent minor streptococcal infection and became carriers of a virulent strain of the Group A streptococcus. The anaesthetist at the Boston Women's Hospital in 1965 (see Chapter 11) was simply a very unusual modern example of the same phenomenon. But before the 1920s, birth attendants had, of course, no way of knowing that the infection they carried was not (or not necessarily) in their clothes, or hands, or equipment, but in the droplets they exhaled directly onto their patients.

Similarly, when the nineteenth-century lying-in hospitals went to very great lengths to fumigate, to lime-wash the walls, and even to close wards for some weeks in the hope of eliminating puerperal fever, it was inevitable that they

---

[31] B. M. Gray, 'Streptococcal Infections', in A. S. Evans, and P. S. Brachman (eds.), *Bacterial Infections in Humans: Epidemiology and Control* (New York, 1991), 639–73.
[32] Topley and Wilson, *Principles of Bacteriology and Immunity* (3rd edn.), 469.

failed. The probable source of infection was not poisons soaked in the fabric of the building but (as they had no way of knowing) the carriers of the Group A streptococcus amongst members of the staff.

The carrier state was probably responsible for the outbreak of surgical wound infection in the wards of Aberdeen hospital that coincided with the town outbreak of puerperal fever in Aberdeen in 1790–2, because there was no direct contact between the birth attendants and the patients in the hospital (Chapter 3). Cross infection between maternity and surgical wards was often reported, most notably in the case of King's College Hospital, where Florence Nightingale closed the maternity ward she had opened on the grounds that a general hospital was far too dangerous a place for women to be delivered.[33] The transfer of infection in hospitals and in home deliveries by infected hands, dressings, or instruments may have been one reason for cross infection. Until the twentieth century it was thought to be the only reason. But a high streptococcal carrier rate amongst doctors and midwives in hospitals may well have been the most important element.

The problem of cross infection was very much in the mind of George Geddes, a general practitioner who worked at first in a country practice in the north of Britain and then moved to a coal-mining area in the industrial Midlands. He wrote two books on puerperal sepsis, one in 1912 and a second in 1926.[34] In his country practice he saw few cases of puerperal fever, but in the industrial area of his second practice he found there were many, especially when the birth attendant was a general practitioner rather than a midwife. Where industrial injuries were common, Geddes believed that general practitioners, who, as part of their daily routine, attended and dressed infected wounds and handled cases of erysipelas, were bound to carry infection to their maternity patients, in spite of careful washing. Midwives, who were usually quite separate from district nurses, never dealt with septic wounds on a regular basis.

The importance of the carrier state was emphasized in 1935 by Ronald Hare:

The work of Smith (1931, 1933), Paine (1931, 1935), Courmont and Sédallian (1931) and Dora Colebrook (1935) indicates very strongly that the vast majority of haemolytic streptococcal infections of the uterus during the puerperium are due to the transfer of organisms to the birth canal from the throats of 'carriers' who were present at or shortly after the time of delivery.[35]

Leonard Colebrook, who estimated in 1936 that 7 per cent of the population were carriers of the Group A streptococcus, believed that 'the haemolytic streptococci of the respiratory tract constitute the chief menace in maternity work; particularly those streptococci associated with recent acute infection of

---

[33] Florence Nightingale, *Introductory Notes on Lying-in Hospitals* (London, 1876).

[34] G. Geddes, *Statistics of Puerperal Sepsis and Allied Infectious Diseases* (Bristol, 1912); *Puerperal Septicaemia: Its Causation, Symptoms, Prevention and Treatment* (Bristol, 1926).

[35] Hare, 'The Classification of Haemolytic Streptococci', 503. A few of the carriers were suffering from sore throats or other minor symptoms, but the majority had no illness and no symptoms.

the respiratory tract'.[36] Gibberd (an obstetric surgeon at Guy's Hospital in London) was one of the first to underline the importance of the carrier state in 1931 when he wrote:

Much more common are cases of infection which can be traced to one individual. Hands and clothing have been blamed in the past but the throat as a source of infection—especially the asymptomatic carrier—has now been recognised. Until recently the use of masks, universal in general surgery, has been omitted in obstetrics. This is a mistake. Masks should always be worn and should be properly constructed with 16 thicknesses of gauze.[37]

Probably, the single most important factor in the causation of streptococcal puerperal fever was not social class, malnutrition, crowded living conditions, or the state of hygiene in the surroundings, but quite simply whether or not the birth attendant was a carrier of the Group A streptococcus, and whether the serotype that was carried was virulent.

Secular Trends and Virulence

In 1992 Katz and Morens published a study of the history of scarlet fever. They noted the same sort of 'spikiness' in the secular trend of scarlet-fever deaths during the nineteenth century as that which occurred in puerperal fever and erysipelas, and they suggested that the 'high scarlet fever attack rates, variable epidemic severity' and other features might have been due to the 'cocirculation of both virulent and avirulent strains [of the Group A streptococcus]'.[38]

Such an explanation might also apply to the history of puerperal fever. The severity of epidemics in hospitals and towns, and the relative or complete absence of severe cases between the epidemics, strongly suggest that from time to time one or more highly virulent serotypes would suddenly appear only to fade away and be replaced by serotypes of low virulence. What would initiate such changes is unknown, although selective pressures have been invoked to explain the appearance and disappearance of different serotypes.

One of the puzzling features of the Group A streptococcus is the undoubted decline in the virulence in or around the time of the Second World War, when, in the words of the late A. B. Christie, the organism seems to have 'lost its epidemic thrust'.[39] Why this happened is uncertain. The use of antibiotics may have played a part, but that is not generally regarded as the whole explanation. Better health, better housing, less overcrowding, and better standards of hygiene are often cited for such declines in infectious diseases, if only for

---

[36] L. Colebrook, 'The Prevention of Puerperal Sepsis', *Journal of Obstetrics and Gynaecology of the British Empire*, 43 (1936), 691–714, at 700.

[37] G. F. Gibberd, 'Streptococcal Puerperal Sepsis', *Guy's Hospital Reports*, 81 (1931), 29–44, at 31.

[38] Katz and Morens, 'Severe Streptococcal Infections', 305.

[39] A. B. Christie, personal communication, 1977. (A. B. Christie was the author of *Infectious Diseases, Epidemiology and Clinical Practice*.)

want of other explanations. But, within the group of diseases associated with the Group A streptococcus, as we shall see, some—notably scarlet fever—had started to decline in severity in the late nineteenth century, and had continued a steady downward decline long before antibiotics were available, while others, such as puerperal fever and erysipelas, showed no signs of a decline in mortality rates until the introduction of the sulphonamides. Indeed, puerperal fever still occurred, sometimes severely, after the introduction of antibiotics, but by the 1970s, if not before, it had become a rare disease.

It is impossible to be sure how mild puerperal fever would have been in the absence of antibiotics, but changes in antiseptic practice are revealing. In the 1920s and first half of the 1930s, when, in retrospect, it seems to have been close to criminal negligence not to wear a mask when delivering a baby, very few doctors or midwives wore masks, let alone sterile gowns, even though puerperal-fever deaths were common. By the late 1930s, with increasing attention to antisepsis and asepsis, wearing masks and gowns was, at any rate in maternity hospitals, accepted practice. Now, however, in the 1980s and 1990s, it has become usual in normal hospital and home deliveries for doctors and midwives not to wear a mask. Although the outbreak of puerperal fever in the Boston Women's Hospital in 1968 reminds us that sudden dangerous epidemics of Group A streptococcal puerperal fever have not totally disappeared, it was an isolated event and in general no harm has come from the abandonment of masks for normal deliveries. That alone may be an eloquent illustration of the decline of the virulence of the Group A streptococcus as far as childbirth is concerned.

Returning to the pre-antibiotic era, it seems likely that the serotypes involved in scarlet fever, on the one hand, and puerperal fever and erysipelas, on the other, were quite different from each other. It is worth looking at that evidence in some detail.

The Relationship of Puerperal Fever to other Streptococcal Diseases

The reader may recall the memorable remark (cited in Chapter 3) of Alexander Gordon of Aberdeen in his treatise of 1795:

That the Puerperal Fever is of the nature of erysipelas, was supposed by Pouteau forty years ago, and has been the opinion of Doctors Young and Home of Edinburgh, since that time. I will not venture positively to assert, that the Puerperal Fever and Erysipelas are precisely of the same specific nature; but that they are connected, that there is an analogy between them, and that they are concomitant epidemics, I have unquestionable proofs. For these two epidemics began in Aberdeen at the same time, and afterwards kept pace together; they both arrived at their *acmè* together, and they both ceased at the same time.[40]

---

[40] Alexander Gordon, *A Treatise on the Epidemic Puerperal Fever of Aberdeen* (London, 1795), 55–6.

We have seen that this was far from being an isolated observation. There is abundant evidence from many sources of an extremely close link between puerperal fever and erysipelas. Whether there was also a close relationship between puerperal fever and necrotizing fasciitis is less sure, mainly because historical accounts of necrotizing fasciitis are few. But the account of the extraordinary epidemic of erysipelas that occurred mainly in New England in the 1840s and 1850s, described in Chapter 4, suggests that, in this epidemic at least, cases of puerperal fever, erysipelas, and necrotizing fasciitis were so closely connected that they may well have been due to the same serotype.[41]

Additional evidence can be found by comparing the secular trends in deaths from puerperal fever and erysipelas, as shown in Figs. 12.4 and 12.5. Although epidemiologists and microbiologists have paid little attention to the history of puerperal fever, when it is mentioned it is usually with the implicit assumption that all streptococcal diseases, including scarlet fever and puerperal fever, were closely related to each other and probably followed the same epidemiological pattern. I believe that assumption is wrong.

In Fig. 12.4, the annual mortality rates for puerperal fever, erysipelas, and scarlet fever during the period of forty years from 1860 to 1899 are shown as percentages of the average rate for each disease throughout the whole period, providing a map of the variations between the good, the average, and the bad years of these three streptococcal diseases. One can see straightaway that the annual variations in mortality rates from puerperal fever and erysipelas followed each other very closely—a fact that is difficult to explain except in terms of the two diseases being caused by the same serotypes of the Group A streptococcus. On the other hand, the variations in the severity of scarlet fever were quite different.

There is other evidence along these lines. In the early decades of the nineteenth century, before death registration was introduced, scarlet fever was known to be a very mild disease with few deaths; yet this was the period in which there were numerous epidemics of puerperal fever with very high mortality and with simultaneous outbreaks of erysipelas. Fig. 12.4 shows the period when scarlet fever was at its most deadly, with epidemics in 1863–4 and 1868–70; but this was a time when mortality from puerperal fever and erysipelas was relatively low. From about 1880, however, mortality from scarlet fever began to decline in quite a dramatic fashion, while mortality from puerperal fever remained at a high level until 1900 and mortality from erysipelas fell only slightly.

---

[41] William Alexander, a surgeon in charge of the maternity wards of a Liverpool workhouse in the 1890s who kept particularly careful records, found that, on the wards, where cases of puerperal fever and erysipelas were common, out of 115 deaths from all causes, 'In four cases, all lock patients, the subject of gonorrhea, &c., phagadenic sloughing of the vulva and vagina set in after labour' (W. Alexander, 'Puerperal Fever', *Liverpool Medico-Chirurgical Journal*, 27 (1894), 354–367, at 356). 'Lock' patients were patients from a venereal disease hospital; the origin of 'lock' in this context is obscure. Phagadena was the nineteenth-century name for what seems to have been necrotizing fasciitis (I. Loudon, 'Necrotising Fasciitis, Hospital Gangrene and Phagadena', *Lancet*, 344 (1994), 1416–18).

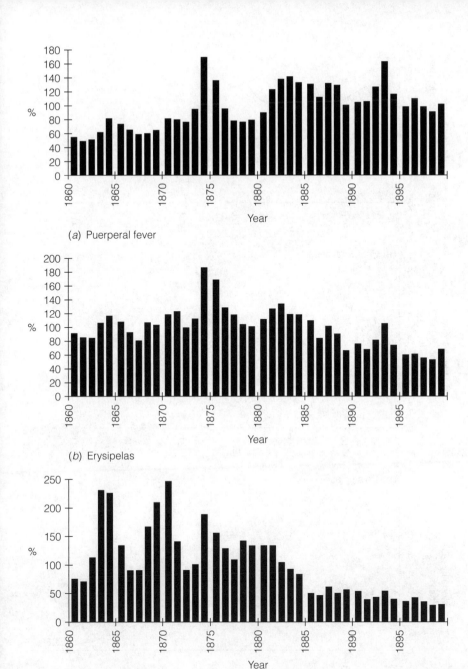

FIG. 12.4 Annual mortality rates due to puerperal fever, erysipelas, and scarlet fever, England and Wales, 1860–1899

Note: For each disease, the annual rate is shown as the percentage of the average annual number of deaths for the whole period of forty years.

Source: *Annual Reports of the Registrar General for England and Wales.*

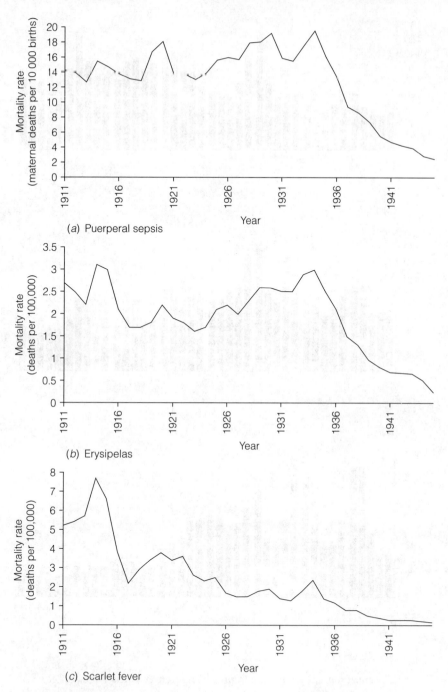

FIG. 12.5 Annual mortality rates due to puerperal fever, erysipelas, and scarlet fever, England and Wales, 1911–1945

Sources: Annual Reports of the Registrar General for England and Wales; Statistical Reviews of the Registrar General for England and Wales.

In the twentieth century the difference is just as remarkable (see Fig. 12.5). The decline in mortality from scarlet fever, which had started in about 1880, continued, falling from 5.2 deaths per 100,000 persons in 1911 to 1.2 in 1936. In the case of erysipelas, the mortality rate per 100,000 stayed high; it was 2.7 in 1911, rising to 3.0 in 1934. Likewise the mortality rate from puerperal fever (per 10,000 births) rose from 14.3 in 1911 to 19.5 in 1934.

It might be that the fall in scarlet-fever mortality was due to a fall in incidence.[42] But the case fatality rate of scarlet fever followed the same downward path as the mortality rate (Fig. 12.6). This suggests that deaths from scarlet fever declined because of a fall in the virulence of the serotypes causing that disease, or an increase in the immunity of children, or both. Whatever the explanation, compared to the mid-nineteenth century, scarlet fever was steadily changing from a deadly disease to a mild one.

In contrast to scarlet fever, the mortality rate and the case fatality rate of erysipelas remained high, suggesting there was no decline in the virulence of the serotypes involved (Fig. 12.6). Probably the case fatality rate of puerperal fever followed the same path as that of erysipelas, but unfortunately it is impossible to be sure. As explained in Chapter 1, the data on notifications of puerperal fever are hopelessly unreliable.

The statistical evidence of the *absence* of a link between puerperal fever and scarlet fever is confirmed by many reports. In 1834 Dr Rigby in London recalled that a mother who had been delivered while she had scarlet fever did not get puerperal fever; and, although there was much scarlet fever in London from June through August 1833, there was not much puerperal fever.[43] In Liverpool in the 1890s, Dr George Johnston stated that he was not satisfied that the existence of scarlet fever in the proximity was the cause of puerperal fever. He mentioned the case of a child who took scarlet fever a few days after its mother had been confined and could not be removed, with the result that both were nursed in the same bed, and the mother did not take puerperal fever.[44]

In his large authoritative text on puerperal fever, published in 1910, Arnold Lea gives chapter and verse for concluding that 'scarlet fever usually runs a normal course in puerperal women and is not directly associated with any infection of the pelvic organs . . . It is very doubtful if any direct causal relationship can be established between infection of the generative tract and the scarlet fever poison.'[45] In 1931 Ruth Tunnicliff showed that the serum of sheep immunized with haemolytic streptococci from the acute stage of scarlet fever protected mice from streptococci from scarlet-fever patients but not against streptococci from other sources.[46] Hektoen found in 1935 that, in contrast to the frequent

[42] Indeed, it has often been argued that mortality from scarlet fever (and other infectious diseases) fell after 1880–1900 because better housing and a falling birth rate led to less crowding and thus to fewer cases.   [43] E. Rigby, 'Midwifery Reports', *London Medical Gazette*, 14 (1834), 400–1.
[44] Alexander, 'Puerperal Fever', 366.   [45] A. Lea, *Puerperal Infection* (London, 1910), 228.
[46] R. Tunnicliff, 'Further Studies on the Specificity of Streptococi', *Journal of the American Medical Association*, 75 (1920), 1339–40.

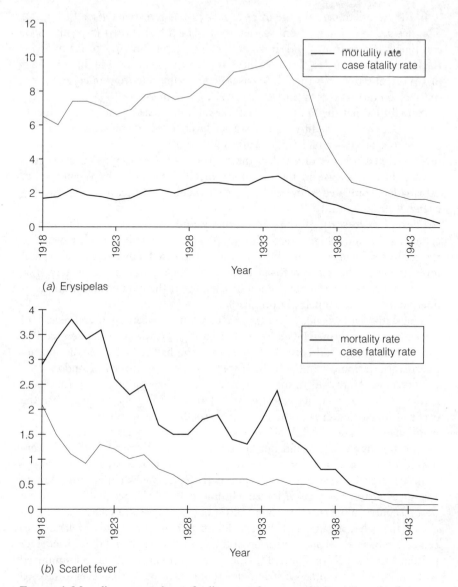

(a) Erysipelas

(b) Scarlet fever

FIG. 12.6 Mortality rates and case fatality rates due to erysipelas and scarlet fever, England and Wales, 1918–1945

Note: Mortality rates measured as deaths per 100,000 persons; case fatality rates measured as deaths as a percentage of notifications.

Sources: *Annual Reports of the Registrar General for England and Wales; Statistical Reviews of the Registrar General for England and Wales.*

coexistence of epidemics of erysipelas and puerperal fever, there were no records of epidemics in which some patients suffered from scarlet fever and some from erysipelas. Scarlet fever was introduced into the Faroe Islands in 1873, where there had been no cases of the disease in the previous fifty-seven years. During the epidemic that followed, 38.3 per cent of the population had scarlet fever but there were no cases of erysipelas.[47]

Another surprising difference between streptococcal diseases was their response to treatment with the sulphonamides. Fig. 12.5 shows that, while the introduction of the sulphonamides caused a sudden downturn in mortality from puerperal fever and erysipelas, the trend in scarlet-fever mortality after the introduction of the sulphonamides continued on the same gently declining path, although sulphonamides were widely used for the treatment of scarlet fever. Many reports in the late 1930s and the 1940s stated that the sulphonamides were 'relatively ineffective' or 'disappointing' in the treatment of scarlet fever.[48]

The best example, because it was a controlled trial, took place in Baltimore in 1938. All cases of scarlet fever admitted to the Sydenham Hospital were allocated to one of three groups, 'no other basis for selection being used other than the order of admission'.[49] One group received scarlet-fever antitoxin; the second received sulfanilamide by mouth, and the third—the control group— received 'the usual symptomatic treatment for their disease'. The three groups were comparable in age and other features. There were no deaths in any group, but in terms of average duration of fever, rash, and stay in hospital there was no difference between any of the three groups. Complication rates were highest in the group receiving sulfanilamides (unexplained fever and sulphanilamide rash), and next highest in the group receiving antitoxin serum (serum sickness). There was no evidence that either serum or sulfanilamide altered the course of scarlet fever.

Many other investigations of the use of sulphonamides in scarlet fever, not only from England,[50] but also from the USA,[51] came to the same general

[47] L. Hektoen, 'The Specificness of Certain Hemolytic Streptococci', *Journal of the American Medical Association*, 105 (1935), 1–2.

[48] W. R. Snodgrass, 'Uses and Abuses of Chemotherapy in Streptococcal Diseases', *Practitioner*, 144 (1940), 16–24; anon., editorial, 'The Medical Use of the Sulphonamides', *Public Health*, 57 (1943), 1–2; Topley and Wilson, *Principles of Bacteriology and Immunity*, 3rd edn., 1477, 1485.

[49] F. F. Schwentker and J. Waghelstein, 'A Note on the Use of Sulfanilamide in Scarlet Fever', *Baltimore Health News*, 15 (1938), 41–6, at 41. I am grateful to Dr Iain Chalmers for drawing my attention to this paper.

[50] J. G. Hogarth, '*p*-benzylaminobenzene sulphonamide in the Treatment of Scarlet Fever', *British Medical Journal* (1937), ii. 1160–2; E. C. Benn, 'Sulfanilamide in the Treatment of Scarlet Fever', *British Medical Journal* (1939), ii. 644–6; A. R. Thompson, 'Chemotherapy and Acute Specific Fevers', *Practitioner*, 144 (1940), 52–60.

[51] F. H. Top and D. C. Young, 'The Treatment of Moderately Severe Scarlet Fever', *Journal of the American Medical Association*, 117 (1941), 2056–60; M. B. Gordon, 'Value of Sulfanilamide and Scarlet Fever Antitoxin in the Treatment of Scarlet Fever', *Journal of the American Medical Association*, 117 (1941), 76–8; C. Wesselhoef, 'Sulfanilamide in the Management of Acute Streptococcal Infection, Particularly Scarlatinal Infections of the Upper Respiratory Tract', *New England Journal of Medicine*, 224 (1941), 221–6; M. J. Fox and N. F. Gordon, 'Treatment of Scarlet Fever', *Archives of Internal*

conclusion: namely, that the sulphonamides were, to quote one paper, 'of no value in the management of the toxic phase of scarlet fever'.[52] One author concluded that scarlet fever was due to a 'haemolytic streptococcus which is not affected by the sulphonamides',[53] although the effectiveness of the sulphonamides against puerperal sepsis and erysipelas was well known. There was some evidence, however, of a reduction (usually slight) of complications of scarlet fever such as adenitis and otitis media in patients treated with the sulphonamides. In contrast, reports from 1944 and later showed that penicillin, if given intramuscularly for a week or so, was highly effective against both the toxic phase of scarlet fever and against the usual complications.[54]

Conclusion

The evidence reviewed in this chapter concerning secular trends in deaths from puerperal fever and erysipelas, on the one hand, and scarlet fever, on the other, suggests that some serotypes were disease specific or rather *diseases* specific. If that is accepted, it may be possible to arrange diseases due to the Group A streptococcus into groups. One group with a common serotype or serotypes might be responsible for puerperal fever, erysipelas, and surgical infections in hospitals. This group might also embrace necrotizing fasciitis, cellulitis, and impetigo, and it may be that this group is associated with acute glomerulonephritis.[55] A second group, associated with different serotypes, might include scarlet fever, pharyngitis, otitis media, and mastoiditis, and probably rheumatic fever.

If this turns out to be true, clearly the groups cannot be defined by their M-antigens alone. There must be other properties that determine which serotypes are associated with one kind of streptococcal disease and which with another. Recent research on the molecular biology of M-proteins has enabled Stollerman to identify the M-serotypes responsible for rheumatic fever, and to show that they are different from M-serotypes associated with glomerulonephritis.[56] It is work such as this that suggests that it may be possible in the future to link certain serotypes with certain kinds of streptococcal disease.

Apart from disease specificity, there is the associated question of what factors lead to changes in streptococcal virulence. As we have seen, the striking feature of nineteenth-century trends in mortality from streptococcal disease was

Medicine, 74 (1944), 1–3; M. B. Gordon *et al.*, 'Value of Sulfanilamide and Scarlet Fever Antitoxin in the Treatment of Scarlet Fever', *Journal of Pediatrics, St Louis*, 19 (1941), 76–8.

[52] Fox and Gordon, 'Treatment of Scarlet Fever', 3.

[53] Hogarth, '*p*-benzylaminobenzene sulphonamide', 1162.

[54] G. J. Thomas, 'Penicillin Treatment of Scarlet Fever', *Journal of the American Medical Association*, 129 (1945), 785–9; Epidemiology Unit No. 82, US Naval Hospital, Treasure Island, 'Penicillin and Scarlet Fever', *American Journal of Medical Sciences*, 211 (1946), 417–20.

[55] These may correspond to what Stollerman has referred to as 'skin-strains' (Stollerman, 'Changing Streptococci', 170).   [56] Ibid. 176.

the 'spikiness' seen in Figs. 12.1–12.4. What was happening to produce such a picture? Were highly virulent serotypes competing with serotypes of low virulence so that first one and then the other predominated? Was there a series of mutations that led to wide changes in virulence? Stollerman asked a similar question when he wrote 'Can epidemic strains emerge de novo through muta-tion, bacteriophage infection, or plasmid-mediated transformation?'[57]

For instance, one of the most curious features of the 'Rosebush-scratch' epidemic in Boston in 1965 (see Chapter 11) was the extreme infectivity, viru-lence, and specificity of the T-type 28 serotype, which suddenly appeared out of the blue and then disappeared. As far as one can tell, of the many people who must have come into contact with the physician-anaesthetist (the source of the infection), only puerperal patients were infected. There seems to be no record of anyone else developing severe streptococcal disease.[58] Has the post-1980 resurgence of invasive Group A streptococcal disease been accompanied by an increase in puerperal sepsis? I have found no records to suggest that this occurred, but it may be that the prompt treatment of any fever in the puer-perium with penicillin has effectively hidden such cases from sight.

These questions of disease specificity and changing virulence are of great interest to the historian of medicine. Why did streptococcal diseases, which were often so lethal in the past, decline in severity during the twentieth cen-tury, especially the second half of the century? How much was this a reflection of social and economic factors? Did the widespread use of antibiotics after the Second World War play a significant part in the decline in streptococcal dis-ease or can the changes be attributed simply to molecular changes in the infec-tive organism? Whatever the answers to these questions, past and present are inextricably linked. I believe that a comprehensive understanding of strepto-coccal disease now, at the end of the twentieth century, is utterly dependent on an understanding of streptococcal disease in the past.

[57] Ibid. 175–6.
[58] The only exception was the two children of one of the cases in the hospital who developed pharyngitis. They may have been infected by their father after a visit to the hospital, or it may have been a coincidental infection.

Select Bibliography

ACKERLEY, R. YATES, 'Remarks on the Nature and Treatment of Puerperal Fever', *London Medical Gazette* (1837–8), ii. 462–6.

ACKERNECHT, E. H., 'Anticontagionism between 1821 and 1867', *Bulletin of the History of Medicine*, 22 (1948), 562–593.

ADAMI, J. G., *Charles White of Manchester (1728–1813), and the Arrest of Puerperal Fever* (Liverpool, 1922).

ALEXANDER, W., 'Puerperal Fever', *Liverpool Medico-Chirurgical Journal*, 27 (1894), 354–67.

ANCELET, G.-P., *Essai historique et critique sur le création et la transformation des maternités à Paris* (Paris, 1896).

Annual Report of the Medical Officer of Health for Manchester for 1907 (Manchester, 1908).

ANON., *An Account of the Rise, Progress and State of the British Lying-in Hospital for Married Women in Brownlow Street, Long Acre* (London, 1757).

ANON., unsigned article, 'On Puerperal Fever and its Treatment', *Medical and Physical Journal*, 1 (1799), 386–9.

ANON., 'Documents relative to the History of the Malignant Puerperal Fever which prevailed in the Lying-in Institution in Vienna from the beginning of August to the middle of November 1819', *Edinburgh Medical and Surgical Journal*, 22 (1824), 83–91.

ANON., 'Critical Analysis: Puerperal Fever', *Edinburgh Medical and Surgical Journal*, 34 (1830), 328–49.

ANON., 'Puerperal Fever' (report of meeting), *Transactions of the College of Physicians of Philadelphia*, 1 (1841–6), 50–62.

ANON., 'Puerperal Fever' (report of an outbreak in Munich Lying-in Hospital), *Medical Times and Gazette*, 1 (1862), 142–3.

ANON., 'Discussion, Fièvre Puerpérale', *Compte-Rendu: Congrès Périodique International des Sciences Médicales*, 4th session (Brussels, 1875).

ANON., 'Communications: Septicémie puerpérale', *Bulletin de L'Académie de Médecine*, 2nd ser., 8 (1879), 238–60, 267–74, 312–26, 481–94, 505–8.

ANON., leading article, 'Puerperal Infection in Private Practice', *Journal of the American Medical Association*, 33 (1902), 1008–9.

ANON., 'Theodore Duka', obituary notice, *Lancet* (1908), i. 1520.

ANON., 'Puerperal Fever and Erysipelas', *Lancet* (1934), ii. 673.

ANON., leading article, 'An Anti-Streptococcal Agent', *Lancet* (1936), i. 269–70.

ANON., leading article, 'The Chemotherapy of Streptococcal Infections', *Lancet* (1936), i. 1303–4.

ANON., editorial, 'The Medical Use of the Sulphonamides', *Public Health*, 57 (1943), 1–2.

ANON., 'A Medical Revolution', *Bayer Review*, special anniversary edition (Mar. 1988), 58–9.

ARMSTRONG, J., *Facts and Observations Relative to the Fever Commonly called Puerperal* (London, 1814).

ARNETH, F. H., 'Evidence of Puerperal Fever Depending upon the Contagious Inoculation of Morbid Matter', *Monthly Journal of Medical Science*, 12 (1851), 505–11.

ASTRUC, JEAN, *Elements of Midwifry with a Short History of the Art of Midwifry*, trans. S. RYLEY (London, 1766).

BACON, C. S., 'The Mortality from Puerperal Infection in Chicago', *American Journal of Obstetrics and Gynaecology*, 8 (1896), 429–46.

BAIRD, D., 'Maternal Mortality in Hospital', *Lancet* (1936), i. 295–8.

—— 'Puerperal Pyrexia', *Practitioner*, 148 (Jan.–June 1942), 869–90.

—— [BAIRD, SIR DUGALD], 'The Evolution of Modern Obstetrics', *Lancet* (1960), ii. 557–64, 609–14.

BANKS, H. S., *Modern Practice in Infectious Fevers* (2 vols.; London, 1951).

BARBOUR, A. H. Freeland, 'Pathology of the Post-Partum Uterus', *Edinburgh Medical Journal*, 31 (1885), 434–44.

BARKER, F., *The Puerperal Diseases* (New York, 1880).

BARNES, R., 'Lectures on Puerperal Fever', *Lancet* (1865), i. 141–2, 169–70, 279–80, 307–8, 443–4, 527–8; (1865), ii. 531–2, 613–15.

—— 'On the Causes, Internal and External, of Puerperal Fever', *British Medical Journal* (1887), ii. 1036–42.

BARNHAM, M., 'ß-Haemolytic Streptococci', in A. M. Emmerson, P. M. Hawkey, and S. H. Gillespie (eds.), *Principles and Practice of Clinical Bacteriology* (London, 1997), 37–71.

BAUDELOCQUE, J.-L., *A System of Midwifery* trans. from the French by J. Heath (London, 1790).

BEECROFT, S., 'Illustrations of the Contagious Nature of Puerperal Fever', *Lancet* (1840–1), i. 684–5.

BELL, A. C., 'The Use of Antistreptococcal Preparations in Obstetrics', *Practitioner*, 139 (Jan.–June 1938), 673–9.

BENN, E. C., 'Sulfanilamide in the Treatment of Scarlet Fever', *British Medical Journal* (1939), ii. 644–6.

BENNETT, E., 'On the Identity of Erysipelas and a Certain Form of Puerperal Fever, and its Contagiousness', *American Journal of the Medical Sciences*, 19 (1850), 376–83.

BERNARDY, E. P., 'Observations on Private Practice in the Past Decade', *Proceedings of the Philadelphia County Medical Society*, 13 (1892), 110–17.

BLACKMORE, E., 'Observations on Puerperal Fever', *Provincial Medical and Surgical Journal*, 9 (1845), 173–8, 210–13, 228–30, 242–5, 321–4, 338–41, 353–5, 369–71, 387–90, 399–401, 638–9.

BLAND, ROBERT, 'Some Calculations of the Number of Accidents or Deaths which Happen in Consequence of Parturition; and of the Proportion of Male to Female Children, as well as of Twins, Monstrous Productions, and Children that are Dead-Born; Taken from the Midwifery Reports of the Westminster General Dispensary', *Philosophical Transactions*, 71 (1781), 355–71.

BLUNDELL, DR, 'Lectures on the Theory and Practice of Midwifery: Puerperal Fever', *Lancet* (1827–8), ii. 641–6.

BONNEY, V., 'The Continued High Mortality of Childbearing', *Proceedings of the Royal Society of Medicine*, 12/3 (1918–19), 75–107.

BOXALL, R., 'Fever in Childbed', *Transactions of the Obstetrical Society of London*, 40 (1890), 219–43, 264–70, 275–303.

—— 'The Mortality of Childbirth', *Lancet* (1893), ii. 9–15.

BRADLEY, DR, 'On an Epidemic of Puerperal Fever', *Medical and Physical Journal*, 28 (1811), 193–201.

BREESE, B., and HALL, C. B., *Beta Hemolytic Streptococcal Diseases* (Boston, 1978).

BRENAN, J., *Thoughts on Puerperal Fever Illustrated by Cases in the Lying-in Hospital, Dublin* (London, 1814).

British Encyclopaedia of Medical Practice (London, 1936).

BROWNE, T. D. O'DONEL, *The Rotunda Hospital, 1745–1945* (London, 1947).

BURNS, J., *The Principles of Midwifery* (9th edn., London, 1837).

BURT-WHITE, H., 'Puerperal Sepsis and Sensitiveness to Streptococcal Toxins', *British Medical Journal* (1928), i. 975–6.

BURTENSHAW, J. H., 'The Fever of the Puerperium (Puerperal Infection)', *New York Journal and Philadelphia Medical Journal*, 79 (1904), 1073–9, 1134–8, 1189–94, 1234–8; 80 (1904), 20–5.

BUTTER, WILLIAM, *An Account of the Puerperal Fevers as they Appear in Derbyshire and Some of the Counties Adjacent* (London, 1775).

BUTTLE, G. A. H., GRAY, W. H., and STEPHENSON, D., 'Protection of Mice against Streptococcal and Other Infections by *p*-aminobenzenesulphonamide and Related Substances', *Lancet* (1936), i. 1286–90.

BYERS, J. W., 'The Prevention of Puerperal Fever in Private Practice', *British Medical Journal* (1887), ii. 1042–4.

BYNUM, W. F., *Science and the Practice of Medicine in the Nineteenth Century* (Cambridge, 1994).

—— and PORTER, R., (eds.), *Companion Encyclopaedia to the History of Medicine* (London, 1993).

CAMPBELL, W., 'Observations on the Disease Usually Termed Puerperal Fever, with Cases' (review), *Edinburgh Medical and Surgical Journal*, 18 (1822), 195–6.

—— *A Treatise of the Epidemic Puerperal Fever as it Prevailed in Edinburgh in 1821–22* (Edinburgh, 1822).

—— 'On Puerperal Fever', *London Medical Gazette*, 9 (1831–2), 353–4.

CARTER, K. CODELL, *I. P. Semmelweis, The Etiology, Concept, and Prophylaxis of Childbed Fever*, trans. and ed. with an introduction (Wisconsin, 1983).

—— 'The Development of Pasteur's Concept of Disease Causation and the Emergence of Specific Causes in Nineteenth-Century Medicine', *Bulletin of the History of Medicine*, 65 (1991), 528–48.

—— and CARTER, B., *Childbed Fever: A Scientific Biography of Ignaz Semmelweis* (Westport, Conn., 1994).

—— and TATE, G. S., 'The Earliest-Known Account of Semmelweis's Initiation of Disinfection at Vienna's Allegemeines Krankenhaus', *Bulletin of the History of Medicine*, 65/2 (1991), 252–7.

—— ABBOTT, S., and SIEBACH, J. L., 'Five Documents Relating to the Final Illness and Death of Semmelweis', *Bulletin of the History of Medicine*, 69 (1995), 255–70.

CEELY, R., 'Account of a Contagious Epidemic Puerperal Fever which Prevailed in Aylesbury and its Vicinity, in the Autumn of 1831', *Lancet* (1834–5), i. 813–18.

CHARTIER, C., and GROSSHANS, E. M., 'Erysipelas', *International Journal of Dermatology*, 29 (1990), 459–67.

CHRISTIE, A. B., *Infectious Diseases, Epidemiology and Clinical Practice* (2nd edn., London, 1974).

CHURCHILL, FLEETWOOD, 'An Historical Sketch of the Epidemics of Puerperal Fever', in Churchill (ed.), *Essays on the Puerperal Fever and Other Diseases Peculiar to Women* (London, 1849), 3–42.

—— (ed.), *Essays on the Puerperal Fever and Other Diseases Peculiar to Women* (London, 1849).

—— *On the Theory and Practice of Midwifery* (London, 1850).

—— 'Report of Private Obstetric Practice for Thirty Nine Years', *Dublin Journal of Medical Science*, 53 (Jan.–June 1872), 525–40.

CLARK, W. R., *At War Within* (Oxford, 1995; paperback edn., 1997).

CLARKE, G. B., 'Observations on Malignant Puerperal Fever', *London Medical Gazette*, NS 5 (1847), 331–4.

CLARKE, JOHN, *Practical Essays on the Arrangement of Pregnancy and Labour and on the Inflammatory and Febrile Diseases of Lying-in Women* (London, 1793; 2nd edn., 1806).

CLARKE, JOSEPH, 'Observations on the Puerperal Fever etc.', *Edinburgh Medical Commentaries*, 15 (1790), 299 ff.; repr. in Fleetwood Churchill (ed.), *Essays on the Puerperal Fever and Other Diseases Peculiar to Women* (London, 1849), 351–62.

CLINE, L. F., *Mea Culpa and the Life and Times of Semmelweis* (London, 1937).

COLEBROOK, L., 'Some Laboratory Investigations in Connexion with Puerperal Fever', *Proceedings of the Royal Society of Medicine*, 19 (1926), section on obstetrics and gynaecology, 31–42.

—— 'The Prevention of Puerperal Sepsis', *Journal of Obstetrics and Gynaecology of the British Empire*, 43 (1936), 691–714.

—— ledger of the cases of puerperal fever treated by Colebrook in 1936, Royal College of Gynaecologists and Obstetricians, Archives.

—— 'The Story of Puerperal Fever, 1800–1950', *British Medical Journal* (1956), i. 247–52.

—— 'Gerhard Domagk', *Biographical Memoirs of Fellows of the Royal Society*, 10 (1964), 38–44.

—— and KENNY, M., 'Treatment of Human Puerperal Infections, and of Experimental Infections in Mice, with Prontosil', *Lancet* (1936), i. 1279–86.

—— —— 'Treatment with Prontosil of Puerperal Infections due to Haemolytic Streptococci', *Lancet* (1936), ii. 1319–22.

—— and PURDIE, A. W., 'Treatment of 106 Cases of Puerperal Fever by Sulphanilamide', *Lancet* (1937), ii. 1237–42, 1291–3.

COLEBROOK, V., 'Leonard Colebrook: Reminiscences on the Occasion of the 25th Anniversary of the Birmingham Burns Unit', *Injury: The British Journal of Accident Surgery*, 2/3 (Jan. 1971), 182–4.

College of Physicians of Philadelphia, 'Discussion', *Transactions of the College of Physicians of Philadelphia*, 1 (1841–6), 50–62.

CONDIE, DR, 'Puerperal Fever', *Transactions of the College of Physicians of Philadelphia*, 1 (1841–6), 50–62.

CONNOR, J. T. H., 'Listerism Unmasked: Antisepsis and Asepsis in Victorian Anglo-Canada', *Journal of the History of Medicine and Allied Sciences*, 49 (1994), 207–39.

COPLAND, J., *Dictionary of Practical Medicine* (3 vols.; London, 1858).

CREIGHTON, C., *History of Epidemics in Britain* (2 vols.; Cambridge 1894; 2nd edn., London, 1965).

CROSS, J., 'Sketches of the Medical Schools of Paris', *London Medical and Physical Journal*, 34 (1815), 478–87.

CROWTHER, A., 'An Influential Doctor', *British Medical Journal* (1996), ii. 1530.

CULLINGWORTH, C. J., *Puerperal Fever: A Preventible Disease* (London, 1888).

—— 'Biographical Note on J. Braxton Hicks', *Transactions of the Obstetrical Society of London*, 40 (1898), 65–78.

—— 'On the Undiminished Mortality from Puerperal Fever in England and Wales', *Transactions of the Obstetrical Society of London*, 40 (1898), 91–114.

—— 'Biographical Note on Étienne Stéphane Tarnier', *Transactions of the Obstetrical Society of London*, 40 (1898), 78–89.

—— *Oliver Wendell Holmes and the Contagiousness of Puerperal Fever* (London, 1906), with an appendix 'Biographical Sketch of Dr. Alexander Gordon of Aberdeen, 1752–99', pp. 33–5.

CUSACK, S., 'On Puerperal Fever', *Dublin Journal of Medical Science*, 9 (1836), 162–5.

DAWSON, P. M., 'Semmelweis, an Interpretation', *Annals of Medical History*, 6 (1924), 258–79.

DELACY, M., 'Puerperal Fever in Eighteenth-Century Britain', *Bulletin of the History of Medicine*, 63 (1989), 521–56.

DENHAM, J., 'On the Recent Epidemic of Puerperal Fever in Dublin', *Dublin Quarterly Journal of Medical Science*, 34 (1862), 317–31.

DENMAN, T., *An Essay on the Puerperal Fever* (London, 1768; 2nd edn., 1773), repr. in Fleetwood Churchill (ed.), *Essays on the Puerperal Fever and Other Diseases Peculiar to Women* (London, 1849), 43–60.

—— *An Essay on Natural Labours* (London, 1786).

—— *An Introduction to the Practice of Midwifery* (2 vols.; London, 1795; 2nd edn., 1801).

DESTOUCHES, L., *La Vie et l'œuvre de Phillipe Ignace Semmelweis (1818–1865)*, thesis for the degree of Doctor of Medicine (state diploma, Rennes, 1924).

DISSE, DR, 'Report on Puerperal Fever', *American Journal of the Medical Sciences*, 330 (1855), 533–4.

DOLÉRIS, J. A., *La Fièvre puerpérale et les organismes inférieurs: Pathogénie et thérapeutique des accidents infectieux des suites de couches* (Paris, 1880).

DOUGLAS, C. E., 'Some Observations on Seventy Years of Country Midwifery Practice', *Journal of Obstetrics and Gynaecology of the British Empire*, 31 (1924), 622–46.

—— and MCKINLAY, P. L., *Report on Maternal Morbidity and Mortality in Scotland* (Edinburgh, 1935).

DOUGLASS, J. C., 'On Puerperal Fever', *Dublin Hospital Reports and Communications*, 3 (1822), 141–60.

DOUTHWAITE, A. H., 'The Use of Antistreptococcal Preparations in General Practice', *Practitioner*, 139 (1937), 661–72.

DRAKE, D., *Systematic Treatise on the Principal Diseases of the Interior Valley of N. America*, 2nd edn., ed. S. H. Smith and F. G. Smith (Philadelphia, 1854).

DUKA, T., 'Childbed Fever, its Cause and Prevention: A Life's History', *Lancet* (1886), ii. 206–8, 246–8.

DUNCAN, J. MATTHEWS, 'The Mortality of Childbed', *Edinburgh Medical Journal*, 15 (1869–70), 399–409.

—— 'Address in Obstetric Medicine', *British Medical Journal* (1874), ii. 213–18.

—— 'Puerperal Fever in Hospitals and Private Practice', *Lancet* (1875), i. 765–6.

DUNN, P., 'Dr Alexander Gordon (1752–99) and Contagious Puerperal Fever', *Archives of Diseases of Children, Fetal and Neonatal Edition*, 78 (1998), 232–3.

EDGAR, I. H., 'I. P. Semmelweis: An Outline for a Biography', *Annals of Medical History*, NS 1 (1939), 74–96.

EDIS, A. W., 'Remarks on the Influence of Obstetric Knowledge on the Mortality of Mothers in Childbed', *British Medical Journal* (1878), ii. 507–11.

EHRLICH, P., 'Chemotherapeutics: Scientific Principles, Methods and Results', *Lancet* (1913), ii. 445–51.

ELKINGTON, F., 'Observations on the Contagiousness of Puerperal Fever', *Provincial Medical and Surgical Journal*, 7 (1844), 287–8.

ERNST, H. C., 'The Etiology of Puerperal Fever', in B. C. Hirst (ed.), *A System of Obstetrics by American Authors* (2 vols.; Edinburgh, 1889), ii. 401–59.

EYLER, J. M., *Victorian Social Medicine: The Ideas and Methods of William Farr* (Baltimore, 1979).

FERGUSON, R. (ed.), *Gooch on Some of the Most Important Diseases of Women* (London, 1859).

FITCH, W. K., 'The Nomenclature and Dosage of New Antistreptococcal Preparations', *Practitioner*, 139 (1937), 680–8.

FITZGERALD, J. A., 'Rosebush Scratch', *New York State Journal of Medicine*, 1 May 1972, 1077–80.

FOTHERGILL, A., 'An Account of an Improved Method of Treating the Puerperal Fever', *London Medical Journal*, 3 (1783), 411–18.

FOTHERGILL, W. E., *Manual of Midwifery* (Edinburgh, 1896).

—— 'Puerperal Pelvic Infection', *British Medical Journal* (1924), i. 773–4.

FOULERTON, A. G. R., 'The Pathology of Puerperal Fevers', *Practitioner* (1905), 387–415.

FOULIS, M. A., and BARR, J. B., 'Prontosil Album in Puerperal Sepsis', *British Medical Journal* (1937), i. 445–6.

FOX, M. J., and GORDON, N. F., 'Treatment of Scarlet Fever', *Archives of Internal Medicine*, 74 (1944), 1–3.

FOX, W. T., 'Puerperal Fever', *Transactions of the Obstetrical Society of London*, 3 (1862), 386–71.

GARIEPY, T. P., 'The Introduction and Acceptance of Listerian Antisepsis in the United States', *Journal of the History of Medicine and Allied Sciences*, 49 (1994), 167–206.

GARRIGUES, H. J., 'On Lying-in Institutions, Especially those of New York', *Transactions of the American Gynaecological Society*, 2 (1878), 593–649.

—— *The Science and Art of Obstetrics* (Philadelphia, 1902).

GARRISON, F. H., *An Introduction to the History of Medicine* (4th edn., Philadelphia, 1929).

GEDDES, G., *Statistics of Puerperal Sepsis and Allied Infectious Diseases* (Bristol, 1912).

—— *Puerperal Septicaemia: Its Causation, Symptoms, Prevention and Treatment* (Bristol, 1926).

GIBBERD, G. F., 'Streptococcal Puerperal Sepsis', *Guy's Hospital Reports*, 81 (1931), 29–44.

—— 'Prontosil in Puerperal Infection', *British Medical Journal* (1937), ii. 229–30.

GODLEE, SIR RICKMAN, *Lord Lister* (3rd edn., Oxford, 1924).

GODWIN, WILLIAM, *Memoirs of the Author of The Rights of Woman* (London, 1798).

GOOCH, R., *An Account of Some of the Most Important Diseases Peculiar to Women* (London, 1831; 2nd edn., 1838).

GOODALL, J. R., *Puerperal Infection* (self-published, 1932).

GORDON, ALEXANDER, *A Treatise on the Epidemic Puerperal Fever of Aberdeen* (London, 1795).

GORDON, M. B., 'Value of Sulfanilamide and Scarlet Fever Antitoxin in the Treatment of Scarlet Fever', *Journal of the American Medical Association*, 117 (1941), 76–8.

GRANSHAW, L., ' "Upon this principle I have based a practice": The Development and Reception of Antisepsis in Britain, 1867–90', in J. V. Pickstone (ed.), *Medical Innovations in Historical Perspective* (Basingstoke, 1992).

GRANVILLE, A. B., 'Reports on the Practice of Midwifery at the Westminster General Dispensary for 1818 and 1819', *London Medical and Physical Journal*, 44 (1820), 231–8; 47 (1822), 282–8, 374–8.

—— 'Phenomena, Facts and Calculations Connected with the Power and Act of Propagation in Females of the Industrial Classes in the Metropolis, Derived from Eleven Years' Experience of Two Lying-in Institutions', *Transactions of the Obstetrical Society of London*, 2 (1860), 139–96.

GRAY B. M., 'Streptococcal Infections' in A. S. Evans and P. S. Brachman (eds.), *Bacterial Infections in Humans: Epidemiology and Control* (New York, 1991), 639–73.

GREENWOOD, D., 'The Quinine Connection', *Journal of Antimicrobial Chemotherapy*, 30 (1992), 417–27.

GROSSHANS, E. M., 'The Red Face Erysipelas', *Clinics in Dermatology*, 11 (1993), 307–14.

HALL, C., and DEXTER, G., 'Account of the Erysipelatous Fever, as it Appeared in the Northern Section of Vermont and New Hampshire, in the Years 1842–43', *American Journal of the Medical Sciences*, 7 (1844), 2–27.

HAMILTON, A., *Outlines of the Theory and Practice of Midwifery* (London, 1791).

HAMILTON, J., *Select Cases in Midwifery Extracted from the Records of the Edinburgh General Lying-in Hospital* (Edinburgh, 1795).

HAMLIN, C., 'Predisposing Causes and Public Health in Early Nineteenth-Century Medical Thought', *Social History of Medicine*, 5/1 (1992), 43–70.

HARE, R., 'Alterations in the Bactericidal Power of the Blood which Occur during Haemolytic Streptococcal Infections in the Puerperium', *Journal of Pathology and Bacteriology*, 41 (1935), 61–76.

—— 'The Classification of Haemolytic Streptococci from the Nose and Throat of Normal Human Beings by Means of Precipitin and Biochemical Tests', *Journal of Pathology and Bacteriology*, 41 (1935), 499–512.

—— *The Birth of Penicillin* (London, 1970).

HAWKINS, F., and STEWART LAWRENCE, J., *The Sulphonamides* (London, 1950).

HEBERDEN, WILLIAM, *Observations on the Increase and Decrease of Different Diseases* (London, 1801).

HEKTOEN, L., 'The Specificness of Certain Hemolytic Streptococci', *Journal of the American Medical Association*, 105 (1935), 1–2.

HEMMINKI, E., and PAAKKULAINEN, Y., 'The Effects of Antibiotics on Mortality from Infectious Diseases in Sweden and Finland', *American Journal of Public Health*, 66 (1976), 1180–4.

HERVIEUX, J.-F.-E., *Traité clinique et pratique des maladies puerpérales* (Paris, 1880).

HERVIEUX, J.-F.-E., 'Revue historique et critique des principales doctrines qui ont régné sur ce qu'on a appelé la fièvre puerpérale', *L'Union médicale*, 2nd ser., 30 (1886), 66–71, 84–7, 97–106.

HEWITT, G., 'On Puerperal Fever in the British Lying-in Hospital', *Transactions of the Obstetrical Society of London*, 10 (1868), 69–92.

HEY, WILLIAM, *A Treatise on the Puerperal Fever Illustrated by Cases which Occurred in Leeds and its Vicinity in the Years 1809–1812* (London, 1815).

HIRSCH, A., *Handbook of Geographical and Historical Pathology* (2nd edn., 1881), trans. C. Creighton (3 vols.; London, 1883).

HIRST, B. C., 'The Death Rate of Lying-in Hospitals in the United States', *Medical News of Philadelphia*, 50 (1887), 253–6.

HOBBS, A. R., 'Puerperal Sepsis', *British Medical Journal* (1928), i. 971–4.

HOERLEIN, H., 'The Development of Chemotherapy for Bacteriological Diseases', *Practitioner*, 139 (1937), 635–49.

—— 'The Chemotherapy of Infectious Diseases Caused by Protozoa and Bacteria', *Proceedings of the Royal Society of Medicine*, 29 (1936), 313–24.

HOGARTH, J. G., '*p*-benzylaminobenzene sulphonamide in the Treatment of Scarlet Fever', *British Medical Journal* (1937), ii. 1160–2.

HÖGBERG, U., *Maternal Mortality in Sweden* (Umeå University Medical Dissertations, NS 156; Umeå, 1985).

—— and Brostrom, G., 'The Impact of Early Medical Technology on Maternal Mortality Rate in Late 19th Century Sweden', *International Journal of Obstetrics and Gynaecology*, 24 (1986), 251–61.

HOLMES, O. W., *Puerperal Fever as a Private Pestilence* (Boston, 1855).

HOLMES, R. S., 'On Erysipelas', *Transactions of the American Medical Association*, 7 (1854), 143–66.

HORROCKS, P., 'An Address on the Midwifery of the Present Day', *British Medical Journal* (1906), i. 541–5.

HRÓBJARTSSON, A., GØTZSCHE, P. C., and GLUUD, C., 'The Controlled Trial Turns 100 Years: Fibiger's Trial of Serum Treatment of Diphtheria', *British Medical Journal*, 317 (1998), 1243–5.

HULME, NATHANIEL, *A Treatise on the Puerperal Fever* (London, 1772); repr. in Fleetwood Churchill (ed.), *Essays on the Puerperal Fever and Other Diseases Peculiar to Women* (London, 1849), 61–116.

HUNTLEY, R. E., 'The Etiology of Puerperal Fever', *British Medical Journal* (1875), i. 271.

HUTCHINSON, R., 'On the Identity of Puerperal Peritonitis and Epidemic Erysipelas', *Lancet* (1839–40), ii. 193–4.

INGLEBY, J. T., 'On Epidemic Puerperal Fever', *Edinburgh Medical and Surgical Journal*, 49 (1838), 412–36.

JELLETT, H., *The Causes and Prevention of Maternal Mortality* (London, 1929).

JEWETT, C., 'The Question of Puerperal Self-Infection', *American Gynaecological and Obstetrical Journal*, 8 (1896), 417–29.

JEWETT, J. F., REID, D. E., SAFON, L. E., and EASTERDAY, C. L., 'Childbed Fever—a Continuing Entity', *Journal of the American Medical Association*, 206/2 (1968), 344–50.

JOHNSON, R. W., 'Prophylactic Use of Sulphonamide Preparations in Obstetric Practice', *British Medical Journal* (1938), i. 562–4.

JUKES, E., 'Some Observations on the Treatment of the Puerperal Fever', *London Medical and Physical Journal*, 45 (1821), 122–8.

KÁPOLNAI, I., 'An Overview of University Education in Obstetrics and Gynaecology in Hungary', in Zoltan Papp (ed.), *Past and Present of the First Department of Obstetrics and Gynaecology of Semmelweis University Medical School* (Ignaz Semmelweis Foundation, Budapest, 1996), 11–66.

KATZ, A. R., and MORENS, D. M., 'Severe Streptococcal Infections in Historical Perspective', *Clinical Infectious Diseases*, 14 (1992), 298–307.

KEELING, J. H., 'An Address on Modern Obstetrics', *British Medical Journal* (1883), ii. 57–60.

KENNEDY, E., 'Zymotic Diseases, as More Especially Illustrated by Puerperal Fever', *Dublin Quarterly Journal of Medical Science*, 47 (1869), 269–307.

—— *Hospitalism and Zymotic Diseases as More Especially Illustrated by Puerperal Fever or Metria . . . Also a Reply to the Criticisms of Seventeen Physicians upon this Paper* (2nd edn., London, 1869).

KIDD, G. H., 'On Puerperal Fever', *British Medical Journal* (1884), ii. 217–21.

KINLOCH, J. P., SMITH, J., and STEPHEN, J. A., *Maternal Mortality: Report on Maternal Mortality in Aberdeen, 1918–1927, with Special Reference to Puerperal Sepsis* (Edinburgh, 1928).

KIRKLAND, THOMAS, *A Treatise on Childbed Fevers, and the Methods of Preventing them* (London, 1774).

KNEELAND, S., 'On the Contagiousness of Puerperal Fever', *American Journal of the Medical Sciences*, 11 (1846), 45–63.

KRAUSE, R. M., 'Dynamics of Emergence', *Journal of Infectious Diseases*, 170 (1994), 265–71.

—— 'Introduction', in R. M. Krause (ed.), *Emerging Infections* (New York, 1998).

LACOMME, DR, 'New Results Obtained in the Trial of a Prophylactic Treatment of Puerperal Infections at the Baudelocque Clinic: Interpretation of Results', *Surgery, Gynaecology and Obstetrics*, 66 (1938), 164. [Originally published in *Bulletin de Société d'Obstetriques et de Gynaecologie de Paris*, 26 (1937), 459.]

LANCASTER, H. O., 'Semmelweis: A Rereading of *Die Aetiologie . . .*', *Journal of Medical Biography*, 2 (1994), 12–21, 84–8.

LE FORT, LÉON, *Des maternités: Études sur les maternités et les institutions charitables d'Accouchement à domicile dans les principaux états de l'Europe* (Paris, 1866).

—— 'Discussion, Fievre Puérperale', in *Compte-Rendu: Congrès Périodique International des Sciences Médicales*, 4th session (Brussels 1875), 331–7.

LEA, A., *Puerperal Infection* (London, 1910).

LEAKE, J., *Practical Observations on the Child-Bed fever* (London, 1772); repr. in Fleetwood Churchill (ed.), *Essays on the Puerperal Fever and Other Diseases Peculiar to Women* (London, 1849), 117–204.

LEASURE, D., 'The Erysipelatous Disease of Lying-in Women', *American Journal of the Medical Sciences*, 31 (1856), 45–9.

LEE, R., *Researches on the pathology and treatment of some of the most important diseases of women* (London, 1833).

—— 'Clinical Reports on Difficult Cases in Midwifery', *London Medical Gazette*, NS 2 (1838–9), 827–32.

—— *Lectures on the theory and practice of midwifery* (London, 1844).

LEE, R. J., 'The Goulstonian Lectures on Puerperal Fever', *British Medical Journal* (1875), i. 267–70, 304–6, 337–9, 371–3, 408–9, 440–2.

LEISHMAN, W., *A System of Midwifery* (2nd edn., Glasgow, 1876).

LISTER, J., 'Discussion on the Relation of Minute Organisms to Unhealthy Processes Occurring in Wounds' (International Medical Congress, 1881), *Lancet* (1881), ii. 548.

LØKKE, A., 'The Antiseptic Transformation of Danish Midwives 1860–1920', in H. Marland and A.-M. Rafferty (eds.), *Midwives, Society and Childbirth: Debates and Controversies in the Modern Period* (London, 1997), 102–33.

LONGSTAFF, G. B., 'On Some Statistical Indications of a Relationship between Scarlatina, Puerperal Fever and Certain Other Conditions', *Transactions of the Epidemiological Society of London*, 4 (1875–81), 421–32.

LOUCHE, J.-L., 'La Maternité de Liège ou cent ans de l'évolution d'un hospice', *Annales de la Société Belge d'Histoire des Hôpitaux et de la Santé Publique*, 22 (1984), 5–25.

LOUDON, I., 'Deaths in Childbed from the Eighteenth Century to 1935', *Medical History*, 30 (1986), 1–41.

—— 'Obstetric Care, Social Class and Maternal Mortality', *British Medical Journal* (1986), ii. 606–8.

—— 'Puerperal Fever, the Streptococcus and the Sulphonamides, 1911–1945', *British Medical Journal* (1987), ii. 485–90.

—— 'Maternal Mortality: 1880–1950. Some Regional and International Comparisons', *Social History of Medicine*, 1/2 (1988), 183–228.

—— 'Obstetrics and the General Practitioner', *British Medical Journal*, 301 (1990), 703–7.

—— *Death in Childbirth: An International Study of Maternal Care and Maternal Mortality 1800–1950* (Oxford, 1992).

—— 'Necrotising Fasciitis, Hospital Gangrene and Phagadena', *Lancet*, 344 (1994), 1416–18.

—— 'Alexander Gordon, Puerperal Fever, and Antisepsis', *Aberdeen University Review*, 56 (1996), 285–300.

—— 'Midwives and the Quality of Maternal Care', in H. Marland and A.-M. Rafferty, *Midwives, Society and Childbirth: Debates and Controversies in the Modern Period* (London, 1997), 180–200.

—— 'The Tragedy of Puerperal Fever', *Health Libraries Review*, 15 (1998), 151–6.

LUSK, W. T., 'The Genesis of an Epidemic of Puerperal Fever', *American Journal of Obstetrics*, 8 (1875), 369–99.

—— *The Science and Art of Midwifery* (3rd edn., London, 1885; 4th edn., 1892).

McCALLUM, D. C., 'Report of the University Lying-in Hospital, Montreal, from Oct. 1 1867 to Oct 1 1875', *Transactions of the Obstetrical Society of London*, 20 (1878), 35–51.

MACFARLANE, A., and MUGFORD, M., *Birth Counts: Statistics of Pregnancy and Childbirth* (2 vols.; London, 1984).

MACFARLANE, G., *Alexander Fleming* (paperback edn., Oxford, 1985).

McKINLAY, P. L., *Maternal Mortality in Scotland, 1911–1945*, extracted from the 91st Annual Report of the Registrar General for Scotland (Edinburgh, 1942).

MACKINTOSH, JOHN, *A Treatise on the Disease Termed Puerperal Fever* (Edinburgh, 1822).

MADDEN, T. M., 'The Prevention and Treatment of Puerperal Fever', *British Medical Journal* (1887), ii. 1045–7.

MARLAND, H. (ed.), *The Art of Midwifery: Early Modern Midwives in Europe* (London, 1993).

—— and RAFFERTY, ANNE-MARIE (eds.), *Midwives, Society and Childbirth. Debates and Controversies in the Modern Period* (London, 1997).

MATTHEWS, J. ROSSER, *Quantification and the Quest for Medical Certainty* (Princeton, NJ, 1995).

MEIGS, C. D., *Females and their Diseases: A Series of Letters to his Class* (Philadelphia, 1848; 2nd edn., 1851).

MELENEY, F. L., ZAU, Z.-D., ZAYTZEFF, H., and HARVEY, H. D., 'Epidemiologic and Bacteriologic Investigations of the Sloane Hospital Epidemic of Hemolytic Streptococcus Puerperal Fever in 1927', *American Journal of Obstetrics and Gynaecology*, 16 (Aug. 1928), 180–94.

MENDENHALL, G., 'On the Mortality in the Lying-in Ward of the Cincinnati Hospital', *Transactions of the Obstetrical Society of London*, 12 (1871), 357–9.

MILNE, G. P., 'The History of Midwifery in Aberdeen', *Aberdeen University Review*, 47 (1978), 293–303.

MINISTRY OF HEALTH, *Interim Report of Departmental Committee on Maternal Mortality and Morbidity* (London, 1930), 32–293.

—— *Final Report of Departmental Committee on Maternal Mortality and Morbidity* (London, 1932), 32–300.

—— *Report of an Investigation into Maternal Mortality* (Cmd. 5422, PP 1936/37 XI; London, 1937).

MINOR, T., 'Erysipelas and Child-Bed Fever', *Practitioner*, 15 (1875), 185–90.

MOSSMAN, G., 'On the Nature and Cure of Puerperal Fever', *London Medical and Physical Journal*, 10 (1803), 11–20.

MOTTRAM, J., 'State Control in Local Context: The Early Years of Midwife Regulation in Manchester, 1900–1914', in H. Marland and A.-M. Rafferty (eds.), *Midwives, Society and Childbirth: Debates and Controversies, in the Modern Period* (London, 1997), 134–52.

MURPHY, E. W., 'Lectures on Lactation and the Disorders Incident to the Puerperal State', *London Medical Gazette*, NS 10 (1850), 485–94.

—— 'Puerperal Fever', *Dublin Quarterly Journal of Medical Science*, 24 (1857), 1–31.

MURPHY, F. P., 'Introduction', in I. P. Semmelweis, 'The Etiology, the Concept and the Prophylaxis of Childbed Fever', trans. by F. P. Murphy, *Medical Classics*, 5/5 (1941), 339–478, 481–589, 591–715, 719–773.

—— 'Ignaz Philipp Semmelweis: An Annotated Biobibliography, *Bulletin of the History of Medicine*, 20 (1946), 653–707.

MURRAY, R. MILNE, 'Presidential Address', *Transactions of the Obstetric Society of Edinburgh*, 26 (1901), 5–23.

MUSSER, M. M., and KRAUSE, R. M., 'The Revival of Group A Streptococcal Diseases with a Commentary on Staphylococcal Toxic Shock Syndrome', in R. M. Krause (ed.), *Emerging Infections* (New York, 1998), 185–218.

NAPIER, A. D. L., *Notes on Puerperal Fever* (Aberdeen, 1875).

NIGHTINGALE, FLORENCE, *Introductory Notes on Lying-in Hospitals* (London, 1876).

NULAND, S. B., 'The Enigma of Semmelweis—an Interpretation', *Journal of the History of Medicine and Allied Sciences*, 34 (1979), 255–72.

Obstetrical Society of London, 'Discussion "On the Relation of Puerperal Fever to the Infective Diseases and Pyaemia"', *Transactions of the Obstetrical Society of London*, 17 (1876), 90–165, 178–209, 217–72.

O'CONNELL, P. A., 'Obstetrics in Vienna', *Boston Medical and Surgical Journal*, 9/20 (1872), 309–12.

OSBORN, W., *Essays on the Practice of Midwifery in Natural and Difficult Labours* (London, 1792).

OXLEY, W. H. F., 'Prevention of Puerperal Sepsis in General Practice', *British Medical Journal* (1934), i. 1017–19.

OZNAN, J. F., *Histoire médicale, générale et particulière des maladies contagieuses et épizootiques* (Lyons, 1835).

PAGET, C. E., *Wasted Records of Disease* (London, 1897).

PAINE, C. G., 'The Aetiology of Puerperal Infection', *British Medical Journal* (1935), i. 243–6.

PARRY, J. S., 'Description of a Form of Puerperal Fever which Occurred at the Philadelphia Hospital Characterized by Diphtheritic Deposits of Wounds of the Genital Passages and by Other Peculiar Phenomena', *American Journal of Medical Sciences*, 69 (1875), 46–76.

PARSONS, G. P., 'The British Medical Profession and Contagion Theory: Puerperal Fever as a Case Study, 1830–1860', *Medical History*, 22 (1978), 138–50.

—— 'Puerperal Fever, Anticontagionists, and Miasmatic Infection, 1840–1860: Toward a New History of Puerperal Fever in America', *Journal of the History of Medicine*, 52 (1997), 424–52.

PASTEUR, L. 'The Germ Theory: Address to the International Medical Congress', *Lancet* (1881), ii. 271–2.

PATTERSON, J., 'Cases of Puerperal Peritonitis', *Dublin Journal of Medical and Chemical Science*, 4 (1834), 170–80.

PEDDIE, DR, 'On the Contagiousness of Puerperal Fever', *London Medical Gazette* (1846), ii. 835–7.

PEEBLES, J. F., 'Facts in Relation to Epidemic Erysipelas, as it Prevailed in Petersburg, Virginia, during the Winter and Spring, 1844–45', *American Journal of the Medical Sciences*, 11 (1846), 23–44.

PENNINGTON, T. H., 'Osteotomy as an Indicator of Antiseptic Surgical Practice', *Medical History*, 38 (1994), 178–88.

—— 'Listerism, its Decline and its Persistence: The Introduction of Aseptic Surgical Techniques in Three British Teaching Hospitals, 1890–99', *Medical History*, 39 (1995), 35–60.

PHILLIPS, H. J., 'Treatment of Puerperal Infection by Intra-Uterine Injections of Glycerine', *Proceedings of the Royal Society of Medicine*, 19 (1926), section on obstetrics and gynaecology, 26–31.

PLAYFAIR, W. S., *A Treatise on the Science and Art of Midwifery* (2 vols.; 5th edn., London, 1884).

—— 'Introduction to a Discussion on the Prevention of Puerperal Fever', *British Medical Journal* (1887), ii. 1034–6.

PLUMPE, G., '125 Years of Bayer—Tradition Means Obligations', unpublished paper (1988).

PORTER, I. A., *Alexander Gordon of Aberdeen, 1752–1799* (Aberdeen University Studies No. 139; Edinburgh, 1958).

PRIESTLY, W. O., 'Notes on a Visit to Some of the Lying-in Hospitals in the North of Europe, and Particularly of the Advantages of the Antiseptic System in Obstetric Practice', *Transactions of the Obstetrical Society of London*, 27 (1885), 197–222.

Public Record Office, Records of the Ministry of Health, MH 55/266, 'Puerperal Pyrexia'.

RAMSBOTHAM, F. H., 'The Eastern District of the Royal Maternity Charity', *London Medical Gazette*, NS 2 (1843–4), 619–25.

RAMSBOTHAM, J., 'On Puerperal Fever', *London Medical and Physical Journal*, 26 (1811), 265–73.

Reports to the Local Government Board on Public Health and Medical Subjects, *Statistics of the Incidence of Notifiable Infectious Diseases in Each Sanitary District in England and Wales during the Year 1911* (London, 1912).

RICHARDSON, W. L., 'The Use of Antiseptics in Obstetric Practice', *Boston Medical and Surgical Journal*, 116 (1887), 73–9.

RIDLEY, R. T. P., 'Cases of Erysipelas which Occurred in Platte County, Missouri, in which there were Marked Evidences of Propagation of the Disease by Contagion', *New York Journal of Medicine*, 10 (1853), 41–8.

RIGBY, E., 'Midwifery Reports', *London Medical Gazette*, 14 (1834), 400–1.

ROBERTON, J., 'Is Puerperal Fever Infectious?' *London Medical Gazette*, 9 (1831–2), 503–5.

—— 'Observations on Parturition', *London Medical Gazette*, 11 (1833), 29–42.

—— *Essays and Notes on the Physiology and Diseases of Women* (London, 1851).

ROLLESTON, J. D., *The History of the Acute Exanthemata: The Fitzpatrick Lectures for 1935 and 1936* (London, 1937).

ROSENBERG, C., *Explaining Epidemics and Other Studies in the History of Medicine* (Cambridge, 1992).

—— and GOLDEN, J. (eds.), *Framing Disease: Studies in Cultural History* (New Brunswick, 1992).

ROSS, P. W., 'Streptococcus and Enterococcus', in D. Greenwood, R. C. B. Slack, and J. F. Peutherer (eds.), *Medical Microbiology* (15th edn., London, 1997), 175–87.

ROUTH, C. H. F., 'On the Causes of the Endemic Puerperal Fever of Vienna', *Medico-Chirurgical Transactions*, 2nd ser. 14 (1849), 27–39.

ROWLING, C. R., 'The History of the Florence Nightingale Lying-in Ward, King's College Hospital', *Transactions of the Obstetrical Society of London*, 10 (1869), 51–6.

ROYSTON, E., and ABOUZAHR, C., 'Measuring Maternal Mortality', *British Journal of Obstetrics and Gynaecology*, 99/7 (1992), 540–2.

RUBINSTEIN, A., 'Subtle Poison: The Puerperal Fever Controversy in Victorian Britain', *Historical Studies*, 20 (1983), 420–38.

RYLE, J. A., and SMITH, R. E., 'The Natural History, Prognosis and Treatment of Streptococcal Fever', *Guy's Hospital Reports*, 81 (1931), 1–28.

SACKS, O., 'Scotomata: Forgetting and Neglect in Science', in R. B. Silvers (ed.), *Hidden Histories of Science* (London, 1997), 141–88.

SCHRÖDER, C., *et al.*, 'Report Prepared by the Puerperal Fever Committee of the Berlin Obstetrical Society, and Laid before the Prussian Minister of Public Health by Dr Falk', trans. from the *Zeitschrift für Geburtshülfe und Gynäkologie*, vol. III, part 1, by Dr Charles E. Underhill, *Edinburgh Medical Journal*, 24 (1878), 435–46.

SCHWENTKER, F. F., and WAGHELSTEIN, J., 'A Note on the Use of Sulfanilamide in Scarlet Fever', *Baltimore Health News*, 15 (1938), 41–6.

SELIGMAN, S. A., 'The Lesser Pestilence: Non-Epidemic Puerperal Fever', *Medical History*, 35 (1991), 89–102.

SELWYN, S., 'Aseptic Rituals Unmasked', leading article in *British Medical Journal* (1984), ii. 1642–3.

SEMMELWEIS, I. P., *Die Aetiologie, der Begriff und die Prophylaxis des Kindbettfiebers* [*Etiology, Concept and Prophylaxis of Childbed Fever*] (Pest, 1861). [It was in fact published in 1860.]

—— 'On the Origin and Prevention of Puerperal Fever', *Medical Times and Gazette* (1862), i. 601–2.

—— 'The Etiology, the Concept and the Prophylaxis of Childbed Fever', trans. with an introduction by F. P. Murphy, *Medical Classics*, 5/5 (1941), 339–478, 481–589, 591–715, 719–773.

—— *The Etiology, Concept, and Prophylaxis of Childbed Fever*, trans. and ed. with an introduction, by K. Codell Carter (Wisconsin, 1983).

SERDUKOFF, M. G., 'The Actual Therapy of Puerperal Fever', *Gynécologie*, 33 (1934), 622.

SEVERN, C., 'Puerperal Fever', *London Medical Gazette*, 8 (1831), 400–1.

SIDEY, C., 'Cases of Puerperal Fever', *Edinburgh Medical and Surgical Journal*, 51 (1839), 91–9.

SIMPSON, J. Y., Correspondence with F. H. Ramsbotham, National Library of Medicine, Bethesda, manuscript collection.

—— 'Report of the Edinburgh Maternity Hospital', *Monthly Journal of Medical Science*, 9 (1848–9), 329–38.

—— 'Some Notes on the Analogy between Puerperal Fever and Surgical Fever', *London and Edinburgh Monthly Journal of Medical Sciences* (Nov. 1850), 414–29.

—— 'Discussion of Arneth's Paper Read to the Edinburgh Medico-Chirurgical Society, April 16, 1851', *Monthly Journal of Medical Science*, 13 (1851), 72–80.

—— *Selected Obstetrical and Gynaecological Works of Sir James Young Simpson Bart.*, ed. J. Watt Black (Edinburgh, 1871).

SINCLAIR, SIR WILLIAM, *Semmelweis, his Life and his Doctrine* (Manchester, 1909).

SKODA, DR, 'On the Causes of Puerperal Fever: Experiments on Animals', *London Medical Journal* (July 1850), 700–3.

SLAUGHTER, F., *Immortal Magyar: Semmelweis, Conquerer of Childbed Fever* (New York, 1950).

SMELLIE, WILLIAM, *A Treatise on the Theory and Practice of Midwifery* (London, 1752).

SMITH, J. BARKER, 'Semmelweis—Physician, Martyr, Pioneer', *Medical Times*, 52 (1924), 38–9, 51–3.

SMITH, J., *Causation and Source of Infection in Puerperal Fever* (Edinburgh, 1931).

—— 'A Further Investigation of Infection in Puerperal Fever', *Journal of Obstetrics and Gynaecology of the British Empire*, 40 (1933), 991.

SMITH, W. TYLER, 'Puerperal Fever', *Lancet* (1856), ii. 503–5, 530–4.

SNODGRASS, W. R., 'Uses and abuses of Chemotherapy in Streptococcal Diseases', *Practitioner*, 144 (1940), 16–24.

—— and ANDERSON, T., 'Prontosil in the Treatment of Erysipelas: A Controlled Trial of 312 Cases', *British Medical Journal* (1937), ii. 101–4.

STAMM, H., *Ein Rückblick auf die Geschichte des Frauenspitals, Basel* (Basle, 1959).

STEELE, A. B., *Maternity Hospitals, their Mortality, and What Should be Done with them* (London, 1874).

STEWART, D. B., and WILLIAMS, J. G., 'Bleeding and Purging: A Cure for Puerperal Fever?', *Journal of Hospital Infection*, 34 (1996), 81–6.

STOLLERMAN, G. H., 'Rheumatogenic Group A Streptococci and the Return of Rheumatic Fever', *Advances in Internal Medicine*, 35/1 (1990), 1–25.

—— 'Changing Streptococci and Prospects for the Global Eradication of Rheumatic Fever', *Perspectives in Biology and Medicine*, 40/2 (1997), 165–87.

STOLLERMAN, G. H., 'Rheumatic Fever', *Lancet* (1997), 935–42.

—— 'The Changing Face of Rheumatic Fever in the 20th Century', *Journal of Medical Microbiology*, 47 (1998), 655–7.

—— 'Streptococcus pyogenes' in S. L. Garbach, J. H. Bartlett, and N. R. Blacklow (eds.), *Infectious Diseases* (2nd edn., Philadelphia, 1998), 1703–19.

STOOKES, DR, 'Some Points in the Puerperal Mortality', *Journal of Obstetrics and Gynaecology of the British Empire*, 23 (1913), 174–6.

STORRS, R., 'Puerperal Fever', *London Medical Gazette*, 3rd. ser. (1845), i. 1087–8.

STROTHER, EDWARD, *Criticon Februm, or a Critical Essay on Fevers* (London, 1716).

TAYLOR, W., and DAUNCEY, M., 'Changing patterns of mortality in England and Wales: II. Maternal Mortality', *British Journal of Preventive and Social Medicine*, 8 (1954), 172–5.

THOMPSON, A. R., 'Chemotherapy and acute specific fevers', *Practitioner*, 144 (1940), 52–60.

TOMALIN C., *The Life and Death of Mary Wollstonecraft* (rev. edn., Harmondsworth, 1985).

TONNELLÉ, M., 'Des fièvres puerpérales observeés à la Maternité de Paris pendant l'année 1829', originally published as four papers in *Archives Générales de Médecin* (Mar., Apr., May, and June 1830); repr. in 'Critical Analysis', *Edinburgh Medical and Surgical Journal*, 34 (1830), 328–49.

TOP, F. H., and YOUNG, D. C., 'The treatment of moderately severe scarlet fever', *Journal of the American Medical Association*, 117 (1941), 2056–60.

TOPLEY, W. W. C., and WILSON, G. S., *Principles of Bacteriology and Immunity* (2nd edn., London, 1936); rev. edn. by G. S. Wilson and A. A. Miles (London, 1946).

TRÖHLER, U., *Tracing Emotions, Concepts and Realities in History: the Göttingen Collection of Perinatal Medicine* (Florence, 1993).

TUNNICLIFF, R., 'Further Studies on the Specificity of Streptococci', *Journal of the American Medical Association*, 75 (1920), 1339–40.

TURK, D. C., PORTER, I. A., DUERDEN, B. I., and REID, T. M. S., *A Short Textbook of Medical Microbiology* (5th edn., London, 1983).

VAN TUESSENBROOEK, CATHARINE, *De Ontwikkeling der Aseptische Verloskunde in Nederland* [*The Development of Aseptic Midwifery in the Netherlands*] (Haarlem, 1911).

VERG, E., *Milestones: The Bayer Story, 1863–1988* (Wilmington, Mass., 1988).

WADDY, J., 'Puerperal Fever', *Lancet* (1845), i. 671–5; (1845), ii. 531–2, 671–2; (1846), i. 38–9, 697–700.

WARD, J. E., and YELL, J. (eds.), 'The Medical Casebook of William Brownrigg MD FRS (1712 and 1800) of the Town of Whitehaven in Cumberland', *Medical History*, suppl. no. 13 (London, 1993).

WARD, L., 'The Cult of Relics: Pasteur Material at the Science Museum', *Medical History*, 38 (1994), 52–72.

WARREN, S. P., 'The Prevalence of Puerperal Septicaemia in Private Practice at the Present Time Contrasted with that of a Generation ago', *American Journal of Obstetrics*, 51 (1905), 301–31.

WATSON, B. P., 'An Outbreak of Puerperal Sepsis in New York City', *American Journal of Obstetrics and Gynaecology*, 16 (1928), 157–79.

WATSON, T., *Lectures on the Principles and Practice of Physic* (1st edn., London, 1843; 4th edn., 1857).

WEATHERALL, M., *In Search of a Cure* (Oxford, 1990).

—— 'Drug Therapies', in W. F. Bynum and R. Porter (eds.), *Companion Encyclopaedia to the History of Medicine* (London, 1993), ch. 39.

WEATHERHEAD, G. H., *An Essay on the Diagnosis between Erysipelas, Phlegmon and Erythema, with an Appendix Touching on the Probable Nature of Puerperal Fever* (London, 1819).

WEINDLING, P., 'The Immunological Tradition', in W. F. Bynum and R. Porter (eds.), *Companion Encyclopaedia to the History of Medicine* (London, 1993), ch. 10.

WELLS, T. SPENCER, 'On the Relation of Puerperal Fever to the Infective Diseases and Pyaemia', *Transactions of the Obstetrical Society of London*, 17 (1876), 90–165.

WESSELHOEF, C., 'Sulfanilamide in the Management of Acute Streptococcal Infection, Particularly Scarlatinal Infections of the Upper Respiratory Tract', *New England Journal of Medicine*, 224 (1941), 221–6.

WEST, T., 'Observations on Some Diseases, Particularly Puerperal Fever, which Occurred in Abingdon and its Vicinity in 1813 and 1814', *London Medical Monthly Journal, Repository and Review*, 3 (1815), 103–5.

WHITBY, L. E. H., 'Questionnaire on Puerperal Sepsis', *Practitioner*, 140 (1938), 324–5.

WHITE, CHARLES, *A Treatise on the Management of Pregnant and Lying-in Women* (London, 1773; repr. with an introduction by Lawrence D. Long (Canton, Mass., 1987)).

—— *An Appendix to the Second Edition of Mr C. White's Treatise on the Management of Pregnant and Lying-in Women* (London, 1777).

WILLIAMS, DR, 'Clinical Observations of Idiopathic Erysipelas', *St Thomas's Hospital Reports*, 1 (1836), 323–38.

WILLIAMS, W., *An Epidemic of Puerperal Septicaemia* (Glamorgan, 1893).

—— 'Puerperal Mortality', *Transactions of the Epidemiological Society of London*, 15 (1895–6), 100–33.

—— *Death in Childbed* (London, 1904).

WILSON, A., *The Making of Man-Midwifery: Childbirth in England, 1660–1770* (Cambridge, Mass., 1995).

WILSON, J., 'Report of the Glasgow Lying-in Hospital for the Year 1851–52 with an Address to the Students Attending the Hospital', *Glasgow Medical Journal*, 1 (1853), 1–10.

WILSON, L. G., 'The Early Recognition of Streptococci as Causes of Disease', *Medical History*, 31/3 (1987), 403–14.

WINCKEL, F., *The Pathology and Treatment of Childbed* (London, 1876).

WORBOYS, M., 'Treatments for Pneumonia in Britain, 1910–1940', in *Medicine and Change: Historical and Sociological Studies of Medical Innovation* (Proceedings of the Symposium INERM held in Paris, 21–23 April, 1992), 317–35.

WYATT, J., 'The Relation of the Haemolytic Streptococcus to Puerperal Infection', *St Thomas's Hospital Reports*, 3 (1938), 81–8.

YOUNG, E. B., 'A Brief Sketch of Semmelweis and his Works on Puerperal Sepsis', *Boston Medical and Surgical Journal*, 52 (1909), 15–17.

YOUNG, J., 'Maternal Mortality from Puerperal Sepsis', *British Medical Journal* (1928), i. 967–71.

Index